The Essential Spinal Cord Injury Medicine Question Bank

Benjamin A. Abramoff
Jing Wang • Christine Krull
Editors

The Essential Spinal Cord Injury Medicine Question Bank

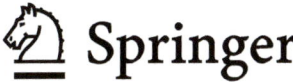 Springer

Editors
Benjamin A. Abramoff
Department of Physical Medicine and
Rehabilitation
University of Pennsylvania - Perelman
School of Medicine
Philadelphia, PA, USA

Jing Wang
Aiken Regional Medical Center
Aiken, SC, USA

Christine Krull
Spinal Cord Injury/Dysfunction Service
VA St. Louis Health Care System
St. Louis, MO, USA

Department of Physical Medicine and
Rehabilitation
Baylor College of Medicine
TIRR Memorial Hermann
Houston, TX, USA

ISBN 978-3-031-07795-1   ISBN 978-3-031-07796-8   (eBook)
https://doi.org/10.1007/978-3-031-07796-8

This Springer imprint is published by the registered company Springer Nature Switzerland AG
The registered company address is: Gewerbestrasse 11, 6330 Cham, Switzerland

Preface

Spinal cord injuries have wide ranging effects on the body and can impact every organ system. Therefore, the mastery of an extensive breadth of material is critical to building a foundation of knowledge to care for individuals who have had spinal cord injuries. One method familiar to those studying medicine to help gain and solidify this knowledge is high-yield question banks.

For learners preparing for spinal cord injury board examinations, we felt that no such question bank existed for spinal cord injury medicine. This left us creating our own questions to test one another and improve our retention of material. Despite this, we felt future students would benefit from a more formal and structured question bank. From this background, *The Essential Spinal Cord Injury Medicine Question Bank* was created.

We want to thank the chapter authors who have spent countless hours developing thought provoking, well-written, and fair questions. Generally, these questions require more than superficial familiarity to answer and test a true understanding of underlying concepts. The detailed explanations and references that the authors provided are as important as the questions and answers themselves. We encourage you to explore these references when you would like to learn more about the concepts addressed in the question.

Although we hope that this question bank will help you gain significant knowledge and feel more comfortable with your upcoming examinations, we recognize that this is just one tool of many including textbooks, review courses, didactics, and most importantly the clinical experience of caring for individuals with spinal cord injury. While we have attempted to include the highest yield topics, we also fully recognize that this text is not exhaustive and lifelong learning is required to master the topics contained in this text.

Our ultimate goal with this question bank is to help individuals feel more comfortable in their clinical care for patients with spinal cord injuries. By feeling comfortable with the clinical knowledge, we hope you have the opportunity to get to know your patients better as unique individuals. To those currently study-ing for your examinations, good luck! We look forward to collaborating with you in the future in our shared mission to improve the lives of those with spinal cord injuries.

Philadelphia, PA, USA   Benjamin A. Abramoff
Aiken, SC, USA   Jing Wang
Houston, TX, USA   Christine Krull

Contents

Contributors

Benjamin A. Abramoff Department of Physical Medicine and Rehabilitation, University of Pennsylvania—Perelman School of Medicine, Philadelphia, PA, USA

Elisabeth K. Acker Spinal Cord Injury and Disorders Service, Central Virginia VA Health Care System, Richmond, VA, USA

Department of Physical Medicine and Rehabilitation, Virginia Commonwealth University, Richmond, VA, USA

Gurtej S. Bajaj Department of Physical Medicine and Rehabilitation, University of Pennsylvania—Perelman School of Medicine, Philadelphia, PA, USA

Samir R. Belagaje Department of Neurology, Emory University, Atlanta, GA, USA

Department of Rehabilitation Medicine, Emory University, Atlanta, GA, USA

Maryam Berri Department of Physical Medicine and Rehabilitation, Michigan Medicine, Ann Arbor, MI, USA

Natasha Bhatia Department of Rehabilitation Medicine, Emory University School of Medicine, Atlanta, GA, USA

Department of Physical Medicine and Rehabilitation, Shirley Ryan AbilityLab, Department of Physical Medicine and Rehabilitation, Northwestern University Feinberg School of Medicine, Chicago, IL, USA

Glendaliz Bosques Department of Neurology, Dell Medical School at University of Texas, Austin, TX, USA

Michael Bush-Arnold Spinal Cord Injury Unit, Rehabilitation Institute of Michigan, Detroit, MI, USA

Carolyn Campbell Department of Physical Medicine and Rehabilitation, University of Washington Hospitals and Clinics, Harborview Medical Center, Seattle, WA, USA

Joel Castellanos Inpatient Rehabilitation, Department of Anesthesiology, UC San Diego Health, San Diego, CA, USA

Wesley Chay Department of Medical Staff, Shepherd Center, Atlanta, GA, USA

Ellia Ciammaichella Department of Physical Medicine and Rehabilitation, Renown Regional Medical Center, Reno, NV, USA

Darby Cruz Department of Respiratory Therapy, TIRR Memorial Hermann, Houston, TX, USA

Joanne M. Delgado-Lebron Department of Physical Medicine & Rehabilitation, Memorial Rehabilitation Institute at Memorial Healthcare System, Hollywood, FL, USA

Michelle M. Didesch Department of Neuro Rehab Physiatry, Confluence Health—Wenatchee Valley Medical Group, Wenatchee, WA, USA

D. Frank Distel Department of Physical Medicine & Rehabilitation, University of Pennsylvania, Philadelphia, PA, USA

James Doan Spinal Cord Injury Division, VA Boston Healthcare System, Boston, MA, USA

Department of Physical Medicine and Rehabilitation, Harvard Medical School/Spaulding Rehabilitation Hospital, Boston, MA, USA

Christina Draganich Physical Medicine and Rehabilitation Department, University of Colorado, Aurora, CO, USA

Lauren Fetsko Department of Pediatrics, University of Wisconsin School of Medicine and Public Health, American Family Children's Hospital, Madison, WI, USA

Karishma Gupta Urology Institute, University Hospitals Cleveland Medical Center, Case Western Reserve University School of Medicine, Cleveland, OH, USA

Beverly Hon Veteran Affairs New Jersey Health Care System, Spinal Cord Injury and Disorders Service, East Orange, NJ, USA

Reuben Horace New York Institute of Technology COM, Old Westbury, NY, USA

Shelly Hsieh, MD Department of Physical Medicine and Rehabilitation, Albert Einstein College of Medicine, Bronx, NY, USA

Burke Rehabilitation Hospital, Montefiore Health System, White Plains, NY, USA

Department of Physical Medicine and Rehabilitation, Rutgers New Jersey Medical School, Newark, NJ, USA

Kessler Institute for Rehabilitation, West Orange, NJ, USA

Donna Huang Spinal Cord Injury Care Line, Michael E. DeBakey VA Medical Center, Houston, TX, USA

H. Ben Taub Department of Physical Medicine and Rehabilitation, Baylor College of Medicine, Houston, TX, USA

Simra Javaid Department of Physical Medicine and Rehabilitation, McGovern Medical School at UTHealth, Houston, TX, USA

Patricia L. Kiefer, MSN, APRN, ACCNS-AG Department of Medicine, Northeast Ohio Veteran Administration Healthcare System, Cleveland, OH, USA

Steven Kirshblum, MD Department of Physical Medicine and Rehabilitation, Rutgers New Jersey Medical School, Newark, NJ, USA

Kessler Institute for Rehabilitation, West Orange, NJ, USA

R. Caleb Kovell Perelman School of Medicine, University of Pennsylvania & The Children's Hospital of Philadelphia, Philadelphia, PA, USA

Christine Krull Spinal Cord Injury/Dysfunction Service, VA St. Louis Health Care System, St. Louis, MO, USA

Department of Physical Medicine and Rehabilitation, Baylor College of Medicine, TIRR Memorial Hermann, Houston, TX, USA

David Leong Physical Medicine and Rehabilitation, MetroHealth Rehabilitation Institute, Cleveland, OH, USA

Audrey Leung Department of Physical Medicine and Rehabilitation, University of Washington Hospitals and Clinics, Harborview Medical Center, Seattle, WA, USA

Aaron J. Lin Department of Physical Medicine and Rehabilitation, University of Texas Medical School at Houston, Houston, TX, USA

John Lin Department of Medical Staff, Shepherd Center, Atlanta, GA, USA

John Lopez, DO Department of Physical Medicine and Rehabilitation, Rutgers New Jersey Medical School, Newark, NJ, USA

Kessler Institute for Rehabilitation, West Orange, NJ, USA

Jennifer E. Mast Department of Physical Medicine and Rehabilitation, OhioHealth Neurological Physicians, Columbus, OH, USA

Chloe McCloskey Department of Physical Medicine & Rehabilitation, University of Pennsylvania, Philadelphia, PA, USA

Jeremiah Nieves, MD Department of Physical Medicine and Rehabilitation, Rutgers New Jersey Medical School, Newark, NJ, USA

Kessler Institute for Rehabilitation, West Orange, NJ, USA

Peter Park Division of Rehabilitation, Department of Neurology, Washington University School of Medicine, Saint Louis, MO, USA

David H. Quan Department of Physical Medicine and Rehabilitation, University of Pennsylvania—Perelman School of Medicine, Philadelphia, PA, USA

Gianna M. Rodriguez Department of Physical Medicine and Rehabilitation, Michigan Medicine, Ann Arbor, MI, USA

Vivian Roy Division of Spinal Cord Injury Medicine, Shirley Ryan Abilitylab, Chicago, IL, USA

Department of Physical Medicine and Rehabilitation, Northwestern University, Chicago, IL, USA

Kendl Sankary Department of Physical Medicine and Rehabilitation, University of Washington Hospitals and Clinics, Harborview Medical Center, Seattle, WA, USA

Kyle A. Scarberry Urology Institute, University Hospitals Cleveland Medical Center, Case Western Reserve University School of Medicine, Cleveland, OH, USA

Sameer Siddiqui Spinal Cord Injury System of Care, Louis Stokes Cleveland VA Medical Center, Cleveland, OH, USA

Department of Physical Medicine and Rehabilitation, Case Western Reserve University, Cleveland, OH, USA

Sushil Singla Division of Spinal Cord Injury Medicine, Shirley Ryan Abilitylab, Chicago, IL, USA

Felicia Skelton H. Ben Taub Department of Physical Medicine and Rehabilitation, Baylor College of Medicine, Houston, TX, USA

Niña Carmela R. Tamayo, DO, MS, MPH Department of Physical Medicine and Rehabilitation, Cleveland Clinic Edwin Shaw Rehabilitation Hospital; Tamayo Physiatry, LLC, Cleveland, OH, USA

Katharine Tam Division of Rehabilitation, Department of Neurology, Washington University School of Medicine, Saint Louis, MO, USA

Spinal Cord Injury and Disorders, Saint Louis VA Healthcare System, Saint Louis, MO, USA

Ryan P. Terlecki Wake Forest University Baptist Health System, Winston-Salem, NC, USA

Heather Theobald, DO, MPH Department of Physical Medicine and Rehabilitation, Mercy Medical Center, Catholic Health Services of Long Island, Rockville Centre, NY, USA

Elizabeth Twist Physical Medicine and Rehabilitation, MetroHealth Rehabilitation Institute, Cleveland, OH, USA

Allison Kessler Division of Spinal Cord Injury Medicine, Shirley Ryan Abilitylab, Chicago, IL, USA

Department of Physical Medicine and Rehabilitation, Northwestern University, Chicago, IL, USA

Lisa Wenzel H. Ben Taub Department of Physical Medicine and Rehabilitation, Baylor College of Medicine, TIRR Memorial Hermann Hospital, Houston, TX, USA

James Wilson Physical Medicine and Rehabilitation, MetroHealth Rehabilitation Institute, Cleveland, OH, USA

Christopher Woolley Pain Medicine, Department of Anesthesiology, UC San Diego, San Diego, CA, USA

Danielle Zheng Pain Medicine, Department of Anesthesiology, UC San Diego, San Diego, CA, USA

Introduction

David H. Quan, Gurtej S. Bajaj, and Benjamin A. Abramoff

This Question Bank

Spinal Cord Injury (SCI) Medicine is a field of medicine that addresses the prevention, diagnosis, and treatment of both traumatic and nontraumatic spinal cord injuries, as well as the management of their various sequelae. SCI medicine has been recognized as a subspecialty by the American Board of Medical Specialties (ABMS) since 1995.

The purpose of this text is to serve as a high-yield resource for fellows and attending physicians preparing for subspeciality certification or recertification through the American Board of Physical Medicine and Rehabilitation (ABPMR) Spinal Cord Injury (SCI) Medicine examination. Medical students and residents may also find these questions useful while preparing for SCI rotations and, in the latter's case, Part I of the ABPMR primary certification examination. In short, this question bank should be of use to anyone wishing to test and expand their knowledge of SCI medicine.

The book is comprised of 22 chapters addressing the full scope of topics tested in the ABPMR SCI Medicine examination. The questions are written by leading experts in the field of SCI medicine and designed to be board-relevant in both content and style. Included with each question is a corresponding in-depth explanation as well as the pertinent citations for the supporting literature. The text has also been edited for clarity and conciseness.

D. H. Quan · G. S. Bajaj · B. A. Abramoff (✉)
Department of Physical Medicine and Rehabilitation, University of Pennsylvania—Perelman School of Medicine, Philadelphia, PA, USA
e-mail: David.quan@pennmedicine.upenn.edu;
Benjamin.Abramoff@pennmedicine.upenn.edu

The Examination

This section provides an overview of the ABPMR SCI Medicine certification examination. The ABPMR is an independent, nonprofit organization that certifies doctors who meet specific educational, training, and professional requirements in this discipline. The ABPMR does not endorse any independent review courses, study guides or other study materials. Questions and items provided in any such materials may not be representative of actual questions on an ABPMR Board examination. For more information on ABPMR board certification and exams, please go to www. abpmr.org.

Purpose of Certification

Currently, the ABPMR offers certification in seven subspecialities of PM&R. The ABPMR has offered certification in SCI Medicine since 1998. Subspecialty certification in SCI medicine both allows physiatrists to demonstrate their competency in the field and ensures the quality of care available to individuals with spinal cord injury. Examinations are administered simultaneously once a year at Pearson Professional Centers nationwide.

Admissibility Requirements

In order to be considered eligible to sit for the examination, applicants must fulfill the following requirements:

1. ABMS Certification—Applicants must be diplomates in good standing of a member board of the ABMS.
2. Licensure—Applicants must have a current, valid, and unrestricted license to practice medicine in at least one jurisdiction in the United States, its territories, or Canada. Physicians must provide evidence of unrestricted licensure in the state or states they practice prior to issuance of the certificate.
3. Training—Applicants must
   • Successfully complete 12 months of an ACGME–accredited SCI Medicine fellowship following their residency,
   • Be evaluated annually by their program director with evaluations submitted directly to ABPMR
   • Be recommended for admissibility to the SCI Medicine Examination by their program director upon completion of their fellowship in SCI medicine.
4. Date of Training Completion—Applicants must complete their SCI Medicine fellowship on or before August 31 of the year of the scheduled examination.

Examination Format

The format of the SCI Medicine Examination should be familiar to candidates who have taken Part I of the ABPMR certification examination. It is a computer-based examination comprised of 280 multiple-choice questions divided into two 3.5-hour sections. All questions are multiple-choice with four options (A–D) with only one best answer. There is a 60-minute break between sections. There is also a tutorial at the beginning of the first section to allow the examinee to familiarize him or herself with the testing software.

On the day of the exam, staff will ask candidates for two forms of identification (ID), including at least one government-issued ID with both their signature and a recent photograph. The other form of ID must also display their signature. Prior to the exam, candidates should ensure that the name listed on both their forms of ID match the name on file with the ABPMR.

Exam results are typically released 6–8 weeks following exam administration. Candidates are notified by email when results become viewable electronically on the ABPMR website.

Examination Outline with Approximate Target Weights

Class 1: Type of Myelopathy
1. Traumatic (55%)
   (a) Cervical
   (b) Thoracic, lumbosacral
   (c) Non-specified/multiple
2. Nontraumatic (25%)
   (a) Motor neuron disorder
   (b) Spondylotic
   (c) Infectious (e.g., epidural abscess, osteomyelitis, HIV, West Nile)
   (d) Immune, inflammatory not including MS (e.g., transverse myelitis)
   (e) Multiple sclerosis
   (f) Tumor
   (g) Vascular (e.g., ischemic myelopathy, arteriovenous malformation, radiation myelopathy)
   (h) Toxic/metabolic/nutritional
   (i) Hereditary and congenital
   (j) Poliomyelitis and post-polio syndrome
3. Myelopathy without specified etiology (20%)

Class 2: Pathophysiology, Evaluation, and Management
1. Prevention of SCI (1%)
2. Applied anatomy, physiology, and kinesiology (3%)
3. Epidemiology, risk factors, and genetics (3%)
4. Neurologic assessment/classification (4%)

5. Acute evaluation and management (medical or surgical) (5%)
6. Spinal orthosis (2%)
7. Imaging of spine or spinal cord (3%)
8. Prognosis/predicting outcome or function (4%)
9. Ethics and professionalism (1%)
10. Electrodiagnostic assessment (2%)
11. Cardiovascular (5%)
    (a) Spinal shock (including neurogenic shock)
    (b) Orthostatic hypotension
    (c) Deep venous thrombosis
    (d) Pulmonary embolism
    (e) Autonomic dysreflexia
    (f) Other autonomic dysfunction
    (g) Other
12. Pulmonary (6%)
    (a) Restrictive pulmonary disease/respiratory impairment
    (b) Invasive and noninvasive ventilation/MIE
    (c) Infection/aspiration/atelectasis
    (d) Sleep disorders
    (e) Other
13. Gastrointestinal (5%)
    (a) Neurogenic bowel
    (b) Swallowing/dysphagia
    (c) Upper GI disorders (e.g., SMA, ileus)
    (d) Other (e.g., pancreatitis, hepatobiliary, appendicitis)
14. Genitourinary (8%)
    (a) Neurogenic bladder
    (b) Infection
    (c) Lithiasis
    (d) Urodynamics
    (e) Renal impairment
    (f) Other
15. Sexuality/reproductive (3%)
    (a) Sexual dysfunction
    (b) Fertility
    (c) Pregnancy
    (d) Other
16. Musculoskeletal (6%)
    (a) Spinal fractures, dislocations, instability
    (b) Contractures/joint complications
    (c) Heterotopic ossification
    (d) Osteoporosis
    (e) Scoliosis and late spine complications
    (f) Overuse injuries
    (g) Fractures (extremities)
    (h) Other

17. Neurological (5%)
    (a) Spasticity
    (b) Late central nervous system complications (hydro, syrinx, tethered cord)
    (c) Peripheral nerve dysfunction
    (d) Traumatic brain injury
    (e) Thermoregulation and sweating
    (f) Neuromodulatory and disease-modifying agents
    (g) Other
18. Pressure injuries (4%)
    (a) Risk factors, prevention
    (b) Staging/assessment/site
    (c) Nonsurgical evaluation and management
    (d) Surgical management
    (e) Other
19. Nutrition, weight management, body composition (1%)
20. Endocrine/metabolic (2%)
    (a) Endocrine
    (b) Lipid metabolism
    (c) Hypercalcemia
    (d) Other metabolic (e.g., hyponatremia)
21. Infection/immune NOS (e.g., sepsis, latex allergy) (2%)
22. Pain (4%)
    (a) Musculoskeletal
    (b) Neuropathic
    (c) Other (e.g., CRPS, nonspecific)
23. Psychological (3%)
    (a) Depression/affective disorder
    (b) Substance disorder
    (c) Cognitive impairment
    (d) Conversion disorder
    (e) Other behavior
24. Healthcare maintenance (2%)
    (a) Immunization
    (b) Preventive health care
    (c) Aging
25. Functional assessment (2%)
26. Exercise and modalities (2%)
    (a) Therapeutic exercise
    (b) Functional electrical stimulation
    (c) Modalities
    (d) Nontraditional therapies
27. Mobility (3%)
    (a) Gait
    (b) Ambulation/lower extremity orthosis
    (c) Wheelchairs, other mobility devices
    (d) Transfers, positioning, and sitting balance

28. Activities of daily living (2%)
    (a) Adaptive equipment/functional orthosis
    (b) Architectural adaptations
    (c) Tendon transfers
    (d) Environmental control technology
29. Speech and communication (1%)
30. Participation/living with SCI (2%)
    (a) Recreation and sports activities
    (b) Community access and driving
    (c) Vocational rehabilitation
    (d) Social issues
31. Healthcare systems (1%)
    (a) Rehabilitation team
    (b) Patient safety
    (c) Medico-legal issues, advocacy
    (d) Practice management
32. Clinical and basic science (3%)
    (a) Research and statistical methods
    (b) Neural injury/regeneration

SCI Medicine Certificate

Upon approval of the application and the candidate's successful completion of the examination, the ABPMR will grant a subspecialty certificate in SCI Medicine. Certificates are mailed approximately three months after notification of results. Note that the certificate is time-limited to a 10-year period, after which a maintenance of certification (MOC) will be necessary. The certificate expires on December 31 of the tenth year of the cycle.

Maintenance of Certification (MOC) in SCI Medicine

To be considered eligible to participate in the SCI Medicine MOC Program, applicants must have a current, valid, and unrestricted license to practice medicine in at least one jurisdiction in the United States, its territories, or Canada. Applying physicians must provide evidence of unrestricted licensure in the state or states in which they practice prior to issuance of the certificate.

MOC requires achieving a passing score on a computer-based, proctored SCI Medicine Examination prior to the certificate expiration date. Applicants may take the examination in years 7–10 of the SCI medicine MOC cycle.

If the subspecialty certificate expires after the 10-year time limit, the physician has a maximum of three years to become recertified (i.e., meet the licensure requirement and pass the subspecialty MOC Examination). After this three-year period, the physician will be required to reapply and meet the application requirements in effect at the time of the new application (i.e., complete another ACGME–accredited SCI medicine fellowship).

Further Reading

American Board of Physical Medicine and Rehabilitation. Subspeciality Certification. Available at: https://www.abpmr.org/Subspecialties. Accessed February 14, 2022.
Sabharwal S, Chiodo AE, Raddatz MM. Administration and performance on the Spinal Cord Injury Medicine Certification Examination over a 10-year period. J Spinal Cord Med. 2019;42(5):606–12. https://doi.org/10.1080/10790268.2018.1475995. Epub 2018 Jun 14

Epidemiology, Risk Factors, and Prevention of Spinal Cord Injury

2

John Lin, Wesley Chay, and Natasha Bhatia

Epidemiology

1. According to data collected from the National Spinal Cord Injury Database (NSCID), between 2005 and 2011, which of the following statements is true regarding the relationship between traumatic spinal cord injury (SCI) and an individual's sex?

   A. Traumatic SCI occurs equally among men and women
   B. Men are twice as likely to have a fall as the etiology of their SCI compared to women
   C. Men are twice as likely to have a gunshot wound as the etiology of their SCI compared to women
   D. Men are twice as likely to have an all-terrain vehicle (ATV) accident as the etiology of their SCI compared to women

   Answer: C.

   Overall, 78.3% of reported traumatic SCIs occurred in men. A gunshot wound as the etiology of SCI was twice as likely in men (11.7%) than in women (5.8%).

J. Lin (✉) · W. Chay
Department of Medical Staff, Shepherd Center, Atlanta, GA, USA
e-mail: John.Lin@Shepherd.org; Wesley.Chay@Shepherd.org

N. Bhatia
Department of Rehabilitation Medicine, Emory University School of Medicine, Atlanta, GA, USA

Department of Physical Medicine and Rehabilitation, Shirley Ryan AbilityLab, Department of Physical Medicine and Rehabilitation, Northwestern University Feinberg School of Medicine, Chicago, IL, USA
e-mail: nbhatia@sralab.org

© The Author(s), under exclusive license to Springer Nature Switzerland AG 2022
B. A. Abramoff et al. (eds.), *The Essential Spinal Cord Injury Medicine Question Bank*, https://doi.org/10.1007/978-3-031-07796-8_2

Fall as the etiology of SCI was approximately equal between men (25.6%) and women (24.2%). ATV accidents as the etiology of SCI was approximately equal between men (1.8%) and women (1.6%). The most common etiology of traumatic SCI in both men and women was automobile accidents (27.9% of injuries in men, and 44.4% of injuries in women).

Chen Y, Tang Y, Vogel LC, Devivo MJ. Causes of spinal cord injury. Top Spinal Cord Inj Rehabil. 2013;19(1):1–8. https://doi.org/10.1310/sci1901-1.

2. According to data collected from the National Spinal Cord Injury Database (NSCID), between 2005 and 2011, what is the most common cause of traumatic spinal cord injury among people older than 45 years in age?

   A. Medical/surgical complications
   B. Automobile accidents
   C. Falls
   D. Gunshot wounds

Answer: C.

Automobile accidents are the leading cause of traumatic spinal cord injury among individuals until age 45 years. At older ages, falls become the leading cause of traumatic SCIs.

Chen Y, Tang Y, Vogel LC, Devivo MJ. Causes of spinal cord injury. Top Spinal Cord Inj Rehabil. 2013;19(1):1–8. https://doi.org/10.1310/sci1901-1.

3. According to a 15-year population-based cohort study between 2002 and 2017, how has the incidence rate of SCI changed over time?

   A. Incidence of SCI in women over age 65 increased significantly over the study period
   B. Incidence of SCI in men over age 65 increased significantly over the study period
   C. Incidence of SCI in women below age 65 increased significantly over the study period
   D. Incidence of SCI in men below age 65 increased significantly over the study period

Answer: A.

Between 2002 and 2017, the incidence of SCI in women in the older age cohort (>65 years) increased on average 4% per year. Incidence of SCI in women in the younger age cohort (<65 years) showed a non-significant decline. There was no change in incidence of SCI in men of all ages over the study period.

Wilson JR, Cronin S, Fehlings MG, Kwon BK, Badhiwala JH, Ginsberg HJ, Witiw C, Jaglal S. Epidemiology and impact of spinal cord injury in the elderly: results of a fifteen-year population-based cohort study. J Neurotrauma. 2020;37(15):1740–51. https://doi.org/10.1089/neu.2020.6985. Epub 2020 May 11.

4. Which spinal cord injury etiology shows the greatest difference in incidence between racial/ethnic groups?

   A. Automobile accidents
   B. Gunshot wounds
   C. Falls
   D. Diving

   Answer: B.

   Gunshot wounds show the greatest difference in etiology profile among racial/ethnic groups, with gunshot wounds causing 33.0% of all SCI in Black individuals, 14.6% in Hispanic individuals, 9.5% in other races, and 3.0% in White individuals.

Chen Y, Tang Y, Vogel LC, Devivo MJ. Causes of spinal cord injury. Top Spinal Cord Inj Rehabil. 2013;19(1):1–8. https://doi.org/10.1310/sci1901-1.

5. Which of the following etiologies is most likely to be associated with a complete (American Spinal Injury Association Impairment Scale [AIS] grade A) injury?

   A. Medical/surgical complications
   B. Diving
   C. Falls
   D. Gunshot wounds

   Answer: D.

   The majority of gunshot wounds (65.6%) and motorcycle crashes (51.8%) resulted in a complete injury. Medical/surgical complications, diving accidents, and falls were comparatively less likely to result in a complete injury (22.4%, 41.8%, and 30.2% respectively).

Chen Y, Tang Y, Vogel LC, Devivo MJ. Causes of spinal cord injury. Top Spinal Cord Inj Rehabil. 2013;19(1):1–8. https://doi.org/10.1310/sci1901-1.

6. Based on SCI Model Systems data between 1973 to 2019, how have the trends of SCI incidence changed over time?

   A. The mean age at time of injury has increased
   B. Probability of injury from falls has decreased

C. Probability of injury from violence and sports has increased
D. The proportion of White individuals sustaining SCI has increased

Answer: A.

The mean age at injury has increased from 28.7 years in 1972–1979 to 43.1 years in 2015–2019. The probability of injury from falls has increased, while the probability of injury from violence and sports has decreased over time. There is a significant trend towards an increasing proportion of non-White individuals sustaining a SCI.

National Spinal Cord Injury Statistical Center, University of Alabama at Birmingham, 2019 Annual Statistical Report—Complete Public Version. https://www.nscisc.uab.edu/Public/2019%20Annual%20Report%20-%20Complete%20Public%20Version.pdf   [Last accessed 29 December 2020].

7. Comparing the data from National Spinal Cord Injury Statistical Center from 2015 to 2019 to that of the preceding fifteen years, which of the following etiologies has increased over time?

   A. Automobile accidents
   B. Falls
   C. Violence
   D. Sports

Answer: B.

The incidence of falls as an etiology of SCI has risen significantly, from 26.8% between 2000 and 2014 to 32% between 2015 and 2019. This is consistent with a proportional increase in the incidence of women with traumatic spinal cord injury above the age of 65. In comparison, the incidence of traumatic spinal cord injury due to automobile accidents, violence and sports has fallen or remained stable.

National Spinal Cord Injury Statistical Center, University of Alabama at Birmingham, 2019 Annual Statistical Report –Complete Public Version. https://www.nscisc.uab.edu/Public/2019%20Annual%20Report%20-%20Complete%20Public%20Version.pdf   [Last accessed 29 December 2020].

8. What is the most common level and severity of spinal cord injury as documented by the National Spinal Cord Injury Statistical Center (NSCISC) from 2015 to 2019?

   A. Complete Paraplegia
   B. Complete Tetraplegia

C. Incomplete Paraplegia
D. Incomplete Tetraplegia

Answer: D.

Incomplete tetraplegia is the most frequent neurological category of SCI (47.2%). The frequency of incomplete paraplegia (19.6%) and complete paraplegia (20.2%) are almost identical. Complete tetraplegia makes up 12.3% of SCIs.

National Spinal Cord Injury Statistical Center, University of Alabama at Birmingham, 2019 Annual Statistical Report –Complete Public Version. https://www.nscisc.uab.edu/Public/2019%20Annual%20Report%20-%20Complete%20Public%20Version.pdf   [Last accessed 29 December 2020].

9. According to model system data, which of the following regarding work and traumatic SCI is true?

A. Most persons sustain spinal cord injuries at work
B. While most injured persons are employed at time of injury, less than half of all individuals with traumatic SCI are employed after injury
C. Of those injured persons who return to work, most return to work within the first year post-injury
D. Jobs in office and administrative support are the most commonly obtained post-injury

Answer: B.

While nearly 60% of all those injured are working at time of injury, less than a third return to work post injury. Since 2001, only 9% of the traumatic spinal cord injuries are related to work. Return-to-work rate for first year post-injury is 12.6%. Injured persons most commonly return to work in management, business, or finance, accounting for about 25% of the total. Jobs in office and administrative support are the second most common, accounting for approximately 11%.

National Spinal Cord Injury Statistical Center, University of Alabama at Birmingham, 2019 Annual Statistical Report—Complete Public Version. https://www.nscisc.uab.edu/Public/2019%20Annual%20Report%20-%20Complete%20Public%20Version.pdf   [Last accessed 29 December 2020].

10. The most common neurological level of injury (NLI) at discharge from inpatient rehabilitation is:

A. C4
B. C6

C. T12
D. L1

Answer: A.

Of the 34,130 injured persons included in the database from National Spinal
Cord Injury Statistical Center, 4931 have NLI at C4. This is followed by 4852
at C5, 3226 at C6, 1949 at T12, 1594 at C7 and 1525 at L1.

National Spinal Cord Injury Statistical Center, University of Alabama at Birmingham,
2019 Annual Statistical Report—Complete Public Version. https://www.nscisc.uab.edu/
Public/2019%20Annual%20Report%20-%20Complete%20Public%20Version.pdf [Last
accessed 29 December 2020].

11. Which risk factor has the greatest association with spinal cord injury secondary
    to gunshot wound?

    A. Having a prior gunshot wound
    B. Having a prior violent injury requiring treatment in the emergency
       department
    C. Having prior involvement in the criminal justice system
    D. Living in rural area

    Answer: C.

    52% of respondents had prior involvement in the criminal justice system. 30%
    had a previous gunshot wound and 16% had another violent injury requiring
    treatment in the emergency department. Gunshot wounds constitute the second
    most common cause of spinal cord injury in urban areas.

Ragucci MV, Gittler MM, Balfanz-Vertiz K, Hunter A. Societal risk factors associated with spinal cord injury secondary to gunshot wound. Arch Phys Med Rehabil.
2001;82(12):1720–3. https://doi.org/10.1053/apmr.2001.26610.

12. All of the following are behavioral factors that have been associated with trau-
    matic spinal cord injury EXCEPT:

    A. Alcohol misuse
    B. Impulsivity
    C. Prescription medication use
    D. Violence

    Answer: C.

    SCI has been associated with impulsivity and risk taking, alcohol misuse, and
    violence. There has not been an association reported between SCI and prescrip-
    tion medication use.

Fordyce WE. Personality characteristics in men with spinal cord injury as related to manner of onset of disability. Arch Phys Med Rehabil. 1964;45:321–5.

Farmer JC, Vaccaro AR, Balderston RA, Albert TJ, Cotler J. The changing nature of admissions to a spinal cord injury center: violence on the rise. J Spinal Disord. 1998;11(5):400–3.

Hawkins DA, Heinemann AW. Substance abuse and medical complications following spinal cord injury. Rehabil Psychol. 1998;(3):219–231. https://doi.org/10.1037/0090-5550.43.3.219

13. In the United States of America, all of the following are true regarding the risk of traumatic spinal cord injury EXCEPT:

    A. Rollover car accidents have a higher rate of SCI compared to non-rollover car accidents
    B. The rate of spinal cord injuries in car accidents is higher than the risk of severe head injury
    C. Being involved in a car accident without a seat belt increases the risk of SCI
    D. Rear-impact car accidents have a lower rate of SCI compared to frontal-impact car accidents

Answer: B.

Rollover crashes, riding without seat belts and frontal impact (as opposed to rear impact) car accidents have all been associated with higher rates of traumatic spinal cord injury in the United States. However, the rate of severe head injuries in car accidents is 13.3 times greater than that of SCI.

Parenteau CS, Viano DC. Spinal fracture-dislocations and spinal cord injuries in motor vehicle crashes. Traffic Inj Prev. 2014;15(7):694–700. https://doi.org/10.1080/1538958 8.2013.867434.

14. The highest incidence of concomitant traumatic brain injuries is seen in which level of spinal cord injuries?

    A. Cervical
    B. Thoracic
    C. Lumbar
    D. Sacral

Answer: A.

A major trend noted in the literature is the increased rate of brain injury associated with higher levels of SCI. Model Systems database of traumatic SCI-traumatic brain injury dual diagnosis include 54.9% in cervical levels, 34.1% in thoracic levels, 7.7% in lumbar levels, and 0% in sacral levels of SCI.

Elovic E, Kirshblum S. Epidemiology of spinal cord injury and traumatic brain injury: the scope of the problem. Top Spinal Cord Inj Rehabil. 1999;5:1–20.

Budisin B, Bradbury CC, Sharma B, Hitzig SL, Mikulis D, Craven C, McGilivray C, Corbie J, Green RE. Traumatic brain injury in spinal cord injury: frequency and risk factors. J Head Trauma Rehabil. 2016;31(4):E33–42. https://doi.org/10.1097/HTR.0000000000000153.

15. With which of the following etiologies of traumatic spinal cord injuries is cervical stenosis/spondylosis most commonly associated?

    A. Automobile accidents
    B. Falls
    C. Sports-related injuries
    D. Acts of violence

Answer: B.

Falls are a particularly important potentially modifiable risk factor for SCI in patients with cervical stenosis/spondylosis. According to Burns (2016), in individuals with tetraplegia due to falls, 40% had cervical stenosis/spondylosis. In comparison, the rate of associated cervical stenosis/spondylosis was lower in other known etiologies of traumatic SCI (25% in MVA, 16.1% in sports, and 10.2% in acts of violence).

Burns SP, Weaver F, Chin A, Svircev J, Carbone L. Cervical stenosis in spinal cord injury and disorders. J Spinal Cord Med. 2016;39(4):471–5. https://doi.org/10.1080/10790268.2015.1114229. Epub 2015 Dec 14.

16. A 20-year-old man with no significant past medical or surgical history presents to the local emergency department with a history of worsening low back pain for the past week. He has developed some increased difficulty walking over the past few days and difficulty controlling his bowel and bladder in the past 24 hours. An MRI of the lumbar spine with contrast demonstrates a fluid collection along the ventral aspect of spinal canal, from L1 to L3, suggestive of an epidural abscess. Which of the following risk factors are most likely present in this patient?

    A. Human immunodeficiency virus
    B. Recent spinal injection
    C. End-stage liver disease
    D. Intravenous (IV) drug abuse

Answer: D.

A 2017 case series found that diabetes was the most common risk factor for spinal epidural abscess occurring in 26.7% of individuals. This was followed by IV drug use (16.8%), spinal injections (5.9%), HIV (5.0%), and end-stage liver disease (5.0%). In a young healthy individual with no significant medical or surgical history, IV drug use is the most likely cause.

Vakili M, Crum-Cianflone NF. Spinal epidural abscess: a series of 101 cases. Am J Med. 2017;130(12):1458–63. https://doi.org/10.1016/j.amjmed.2017.07.017. Epub 2017 Aug 7.

17. In the United States of America, the largest percentage of sports-related spinal cord injuries are due to which sport?

    A. Wrestling
    B. Diving
    C. Cycling
    D. Horseback riding

Answer: B.

Sport-related spinal cord injuries in the USA are most commonly due to diving, followed by cycling, horseback riding, and wrestling. In a global systematic review, diving was also the sport causing the greatest number of SCI's worldwide.

Chan CW, Eng JJ, Tator CH, Krassioukov A; Spinal Cord Injury Research Evidence Team. Epidemiology of sport-related spinal cord injuries: A systematic review. J Spinal Cord Med. 2016;39(3):255–64. https://doi.org/10.1080/10790268.2016.1138601. Epub 2016 Feb 18.

18. Which of the following factors has the greatest association with SCI secondary to a fall compared to SCI from a non-fall etiology?

    A. Older age
    B. African-American race
    C. Lumbar level injury
    D. American Spinal Injury Association Impairment Scale (AIS) A classification

Answer: A.

The rate of SCI as a result of a fall has increased over the last four decades. SCI due to fall is especially common among the elderly. Of people 76 years of age and older with an SCI, 75% are due to falls. Persons with a fall-induced SCI are more likely to be white. They are more likely to have a cervical injury and an AIS D classification.

Chen Y, Tang Y, Allen V, DeVivo MJ. Fall-induced spinal cord injury: External causes and implications for prevention. J Spinal Cord Med. 2016;39(1):24–31. https://doi.org/10.1179/2045772315Y.0000000007. Epub 2015 Apr 1.

19. Which of the following etiologies is the most common cause of non-traumatic spinal cord injuries?

    A. Neoplasm
    B. Infection
    C. Ischemic
    D. Spinal stenosis

    Answer: D.

    In a study conducted at a Level I trauma center of a Regional SCI Model System, 54% of non-traumatic SCI was due to spinal stenosis, followed by tumors (22%), ischemia (8%), and infection (7%).

    McKinley WO, Seel RT, Hardman JT. Nontraumatic spinal cord injury: incidence, epidemiology, and functional outcome. Arch Phys Med Rehabil. 1999;80(6):619–23. https://doi.org/10.1016/s0003-9993(99)90162-4.

20. A 65-year-old individual presents to your rehabilitation facility with spinal cord injury following a fall. The most likely cause of her fall-induced spinal cord injury was a fall:

    A. On the ground/same level
    B. Off a ladder
    C. Down stairs and steps
    D. From a building

    Answer: A.

    A 2016 analysis of epidemiological data from the 21 SCI Model Systems Centers in the United States showed that same level falls (e.g. slipping, tripping, and stumbling) contributed to 20% of fall-induced SCI. This was followed by falls from building (16%), stairs and steps (16%), and ladder (9%).

    Chen Y, Tang Y, Allen V, DeVivo MJ. Fall-induced spinal cord injury: External causes and implications for prevention. J Spinal Cord Med. 2016;39(1):24–31. https://doi.org/10.1179/2045772315Y.0000000007. Epub 2015 Apr 1.

21. In order to decrease fall risk and subsequent risk of spinal cord injury, which one of the following recommendations would you NOT make for the home environment to improve safety?

    A. Removing clutter and power cords from the floor
    B. Placement of throw rugs
    C. Maintaining good lighting
    D. Installing handrails and grab bars

Answer: B.

Living environments can be improved by removing clutter, loose carpets, uneven floor surfaces and by providing good lighting, handrails, and appropriate toilets and beds.

Chen Y, Tang Y, Allen V, DeVivo MJ. Aging and Spinal Cord Injury: External Causes of Injury and Implications for Prevention. Top Spinal Cord Inj Rehabil. 2015;21(3):218–26. https://doi.org/10.1310/sci2103-218. Epub 2015 Jul 29.

22. A 67-year-old male inquires about fall prevention strategies as a friend recently sustained a spinal cord injury from a fall. To prevent falls in the elderly and thereby minimize the risk of associated spinal cord injury, the Center for Disease Control (CDC) advises:

A. Consumption of heart healthy diet
B. Reduction in weight
C. Participation in strength and balance exercises
D. Adherence to immunization recommendations

Answer: C.

Citing a 30% increase over ten years (2007–2016) in the death rate stemming from falls, CDC recommends strength and balance exercises along with vision evaluation and house fall safety optimization (e.g. removal of objects that may lead to tripping, addition of grab bars in the bathroom, addition of stairway railings, and improving lighting inside the house).

Older Adult Fall Prevention: Important Facts about Falls. http://www.cdc.gov/HomeandRecreationalSafety/Falls/adultfalls.html [Cited 2020 December 20.]

23. Rule changes by the American football community in which of the following have resulted in reduction of spinal cord injuries?

A. Lengthening the distance of kicking attempts for points after touchdowns
B. Banning head-down tackling
C. Penalizing blocks to the side and below the waist of all offensive players
D. Removal of players from the game for suspected head trauma

Answer: B.

After banning the technique of head-down tackling, the incidence of related catastrophic SCI injuries reduced from 32 persons in 1975 to 8 in 2007. Rule changes to mitigate repetitive concussive injuries may have secondary benefits associated with preventing spinal cord injury although this has not been shown to be as effective as implementation of head-up tackling. Low blocks are implemented to minimize injuries to the lower limbs. Lengthening the distance of kicking attempts for points after touchdowns was designed to improve the competitiveness of the game.

Chao S, Pacella MJ, Torg JS. The pathomechanics, pathophysiology and prevention of cervical spinal cord and brachial plexus injuries in athletics. Sports Med. 2010;40(1):59–75. https://doi.org/10.2165/11319650-000000000-00000.

24. A mother accompanies her teenage daughter to a visit with you. She asks you how to prevent a spinal cord injury for her child at a pool-side party next weekend. What is the best advice you can give the mother?

    A. Have her request to have the party held at a private pool instead of a public pool
    B. Encourage her to make sure there is a lifeguard present at the party enforcing no-diving rules
    C. Request to have signs posted warning against diving
    D. Educating her child regarding association of spinal cord injury and illicit substance abuse at the pool party

    Answer: B.

    Up to 87% of swimming pool related spinal cord injuries are associated with diving, with 95% of these occurring at depth below 8 feet. A person trained in water safety enforcing no-diving rule can mitigate these injuries as 94% of all these spinal cord injuries occur without a lifeguard on duty. This approach has been advocated by national pediatric organizations. Although almost all injuries (87%) occur in private/residential pools, not all public access swimming pools are staffed with lifeguards. While most injuries occur in a setting without warning signs, 13% of injuries occur in spite of posted warning signs. As a passive intervention for prevention, signs are likely to be less effective than the active intervention of a lifeguard. Drug use has only been associated in 2% of these injuries.

DeVivo MJ, Sekar P. Prevention of spinal cord injuries that occur in swimming pools. Spinal Cord. 1997;35(8):509–15. https://doi.org/10.1038/sj.sc.3100430.

Spinal cord injury awareness: Prevention begins with awareness. https://www.shrinershospitalsforchildren.org/shc/spinal-cord-injury-awareness?srcaud=SHC [Cited 2020 December 20.]

25. To prevent and minimize ischemic spinal cord injury associated with thoracic aortic repair, which of the following strategies has been shown to be most effective?

    A. Performing the repair using open surgery as opposed to thoracic endovascular aortic repair (TEVAR)
    B. Routine prophylactic cerebrospinal fluid drain placement

C. Routine neurophysiological monitoring using transcranial motor-evoked potentials or somatosensory-evoked potentials during TEVAR
D. Maintenance of mean arterial pressure above 80 mmHg after detection of ischemic spinal cord injury

Answer: D.

Due to the association of the high incidence of intra- and post-operative decrease in mean arterial pressure (MAP) and spinal cord ischemia, maintenance of MAP above 80 mmHg is recommended after detection of ischemic spinal cord injury.

Greenberg (2008) reported no statistical difference regarding ischemic spinal cord injury using either open or endovascular aortic repair. While there are specified indications for cerebrospinal fluid drain placement, Keith (2012) reported a comparable spinal ischemic rate of 3.2 versus 3.5 percent in routine versus no routine drain placement. Although neurophysiological monitoring has shown the ability to detect SCI, it is unclear if changes in neurophysiological monitoring signals would actually manifest postoperative SCI in the absence of intervention.

Greenberg RK, Lu Q, Roselli EE, Svensson LG, Moon MC, Hernandez AV, Dowdall J, Cury M, Francis C, Pfaff K, Clair DG, Ouriel K, Lytle BW. Contemporary analysis of descending thoracic and thoracoabdominal aneurysm repair: a comparison of endovascular and open techniques. Circulation. 2008;118(8):808–17. https://doi.org/10.1161/CIRCULA-TIONAHA.108.769695. Epub 2008 Aug 4.

Keith CJ Jr, Passman MA, Carignan MJ, Parmar GM, Nagre SB, Patterson MA, Taylor SM, Jordan WD Jr. Protocol implementation of selective postoperative lumbar spinal drainage after thoracic aortic endograft. J Vasc Surg. 2012;55(1):1–8; discussion 8. https://doi.org/10.1016/j.jvs.2011.07.086. Epub 2011 Oct 6.

Weigang E, Hartert M, Siegenthaler MP, Pitzer-Hartert K, Luehr M, Sircar R, von Samson P, Beyersdorf F. Neurophysiological monitoring during thoracoabdominal aortic endovascular stent graft implantation. Eur J Cardiothorac Surg. 2006;29(3):392–6. https://doi.org/10.1016/j.ejcts.2005.11.039. Epub 2006 Jan 24.

Etz CD, Di Luozzo G, Zoli S, Lazala R, Plestis KA, Bodian CA, Griepp RB. Direct spinal cord perfusion pressure monitoring in extensive distal aortic aneurysm repair. Ann Thorac Surg. 2009;87(6):1764–73; discussion 1773–4. https://doi.org/10.1016/j.athoracsur.2009.02.101.

Etz CD, Weigang E, Hartert M, Lonn L, Mestres CA, Di Bartolomeo R, Bachet JE, Carrel TP, Grabenwöger M, Schepens MA, Czerny M. Contemporary spinal cord protection during thoracic and thoracoabdominal aortic surgery and endovascular aortic repair: a position paper of the vascular domain of the European Association for Cardio-Thoracic Surgery†. Eur J Cardiothorac Surg. 2015;47(6):943–57. https://doi.org/10.1093/ejcts/ezv142.

26. Regarding prevention and mitigation of spinal cord injury related to trampoline use, which of the following is true?

A. There has been a decrease in injuries related to public trampoline facilities
B. Keeping children under the age of 6 from using trampolines will prevent most pediatric injuries

C. For adults, trampoline injury prevention strategies should be focused primarily on mitigation of injuries to the upper extremities

D. Competent supervision is still needed even if there is netting present

Answer: D.

The primary prevention strategy for trampoline-related SCI is supervision. While netting is helpful in reducing injuries, it is not an adequate substitution for competent supervision. There has been an alarming increase in injuries occurring at public trampoline facilities over the last ten years. Two-thirds of injuries reported in children occur between the ages of 6 and 14 years. In one series examining trampoline related injuries in adults, Arora (2015) noted significantly more spinal injuries compared to upper extremity injuries. However, there were less spinal injuries compared to lower extremity injuries.

Bellon K, Kolakowsky-Hayner SA, Chen D, McDowell S, Bitterman B, Klaas SJ. Evidence-based practice in primary prevention of spinal cord injury. Top Spinal Cord Inj Rehabil. 2013;19(1):25–30. https://doi.org/10.1310/sci1901-25.

Fitzgerald RE, Freiman SM, Kulwin R, Loder R. Demographic changes in US trampoline-related injuries from 1998 to 2017: cause for alarm. Inj Prev. 2021;27(1):55–60. https://doi.org/10.1136/injuryprev-2019-043501. Epub 2020 Mar 9.

Arora V, Kimmel LA, Yu K, Gabbe BJ, Liew SM, Kamali Moaveni A. Trampoline related injuries in adults. Injury. 2016;47(1):192–6. https://doi.org/10.1016/j.injury.2015.09.002. Epub 2015 Sep 11.

27. Regarding motor vehicle-related spinal cord injuries, which of the following is true?

A. Motor vehicle-related spinal cord injuries are not reduced by supplemental restraint system

B. Recent improvements in car seats have primarily focused on comfort as opposed to safety

C. Engineering and equipment innovations have played a significant role in tertiary prevention of motor vehicle-related spinal cord injuries

D. Education and awareness are essential in primary prevention of motor vehicle-related spinal cord injuries

Answer: D.

Education, awareness, and engineering and equipment innovations have all played a vital role in primary prevention of motor vehicle-related spinal cord injuries. Improvements in car seats and airbags have reduced the incidence of motor vehicle-related spinal cord injuries. Secondary injury prevention is the responsibility of the entire health care system and includes first aid, retrieval, and acute hospitalization of the injured person. Tertiary prevention measures focus on prevention of long-term disability.

Tator C. Current primary to tertiary prevention of spinal cord injury. Top Spinal Cord Inj Rehabil. 2004;10(1):1–14.

28. The Stopping Elderly Accidents, Deaths and Injuries (STEADI) toolkit is a resource created by the CDC for health care providers to use in assessing and addressing which of the following?

    A. Motor vehicle safety in elderly drivers
    B. Fall risk in older individuals
    C. Drug overdose safety
    D. Violence prevention with elder abuse

Answer: B.

The STEADI toolkit is a resource created by the CDC for health care providers to use in assessing and addressing fall risk in older individuals. These resources include basic information about falls, screening options, information on medications linked to falls, standardized gait and balance assessment tests, and online training.

STEADI—Older Adult Fall Prevention. https://www.cdc.gov/steadi/materials.html [Cited 2020 December 20.]

Anatomy, Physiology and Imaging of the Spinal Cord

3

Joanne M. Delgado-Lebron

Questions

1. The main difference between meningeal coverings of the spinal cord compared to the brain is:

   A. The spinal cord is covered only by two meningeal layers
   B. The spinal epidural space is an actual space
   C. Cerebral spinal fluid circulates in the subarachnoid space.
   D. The spinal dura consists of both a meningeal and a periosteal layer

   Answer: B.

   As in the cranium, three layers of meninges surround the spinal cord for its entire length. The cranial dura consists of two tightly adherent layers, and the cranial epidural space is bound by periosteum outwardly and the two-layered dura inwardly. In the spinal canal (beginning at the foramen magnum), the dura only has a meningeal layer. The periosteal dural layer separates from the inner layer, creating an anatomical epidural space. The spinal epidural space is an actual space that contains veins and fatty tissue, which serves as a useful landmark on MRI. Additionally, anesthesia can be used in the spinal epidural space for a segmental or regional block. Similar to the brain, cerebral spinal fluid circulates in the subarachnoid space.

J. M. Delgado-Lebron (✉)
Department of Physical Medicine & Rehabilitation, Memorial Rehabilitation Institute at Memorial Healthcare System, Hollywood, FL, USA
e-mail: jdelgadolebron@mhs.net

Cho TA. Spinal cord functional anatomy. Continuum (Minneap Minn). 2015;21(1 Spinal Cord Disorders):13–35. https://doi.org/10.1212/01.CON.0000461082.25876.4a.

2. The spinal cord is anchored by all of the following EXCEPT:

   A. Dentate ligaments
   B. Ligamentum flavum
   C. Filum terminale
   D. Coccygeal ligament

Answer: B.

The spinal cord is anchored rostrally at the cervicomedullary junction by dentate ligaments and caudally by the filum terminale (an extension of the pia at the conus medullaris, which attaches to the first coccygeal segment through the sacral dura). At the level of the 2nd sacral vertebra the spinal dura becomes a thin extension called the coccygeal ligament (or the filum terminale externum) and serves to anchor the spinal dura to the coccyx. The pia mater invests the spinal cord intimately and on either side of the cord, a pial thickening and extension between the ventral and dorsal nerve roots form the paired dentate ligaments, which tether it to the dura mater laterally. Caudally, another pial thickening forms the filum terminale, which anchors the conus medullaris to the bony sacrum. The ligamentum flavum consists of a series of ligaments that connects the anterior aspects of adjacent laminae.

Cho TA. Spinal cord functional anatomy. Continuum (Minneap Minn). 2015;21(1 Spinal Cord Disorders):13–35. https://doi.org/10.1212/01.CON.0000461082.25876.4a.
Miele VJ, Panjabi MM, Benzel EC. Anatomy and biomechanics of the spinal column and cord. Handb Clin Neurol. 2012;109:31–43. https://doi.org/10.1016/B978-0-444-52137-8.00002-4.

3. Regarding the nerve roots, which of the following is true?

   A. Afferent neurons enter the spinal cord through the dorsal root
   B. Lumbar roots run at right angles compared to cervical roots which runs more obliquely
   C. There are two total branches arising from each common spinal nerve trunk
   D. Efferent nerve roots leave the spinal canal through the anterior neural (intravertebral) foramen, afferent nerve roots enter through posterior neural (intravertebral) foramen.

Answer: A.

The dorsal roots consist of several types of afferent fibers that are organized somatotopically. The anterior root bundles constitute the motor output from the spinal cord. Usually the following four branches (rami) arise from the common spinal nerve trunk: dorsal ramus, ventral ramus, meningeal branch, ramus communicans. Lower in the spinal column of adults, the bony elements and neural elements become less directly in line, and the angle of the roots becomes less perpendicular compared to the more caudal/cervical segments. There is no such thing as anterior and posterior neural foramen (only a single one exists on both sides).

Bican O, Minagar A, Pruitt AA. The spinal cord: a review of functional neuroanatomy. Neurol Clin. 2013;31(1):1–18. https://doi.org/10.1016/j.ncl.2012.09.009.
Sapru HN. Spinal cord anatomy, physiology and pathophysiology. In: Kirshblum S, Campagnolo DI, editors. Spinal cord medicine. 2nd ed. Philadelphia: Lipincott Williams & Wilkins; 2011. pp. 6–30.

4. Which of the following is true about the spinal nerves?

   A. They contain sensory nerve fibers
   B. There are 8 cervical, 12 thoracic, 5 lumbar, 5 sacral and 1 coccygeal.
   C. In the cervical segments all the spinal roots exit the foramina caudal to the same level vertebra
   D. Myotomes are the area of sensory innervation of each spinal nerve.

   Answer: B.

   31 pairs of spinal nerves exist, including 8 cervical, 12 thoracic, 5 lumbar, 5 sacral and 1 coccygeal. By convention, spinal nerves in the cervical region exit above their corresponding vertebra with the exception of C8, which exists above T1 due to lack of C8 vertebrae. They are mixed nerves containing both sensory and motor nerve fibers. Myotomes are the muscles innervated by one spinal nerve while dermatomes are the areas of sensory innervation for each spinal nerve.

Diaz E, Morales H. Spinal cord anatomy and clinical syndromes. Semin Ultrasound CT MR. 2016;37(5):360–71. https://doi.org/10.1053/j.sult.2016.05.002. Epub 2016 May 6.
Cho TA. Spinal cord functional anatomy. Continuum (Minneap Minn). 2015;21(1 Spinal Cord Disorders):13–35. https://doi.org/10.1212/01.CON.0000461082.25876.4a.

5. Each of the spinal cord segments always have a pair of sensory and motor roots EXCEPT for:

   A. C1
   B. T1
   C. L1
   D. S1

   Answer: A.

   There are 31 spinal cord segments (eight cervical, one thoracic, five lumbar, five sacral, and one coccygeal). Except for C1, which has no sensory nerve root, each segment always has a pair of dorsal (sensory) and ventral (motor) roots that join to form a mixed spinal nerve just as they enter the dural sleeve and neural foramina. C1 has a small meningeal branch that supplies the dura around the foramen magnum. The dorsal root and ganglion of C1 may be absent. Each spinal nerve corresponds to a vertebra, except for C8, which has no corresponding vertebra.

Cho TA. Spinal cord functional anatomy. Continuum (Minneap Minn). 2015;21(1 Spinal Cord Disorders):13–35. https://doi.org/10.1212/01.CON.0000461082.25876.4a.

6. All of the following are true about the lumbar cistern EXCEPT:

    A. It is found between the 2nd lumbar vertebra and 2nd sacral vertebra
    B. It contains the widest subarachnoid space
    C. It is considered the target for lumbar punctures
    D. It contains the lowest part of the spinal cord and the conus medullaris.

Answer: D.

The lumbar cistern is the area of the dural sac that extends distal to the conus medullaris (between the 2nd lumbar vertebra and the 2nd sacral vertebra). It contains CSF and is the target for lumbar punctures as well as the widest subarachnoid space.

Sapru HN. Spinal cord anatomy, physiology and pathophysiology. In: Kirshblum S, Campagnolo DI, editors. Spinal cord medicine. 2nd ed. Philadelphia: Lipincott Williams & Wilkins; 2011. pp. 6–30.

7. All of the following are true regarding the gray matter of the spinal cord EXCEPT:

    A. In the thoracic levels the amount of gray matter is less than in the cervical levels.
    B. The lateral horns contain preganglionic cells of the autonomic neurons.
    C. The posterior horn contains the gamma motor neurons.
    D. The anterior horn is organized somatotropically with neurons controlling more distal muscles located more laterally.

Answer: C.

The ratio of gray substance to white matter varies markedly at different levels of spinal cord. In the thoracic levels the amount of gray matter is less than that in the cervical and lumbosacral enlargements. The anterior horn contains alpha and gamma motor neurons, and it is organized somatotopically (the neurons controlling the axial muscles are most medially placed, the neurons controlling the proximal limb muscles are in between, and the neurons controlling the distal limbs are most laterally placed). The lateral column contains preganglionic cells for the autonomic nervous system in the thoracic and upper lumbar areas.

Bican O, Minagar A, Pruitt AA. The spinal cord: a review of functional neuroanatomy. Neurol Clin. 2013;31(1):1–18. https://doi.org/10.1016/j.ncl.2012.09.009 .

Cho TA. Spinal cord functional anatomy. Continuum (Minneap Minn). 2015;21(1 Spinal Cord Disorders):13–35. https://doi.org/10.1212/01.CON.0000461082.25876.4a.

8. The vast majority of motor neurons in the gray matter are located in which lamina?

    A. II
    B. IV
    C. VII
    D. IX

Answer: D.

Lamina II corresponds to the substantia gelatinosa of Rolando, which is involved with the transmission and modulation of pain and temperature. Lamina IV contains the proper sensory nucleus and relays sensory and motor information. Lamina VII occupies most of the intermediate gray matter, which contains the nucleus of Clarke (involved in unconscious proprioception) as well as autonomic neurons. Lamina IX contain the various columns of descending motor neurons that innervates skeletal muscle.

Schoenen J Clin Anat Spinal Cord Neurol Clin. 1991;9(3):503–32.

Sapru HN. Spinal cord anatomy, physiology and pathophysiology. In: Kirshblum S, Campagnolo DI, editors. Spinal cord medicine. 2nd ed. Philadelphia: Lipincott Williams & Wilkins; 2011. pp. 6–30.

9. The fibers carrying information about pain and temperature are located in which tract?

    A. Spinocerebellar tract
    B. Spinothalamic tract
    C. Dorsal column pathway
    D. Corticospinal tract

Answer: B.

The spinothalamic tract carries information on pain, temperature, and crude touch. The spinocerebellar carries information mostly involved in unconscious proprioception. The dorsal column pathway carries information on fine touch, vibration and proprioception. The corticospinal tract is the main descending pathway involved in voluntary motor control.

Cho TA. Spinal cord functional anatomy. Continuum (Minneap Minn). 2015;21(1 Spinal Cord Disorders):13–35. https://doi.org/10.1212/01.CON.0000461082.25876.4a.

10. The fibers of the spinothalamic tract originate in the dorsal horn and ascend in the spinal cord through:

    A. Ipsilateral spinothalamic tract, before pyramidal decussation
    B. Ipsilateral spinothalamic tract, mostly uncrossed
    C. Contralateral spinothalamic tract, mostly uncrossed
    D. Contralateral spinothalamic tract, after anterior commissure decussation

Answer D.

The spinothalamic tract, along with several other less clinically significant tracts, constitute the anterolateral system, in which the initial synapse occurs in the dorsal horn gray matter. Second-order neurons then send axons across the anterior commissure (anterior to the central canal) to ascend in the contralateral anterolateral pathway. This decussation is usually two to three segments proximal to the initial synapse, so that lesions affecting the anterolateral tract at a given spinal cord level will have a contralateral sensory deficit two to three levels lower to the lesion. For those two to three segments, the sensory deficit will be ipsilateral.

Cho TA. Spinal cord functional anatomy. Continuum (Minneap Minn). 2015;21(1 Spinal Cord Disorders):13–35. https://doi.org/10.1212/01.CON.0000461082.25876.4a.

11. The fasciculus gracilis of the spinal cord carries information about:

    A. Ipsilateral voluntary motor control of the upper extremities
    B. Contralateral voluntary motor control of the upper extremities
    C. Ipsilateral vibration and position sense of the lower extremities
    D. Contralateral vibration and position sense of the lower extremities

Answer: C.

The dorsal column pathway is responsible for the transmission of sensations of vibration, proprioception (position sense), and 2-point discrimination from the skin and joints. The fasciculus gracilis, part of this pathway, is located medially and transmits sensation from the lower half of the body, whereas the fasciculus cuneatus, which is located more laterally at levels rostral to T5, carries proprioceptive input from the upper thorax through the upper half of the body.

Bican O, Minagar A, Pruitt AA. The spinal cord: a review of functional neuroanatomy. Neurol Clin. 2013;31(1):1–18. https://doi.org/10.1016/j.ncl.2012.09.009.

12. The dorsal column pathway originates in the dorsal horn and ascend in the spinal cord through:

A. Ipsilateral dorsal columns uncrossed
B. Ipsilateral dorsal columns after anterior commissure decussation
C. Contralateral dorsal columns prior to pyramidal decussation
D. Contralateral dorsal columns after anterior commissure decussation

Answer: A.

Fibers entering the posterior column system ascend the entire length of the spinal cord before synapsing with second-order neurons in the medulla. Axons carrying vibration and proprioception from the lower extremities and lower trunk enter the ipsilateral gracile fasciculus medially, while fibers from the upper extremities and neck are added on laterally to form the cuneate fasciculus. Both gracile and cuneate pathways synapse in the medulla, where second-order neurons in their respective nuclei finally send projections across the midline via internal arcuate fibers to the contralateral medial lemniscus and then to the thalamic ventral posterolateral (VPL) nucleus.

Cho TA. Spinal cord functional anatomy. Continuum (Minneap Minn). 2015;21(1 Spinal Cord Disorders):13–35. https://doi.org/10.1212/01.CON.0000461082.25876.4a.

13. Which of the following is correct?

A. The fasciculus gracilis is laterally located in the dorsal columns and carries sensory information from lower extremities.
B. The fasciculus cuneatus is laterally located in the dorsal columns and carries sensory information from upper extremities.
C. The fasciculus gracilis is medially located in the dorsal columns and carries sensory information from upper extremities.
D. The fasciculus cuneatus is medially located in the dorsal columns and carries sensory information from upper extremities.

Answer: B.

Axons carrying vibration and proprioception (conscious and unconscious) from the lower extremities and lower trunk enter the ipsilateral gracile fasciculus and are located medially, while fibers from the upper extremities and neck are added on laterally to form the cuneate fasciculus.

Cho TA. Spinal cord functional anatomy. Continuum (Minneap Minn). 2015;21(1 Spinal Cord Disorders):13–35. https://doi.org/10.1212/01.CON.0000461082.25876.4a.

14. Unconscious proprioception information is carried afferently in the spinal cord in which tract?

    A. Rubrospinal Tract
    B. Paleospinothalamic tract
    C. Reticulospinal tract
    D. Spinocerebellar Tracts

Answer: D.

Unconscious proprioception information from the lower extremities and lower trunk travels alongside conscious proprioception in the gracile fasciculus, before collateral fibers exit to synapse on the thoracic posterior (Clarke) nucleus. Secondary neurons send fibers through the ipsilateral posterior spinocerebellar tracts to the cerebellum via the inferior cerebellar peduncle. Analogous collaterals carrying upper extremity and trunk unconscious proprioception exit the cuneate fasciculus to synapse in the medullary accessory cuneate nucleus, which sends signals to the ipsilateral inferior cerebellar peduncle. The rubrospinal tract carries descending signals that modulate proximal, largely flexor movements of the upper limb. The paleospinothalamic tract is an element of the spinothalamic tract which is involved in transmitting pain information (particularly C-fiber mediated dull, burning pain). The reticulospinal tract consists of two pathways and influences muscle tone, reflexes, respiration, and autonomic function.

Cho TA. Spinal cord functional anatomy. Continuum (Minneap Minn). 2015;21(1 Spinal Cord Disorders):13–35. https://doi.org/10.1212/01.CON.0000461082.25876.4a.

15. Which of the following best describes the corticospinal tract?

    A. Originates primarily from the primary motor cortex, descends ipsilaterally in the brain until fibers decussate in the pyramids at the level of the medulla and descend in the lateral column of the spinal cord.
    B. Originates in the dorsal root ganglion, synapses in the dorsal horn, crossed over contralaterally at the level of the cord and ascend in the contralateral white matter.
    C. 100% of the corticospinal fibers decussate
    D. Fibers carrying information from more caudal segments are more medially located, whereas fibers carrying information from rostral segments are more laterally located.

Answer: A.

The corticospinal tract (CST) is a descending motor tract that controls fine movements and the most important motor pathway in humans. It consists of axons from upper motor neurons (UMNs), more than 50% of which arise from the primary motor cortex, with the remainder contributed by the premotor cortex, supplementary motor area, and sensory cortex. These fibers descend through the cerebral white matter, posterior limb of the internal capsule, cerebral peduncle, and ventral pons. In the medulla, 75%–90% of the fibers in the CST decussate in the pyramid and continue as the lateral CST in the lateral column. The neurons of the lateral CST synapse in the ventral horn before exiting the cord. Ten percent of the axons do not decussate but rather continue as the anterior CST, crossing over to the opposite side in each spinal cord segment supplying motor neurons in the ventral horn. Fibers synapsing in more rostral (cervical) areas are situated medially and fibers synapsing to caudal (sacral) regions are situated laterally. Option B describes spinothalamic tract.

Kunam VK, Velayudhan V, Chaudhry ZA, Bobinski M, Smoker WRK, Reede DL. Incomplete cord syndromes: clinical and imaging review. Radiographics. 2018;38(4):1201–1222. https://doi.org/10.1148/rg.2018170178.

Cho TA. Spinal cord functional anatomy. Continuum (Minneap Minn). 2015;21(1 Spinal Cord Disorders):13–35. https://doi.org/10.1212/01.CON.0000461082.25876.4a.

16. A 25-year-old female patient with new diagnosis of multiple sclerosis presenting as a Brown Sequard Syndrome will demonstrate all of the following neurologic deficits EXCEPT:

    A. Ipsilateral lower motor neuron weakness at the level of the lesion
    B. Ipsilateral upper motor neuron weakness below the level of the lesion
    C. Contralateral loss of vibration and position sense below the level of the lesion
    D. Contralateral loss of pain and temperature two levels below the level of the lesion

    Answer: C.

    Brown Sequard is characterized by ipsilateral lower motor neuron weakness at the level of the lesion, ipsilateral upper motor neuron weakness below the level of the lesion, ipsilateral loss of vibration and position sense below the level of the lesion and contralateral loss of pain and temperature two levels below the level of the lesion.

Cho TA. Spinal cord functional anatomy. Continuum (Minneap Minn). 2015;21(1 Spinal Cord Disorders):13–35. https://doi.org/10.1212/01.CON.0000461082.25876.4a.

17. Which of the following is true regarding the rubrospinal tract?

    A. It is an ascending tract involved in conscious proprioception
    B. It is a descending tract involved in modulating flexor muscles of upper extremities

C. It originates in the precentral motor cortex
D. Decussates obliquely across 2–3 levels on the spinal cord.

Answer: B.

The rubrospinal tract originates in the contralateral red nucleus in the brainstem and descends just anterior to the corticospinal tract, projecting to interneurons that modulate proximal, largely flexor movements of the upper limb. Conscious proprioception is controlled by the dorsal columns. The corticospinal tract is also a descending tract that originates in the precentral motor cortex and is involved in motor control of axial and limb muscles. The spinothalamic tract is an ascending pathway involved in pain and temperature sensory modalities and it decussates at the level of the cord spanning 2–3 levels.

Bican O, Minagar A, Pruitt AA. The spinal cord: a review of functional neuroanatomy. Neurol Clin. 2013;31(1):1–18. https://doi.org/10.1016/j.ncl.2012.09.009.

18. A 55 y/o healthy male patient was moving some heavy boxes at home when he felt an acute severe sharp pain in his back, radiating down both legs. He decided to stay home and rest until the next day, when he started noticing bilateral leg weakness and difficulty with urination. On evaluation in the Emergency Department, the patient was found to have bilateral leg weakness, normal patellar reflexes and brisk Achilles deep tendon reflexes bilaterally, urinary retention, and hypoesthesia in his buttocks, perineum and inner thighs. This patient's injury most likely is located at what vertebral level?

A. T4
B. T9
C. T12
D. S1

Answer: C.

This patient presents with a characteristic scenario of conus medullaris syndrome (CMS) secondary to an acute herniated disc at the level of T12. Injuries involving segments from T12 to L2 can lead to CMS. One possible etiology is compression of the conus medullaris due to herniated disc. Classic clinical features include severe back pain, lower extremity weakness (many times with mixed upper motor neuron (UMN) and lower motor neuron (LMN) signs), saddle anesthesia, bladder/bowel dysfunction and erectile dysfunction. CMS can many times overlap with cauda equina syndrome (such as what may be seen with a L5 disc herniation), with the main difference of UMN deficits present in CMS.

Kunam VK, Velayudhan V, Chaudhry ZA, Bobinski M, Smoker WRK, Reede DL. Incomplete cord syndromes: clinical and imaging review. Radiographics. 2018;38(4):1201–1222. https://doi.org/10.1148/rg.2018170178.

19. Sympathetic preganglionic neurons are located at:

   A. Anterior horn at T1–L2
   B. Dorsal horn at T1–L2
   C. Intermediolateral cell column at T1–L2
   D. Central column at S2–S4 segments

Answer: C.

In the thoracic region, the posterolateral portion of the anterior column is called the lateral (intermediolateral) column. This lateral column contains preganglionic cells for the autonomic nervous system in the thoracic and upper lumbar areas. From T1 to L2 spinal segments, preganglionic sympathetic neurons within the intermediolateral gray column give rise to sympathetic axons, which leave the spinal cord through the anterior roots and travel to the adjacent sympathetic ganglia through white rami communicans. The anterior horn contains alpha and gamma motor neurons.

Bican O, Minagar A, Pruitt AA. The spinal cord: a review of functional neuroanatomy. Neurol Clin. 2013;31(1):1–18. https://doi.org/10.1016/j.ncl.2012.09.009.

20. Parasympathetic preganglionic neurons in the spinal cord are located at:

   A. Anterior horn at T1–L2
   B. Dorsal horn at T1–L2
   C. Intermediolateral cell column at T1–L2
   D. Intermediolateral cell column at S2–S4 segments

Answer: D.

Parasympathetic preganglionic neurons arise from the spinal segments S2, S3, and S4 within the intermediolateral gray column. These neurons leave the spinal cord through ventral roots and, after projecting to the viscera, synapse on postganglionic parasympathetic ganglia. Parasympathetic preganglionic neurons pass through the vagus nerve through the level of the splenic flexure of the colon.

Bican O, Minagar A, Pruitt AA. The spinal cord: a review of functional neuroanatomy. Neurol Clin. 2013;31(1):1–18. https://doi.org/10.1016/j.ncl.2012.09.009.

21. The main spinal cord arterial supply consists of:

    A. 1 anterior and 1 posterior spinal arteries
    B. 1 anterior and 2 posterior spinal arteries
    C. 2 anterior and 2 posterior arteries
    D. 2 anterior and 1 posterior arteries

Answer: B.

Arterial systems identified at the surface of the spinal cord include the longitudinal arterial trunks that extend along the long axis of the spinal cord and are constituted by the anterior spinal artery and two posterior spinal arteries.

Santillan A, Nacarino V, Greenberg E, Riina HA, Gobin YP, Patsalides A. Vascular anatomy of the spinal cord. J Neurointerv Surg. 2012;4(1):67–74. https://doi.org/10.1136/neurintsurg-2011-010018. Epub 2011 May 2.

22. Which of the following is true about the artery of Adamkiewicz?

    A. Almost always arises in the cervicothoracic region
    B. Feeds to the posterior spinal arteries and occlusion can result in loss of vibration and proprioception
    C. Is the most inferior radicullomedulary artery
    D. Feeds into the anterior spinal artery and occlusion can result in flaccid paraplegia.

Answer: D.

The most important anterior radicular artery and the one most easily recognized in angiography is the artery of Adamkiewicz (AKA). It almost always arises in the thoracolumbar region, between T8 and L2 in 75% of cases. The AKA forms the classic 'hairpin' loop when it anastomosis with the anterior spinal artery (ASA) and gives off a thin ascending branch and a larger descending branch. Portions of the thoracic and upper lumbar spinal cord are extremely vulnerable to ischemic compromise as there is minimal collateral supply to the spinal cord inferior to the junction of the AKA and ASA. Lesions to the AKA typically affects the anterior two-thirds of the cord and spare the dorsal columns. The most common cause of this vascular insufficiency is spinal cord ischemia or infarction. Patients typically present with complete motor deficiency below the level of the lesion due to involvement of the corticospinal tract and anterior horn cells, as well as loss of pain, temperature and bladder/bowel dysfunction. The sensations of fine touch, proprioception, and vibration are often preserved.

Santillan A, Nacarino V, Greenberg E, Riina HA, Gobin YP, Patsalides A. Vascular anatomy of the spinal cord. J Neurointerv Surg. 2012;4(1):67–74. https://doi.org/10.1136/neurintsurg-2011-010018. Epub 2011 May 2.

Kunam VK, Velayudhan V, Chaudhry ZA, Bobinski M, Smoker WRK, Reede DL. Incomplete cord syndromes: clinical and imaging review. Radiographics. 2018;38(4):1201–22. https://doi.org/10.1148/rg.2018170178.

23. Characteristic MRI findings of occlusion to the artery of Adamkiewicz include:

   A. Diffusion restriction in the anterior two-thirds of the cord on diffusion weighted images
   B. Fluid filled cavity involving the central portion of the cord
   C. Edema and T2 increased signal involving the posterior two thirds of the cord
   D. T2 increased signal involving the left side of the cord

   Answer: A.

   Characteristic MRI imaging features of acute spinal cord ischemia include diffusion restriction in the ASA territory on diffusion-weighted images and a pencil-like hyperintense signal on sagittal T2-weighted images, with or without cord enlargement. Axial MRI images will show a central T2-hyperintense signal on either side of the median fissure because there is relative sparing of the peripheral and posterior cords due to collateral vessels from the vascular pial plexus and both posterior spinal arteries. A central T2-hyperintense signal resembling snake eyes is sometimes seen in the anterior spinal cord on either side of the median fissure. A fluid filled cavity involving the central portion of the cord can be seen in syringomyelia, resulting more in a central cord-like syndrome or loss of pain and temperature. T2 increased signal involving a hemisection of the cord is characteristic of Brown Sequard syndrome.

Kunam VK, Velayudhan V, Chaudhry ZA, Bobinski M, Smoker WRK, Reede DL. Incomplete cord syndromes: clinical and imaging review. Radiographics. 2018;38(4):1201–22. https://doi.org/10.1148/rg.2018170178.

24. All of the following are true regarding imaging of the spine and spinal cord EXCEPT:

   A. Plain radiographs are limited by patient positioning and poor visualization of craniocervical junction.
   B. CT scan is superior to plain radiographs in a patient with suspected traumatic cervical spine injury with or without neurological deficits.

C. CT scan is more readily available and provides faster results compared to MRI
D. CT scan is the preferred imaging modality for assessment of ligaments and intervertebral discs integrity

Answer: D.

In detection of ligamentous injuries, MRI has high sensitivity and specificity with reported rates of 91% and 100%, respectively. An article by Jo et al. (2018) recommends that additional MRI evaluation be undertaken in (1) those with no visible injury morphology on CT with persistent pain or neurologic deficits, (2) patients who will not be examinable for at least 48 h, (3) for the purposes of treatment planning in mechanically unstable spine, (4) those with clinical or imaging findings suggestive of ligamentous injuries, and (5) those with significant injury morphology on CT.

Jo AS, Wilseck Z, Manganaro MS, Ibrahim M. Essentials of spine trauma imaging: radiographs, CT, and MRI. Semin Ultrasound CT MR. 2018;39(6):532–550. https://doi.org/10.1053/j.sult.2018.10.002. Epub 2018 Oct 26.

25. The most sensitive view in plain radiographs to assess for a C2 fracture is:

A. Regular anterior-posterior (AP) view
B. AP open mouth view
C. Regular lateral view
D. Swimmer's view

Answer: B.

On the AP open-mouth view, the odontoid (dens), body of C2, lateral masses of C1 and C2, and the C1–C2 apophyseal joint should be clearly visible and neither the teeth nor the skull base should obstruct the dens. Lateral view and specifically a modified lateral view also known as swimmer's view is the preferred for assessing cervicothoracic junction. The lateral view is the most sensitive at demonstrating traumatic abnormalities of the cervical spine below C2. A well-performed lateral view will image from the C1 to the C7–T1 junction. If C7 and/or the C7–T1 junction is not well visualized, additional swimmer's view can be obtained.

Jo AS, Wilseck Z, Manganaro MS, Ibrahim M. Essentials of spine trauma imaging: radiographs, CT, and MRI. Semin Ultrasound CT MR. 2018;39(6):532–50. https://doi.org/10.1053/j.sult.2018.10.002. Epub 2018 Oct 26.

26. What type of injury is demonstrated in the image below?

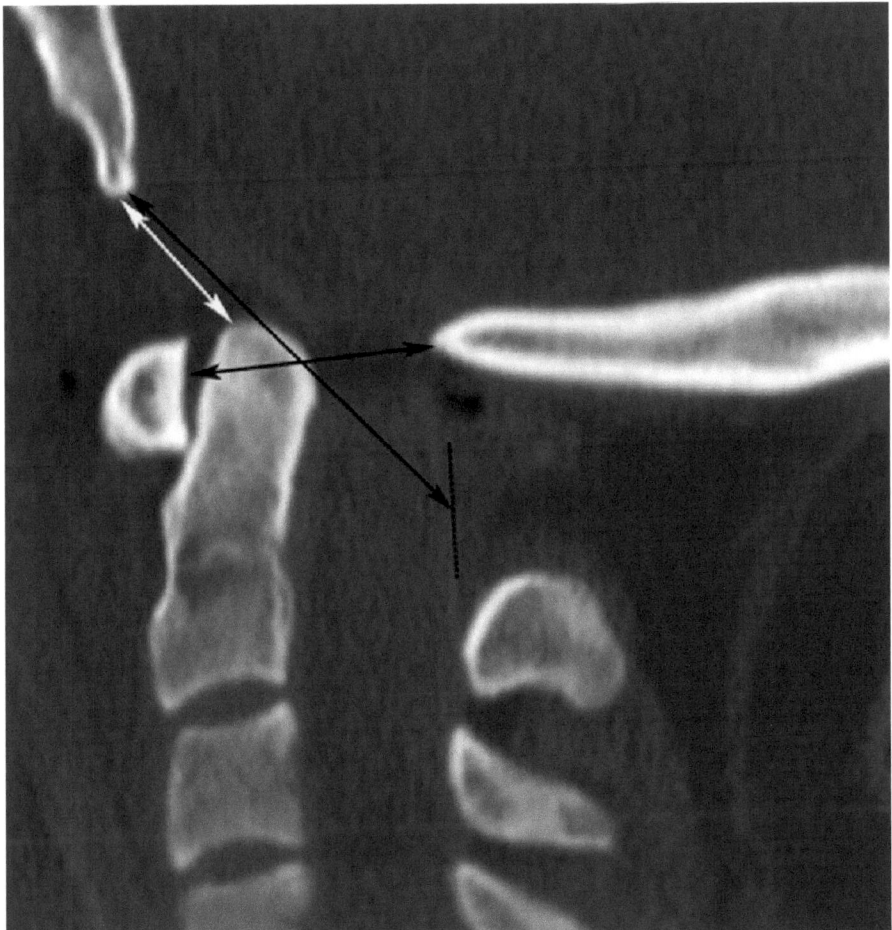

   A. Atlantoaxial dissociation
   B. Atlanto-occipital dissociation
   C. Jefferson fracture
   D. Hangman's fracture

Answer: B.

This is a CT image showing atlanto-occipital dissociation. White double-sided arrow shows increased basion-dens interval and the black double-sided arrows show an increased powers ratio.

Jo AS, Wilseck Z, Manganaro MS, Ibrahim M. Essentials of spine trauma imaging: radiographs, CT, and MRI. Semin Ultrasound CT MR. 2018;39(6):532–50. https://doi.org/10.1053/j.sult.2018.10.002. Epub 2018 Oct 26.

27. A 32-year-old male football player complained of acute neck pain after a witnessed tackle against another player during a game. Neurological exam on the scene was negative. Initial CT scan done showed the following findings.

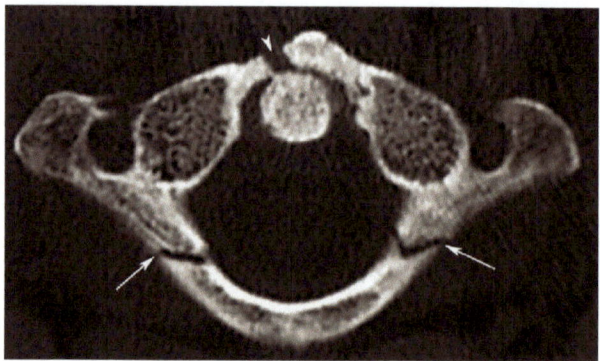

This type of injury is also known as:

    A. Jefferson Fracture
    B. Hangman's fracture
    C. Atlantoaxial instability
    D. Atlantooccipital dislocation

Answer: A.

This is a CT image of a C1 or atlas fracture. The most common fracture pattern affecting C1 is a burst fracture also known as Jefferson's fracture. Jefferson fracture is characterized by 2–4 part fracture with unilateral or bilateral fractures through the anterior and posterior arches. Fracture of C1 is usually the result of severe hyperextension or excessive axial loading.

Jo AS, Wilseck Z, Manganaro MS, Ibrahim M. Essentials of spine trauma imaging: radiographs, CT, and MRI. Semin Ultrasound CT MR. 2018;39(6):532–50. https://doi.org/10.1053/j.sult.2018.10.002. Epub 2018 Oct 26.

28. Which of the following MRI findings have NOT been correlated with poor prognosis for neurological recovery after a traumatic spinal cord injury?

    A. Parenchymal hemorrhage
    B. Cord transection
    C. Cord edema
    D. Longer lesion length

Answer: C.

MRI findings including parenchymal hemorrhage, cord transection, and longer lesion length have all been correlated with less favorable neurological outcome. Cord edema generally has a more favorable prognosis.

Lammertse D, Dungan D, Dreisbach J, Falci S, Flanders A, Marino R, Schwartz E; National Institute on Disability and Rehabilitation. Neuroimaging in traumatic spinal cord injury: an evidence-based review for clinical practice and research. J Spinal Cord Med. 2007;30(3):205–14. https://doi.org/10.1080/10790268.2007.11753928.

29. Clay-Shoveler's fracture is characterized by:

    A. Axial loading or hyperflexion injury to the anterior vertebral body
    B. Facet dislocation of mid-cervical vertebrae
    C. Avulsion fracture of the spinous process of lower cervical or upper thoracic vertebra
    D. Associated severe neurological deficits

Answer C.

A clay-shoveler's fracture is stress-type avulsion fracture of the lower cervical or upper thoracic spinous processes. Most commonly, the spinous processes of the C7 and T1 vertebrae are affected. The mechanism of trauma is the repetitive, forceful shear pull of the upper back muscles (like that seen on clay shoveler's) on the relatively long and slender spinous processes at this level, ultimately leading to fatigue fractures. These fractures are usually stable and rarely accompanied by neurological deficits. Axial loading or hyperflexion injury to the anterior vertebral body can result in a wedge compression fracture. Facet dislocation is not typically associated with a Clay-Shoveler's fracture.

Posthuma de Boer J, van Wulfften Palthe AF, Stadhouder A, Bloemers FW. The clay Shoveler's fracture: a case report and review of the literature. J Emerg Med. 2016;51(3):292–7. https://doi.org/10.1016/j.jemermed.2016.03.020. Epub 2016 Jun 1.

30. Based on Denis' concept of spine stability, fractures with evidence of which of the following are considered the most unstable?

    A. Posterior longitudinal ligament
    B. Anterior longitudinal ligament
    C. Anterior half of vertebral body
    D. Ligamentum flavum

Answer: A.

Denis (1976) developed a three-column system to classify thoracolumbar spinal fractures as mechanically stable and unstable. Anterior column includes the anterior longitudinal ligament, anterior half of the vertebral body and anterior half of the anterior disc annulus. The middle column includes the posterior half of the vertebral body, the posterior annulus fibrosus and the posterior longitudinal ligament. The posterior column includes pedicles, facets, ligamentum flavum, lamina, spinous process, interspinous and supraspinous ligaments. Injuries involving two or more fractures or those involving the middle column are considered the most unstable.

Denis F. The three-column spine and its significance in the classification of acute thoraco-lumbar spinal injuries. Spine (Phila Pa 1976). 1983;8(8):817–31. https://doi.org/10.109 7/00007632-198311000-00003. pine concept in acute spinal trauma. Clin Orthop Relat Res. 1984;(189):65–76.

31. The following image is an example of what type of odontoid fracture?

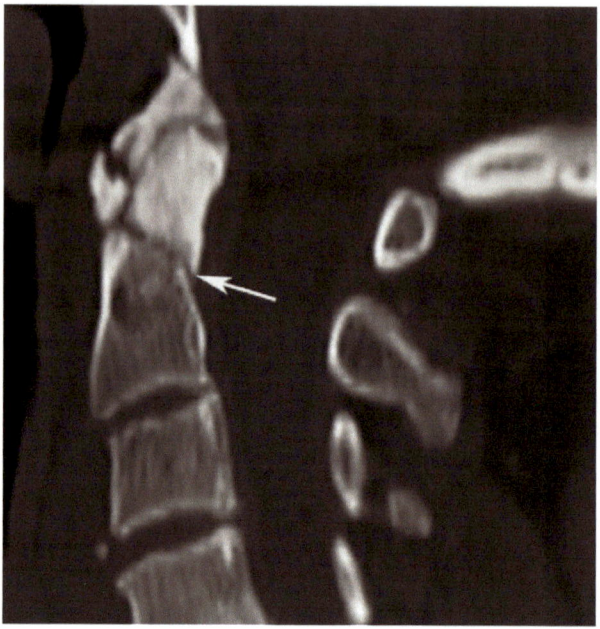

A. Type I
B. Type II
C. Type III
D. Type IV

Answer: B.

The Anderson and D'Alonzo classification describes 3 different types of odontoid fractures: Type I is fracture of the tip of the odontoid, Type II is fracture at the junction of the odontoid and the C2 body (like the one shown in the image), and Type III is the fracture through the C2 body. There is no type IV.

Jo AS, Wilseck Z, Manganaro MS, Ibrahim M. Essentials of spine trauma imaging: radiographs, CT, and MRI. Semin Ultrasound CT MR. 2018;39(6):532–50. https://doi.org/10.1053/j.sult.2018.10.002. Epub 2018 Oct 26.

32. SCIWORA is best characterized by:

A. Traumatic injury to the cervical spine with no neurological deficits
B. Neurological deficits after a traumatic event with no abnormal findings on MRI
C. Neurological deficits after a traumatic injury with no abnormal findings on x-ray or and CT scan
D. Neurological deficits after a traumatic injury to the spine with no abnormal findings on x-ray but evidence of bone fracture and ligament injury in CT scan

Answer: C.

"Spinal Cord Injury Without Radiographic Abnormality" (SCIWORA) is a term used when there are objective clinical signs of traumatic spinal cord injury, but there is no evidence of fracture or malalignment on x-rays or CT scan of the spine. It is most commonly seen in children with a predilection for the cervical spinal cord due to the increased mobility of the cervical spine, the inherent ligamentous laxity, and the large head-to-body ratio during childhood. However, it can also be seen in adults affecting the thoracolumbar spinal cord. It is becoming less common with advancing imaging modalities. MRI is the preferred diagnostic tool in patients with SCIWORA because of its superior ability to identify soft tissue lesions such as cord edema, hematomas and transections, and discoligamentous injuries that may not be visualized in x-rays and CT.

Atesok K, Tanaka N, O'Brien A, Robinson Y, Pang D, Deinlein D, Manoharan SR, Pittman J, Theiss S. Posttraumatic spinal cord injury without radiographic abnormality. Adv Orthop. 2018;4;2018:7060654. https://doi.org/10.1155/2018/7060654.

Assessment, Classification, and Prognosis in Spinal Cord Injuries

4

Donna Huang, James Doan, and Sameer Siddiqui

Questions

1. When testing pin prick sensation using the International Standards for Neurological Classification of Spinal Cord Injury (ISNCSCI), what number of correct out of ten attempts is considered accurate when assessing whether a patient can discriminate between sharp and dull stimuli?

   A. 6
   B. 7
   C. 8
   D. 9

   Answer: C.

D. Huang (✉)
Spinal Cord Injury Care Line, Michael E. DeBakey VA Medical Center, Houston, TX, USA

H. Ben Taub Department of Physical Medicine and Rehabilitation, Baylor College of Medicine, Houston, TX, USA
e-mail: donna.huang@bcm.edu

J. Doan
Spinal Cord Injury Division, VA Boston Healthcare System, Boston, MA, USA

Department of Physical Medicine and Rehabilitation, Harvard Medical School/Spaulding Rehabilitation Hospital, Boston, MA, USA
e-mail: james.doan@va.gov

S. Siddiqui
Spinal Cord Injury System of Care, Louis Stokes Cleveland VA Medical Center, Cleveland, OH, USA

Department of Physical Medicine and Rehabilitation, Case Western Reserve University, Cleveland, OH, USA
e-mail: sameer.siddiqui2@va.gov

© The Author(s), under exclusive license to Springer Nature Switzerland AG 2022
B. A. Abramoff et al. (eds.), *The Essential Spinal Cord Injury Medicine Question Bank*, https://doi.org/10.1007/978-3-031-07796-8_4

When it is unclear whether a patient can distinguish between sharp and dull stimuli, 8 out of 10 correct responses is considered accurate. This reduces the chance of guessing the stimuli correctly to less than 5%.

American Spinal Injury Association. International standards for neurological classification of spinal cord injury. Richmond, VA: American Spinal Injury Association; 2019.

2. Which of the following is not a component of the International Standards for Neurological Classification of Spinal Cord Injury?

   A. Pinprick sensation
   B. Deep anal pressure
   C. Deep tendon reflexes
   D. Manual muscle testing

Answer: C.

The components of the ISNCSCI are the sensory examination, motor examination, deep anal pressure, and voluntary anal contraction. The sensory examination consists of testing 28 key sensory points on both sides of the body for pin prick as well as light touch. The required components of the motor examination include testing 10 key muscles, 5 in the upper limbs and 5 in the lower limbs, on both sides of the body. A number of optional muscles may be tested and may be helpful in determining motor incomplete injuries. Although deep tendon reflexes are not part of the ISNCSCI exam, they may be useful to assess along with sacral reflexes (anal wink and bulbocavernosus reflex) to identify the resolution of spinal shock and to distinguish between upper and lower motor neuron patterns of injury.

American Spinal Injury Association. International standards for neurological classification of spinal cord injury. Richmond, VA: American Spinal Injury Association; 2019.

3. A complete spinal cord injury is defined by:

   A. The absence of sacral sparing
   B. The absence of sensory function below the neurologic level of injury
   C. Complete transection of the spinal cord on imaging
   D. The absence of motor function greater than three levels below the neurologic level of injury

Answer: A.

A complete spinal cord injury is defined by the absence of motor (voluntary anal contraction) or sensory function in the sacral segments (S4–5 or deep anal pressure). Preservation of motor or sensory function in the sacral segments is also known as sacral sparing.

American Spinal Injury Association. International standards for neurological classification of spinal cord injury. Richmond, VA: American Spinal Injury Association; 2019.

4. You are testing pinprick sensation on the dorsal aspect of the proximal phalanx of the third digit. When a sharp stimulus is applied, the patient reports feeling a sharp sensation that is more intense than that of the face. When a dull stimulus is applied, the patient reports feeling a dull sensation. He is able to distinguish accurately between the sharp and dull sensation with multiple trials. How would you score this finding?

A. Score of 1 in the C6 dermatome
B. Score of 2 in the C6 dermatome
C. Score of 0 in the C7 dermatome
D. Score of 1 in the C7 dermatome

Answer: D.

When assessing pin prick sensation, a clean safety pin is used, and sensation at each of the key sensory points is compared to that of the face. A score of 2 is given if the sensation that is perceived at that sensory point is the same as the face and the ability to distinguish between sharp and dull is intact. A score of 1 is given if there is altered sensation, whether hypo- or hyperesthesia, compared to the face and the ability to distinguish between sharp and dull is intact. A score of 0 is given if there is absent sensation or if there is sensation, but the ability to distinguish between sharp and dull is absent. The key sensory point for the C7 dermatome corresponds with the proximal phalanx of the third digit, while the key sensory point for the C6 dermatome corresponds with the proximal phalanx of the first digit.

American Spinal Injury Association. International standards for neurological classification of spinal cord injury. Richmond, VA: American Spinal Injury Association; 2019.

5. Which muscle action is tested to determine motor function in the T1 myotome?

A. Distal interphalangeal joint flexion of the third finger
B. Elbow extension
C. Abduction of the fifth finger
D. Wrist extension

Answer: C.

Motor function of the T1 myotome is assessed by abduction of the fifth finger. DIP flexion of the third finger is used to test the C8 myotome. Elbow extension (triceps) is the key muscle group used to test the C7 myotome. The C6 myotome is assessed by wrist extension.

American Spinal Injury Association. International standards for neurological classification of spinal cord injury. Richmond, VA: American Spinal Injury Association; 2019.

6. When should non-key muscle groups be tested in order to potentially change ASIA classification?

A. When the patient has a complete injury
B. When there is evidence of spinal cord edema on MRI
C. When there is suspicion of functional neurologic disorder
D. When the patient appears to have a sensory incomplete/motor complete injury

Answer: D.

Non-key muscle groups should be tested when a patient has an apparent American Spinal Injury Impairment Scale (AIS) B (sensory incomplete/motor complete) classification. Presence of motor function in non-key muscle groups can distinguish between an apparent sensory incomplete/motor complete injury (AIS B) and a sensory incomplete/motor incomplete (AIS C) injury.

American Spinal Injury Association. International standards for neurological classification of spinal cord injury. Richmond, VA: American Spinal Injury Association; 2019.

7. A patient has intact pin prick and light touch sensation on tested dermatomes through the axilla bilaterally. He has 3/5 strength in the triceps bilaterally with 5/5 strength in bilateral biceps and wrist extension. He has 0/5 strength in his hands and lower extremities. Deep anal pressure and voluntary anal contraction are present. What is the ISNCSCI classification of this patient's spinal cord injury?

A. C6 American Spinal Injury Impairment Scale (AIS) C
B. C6 AIS B
C. C7 AIS C
D. C7 AIS B

Answer: C.

The ISNCSCI classification of the patient with the physical exam described is C7 AIS C. The patient's sensory level is T2 (intact through the axilla). The sensory level is defined as the most caudal level at which both light touch and pin prick sensation are intact bilaterally. The motor level is determined by the lowest level at which the key muscle group strength is at least 3/5 with all preceding key muscle groups rostral to this level judged to be intact (5/5). In this case, that is C7 (triceps). Of note, in regions where there are no testable muscles, the motor level is presumed to be the same as the sensory level as long as rostral testable muscles are intact. Sensory incomplete status is determined by preservation of sensation in the sacral segments, in this case as evidenced by the presence of deep anal pressure. Motor incomplete status is defined as preservation of motor function >3 levels below the motor level on each side of the body OR preservation of voluntary anal contraction, as is true in this case. In order to achieve an AIS D rating, the individual would have to have ≥50% (half or more) of the testable key AIS muscles below the neurologic level of injury with at least 3/5 strength or greater.

American Spinal Injury Association. International standards for neurological classification of spinal cord injury. Richmond, VA: American Spinal Injury Association; 2019.

8. What is the typical recovery pattern from earliest to latest in a person with central cord syndrome?

A. Proximal upper extremities, distal upper extremities, bowel and bladder, lower extremities
B. Lower extremities, bowel and bladder, proximal upper extremities, distal upper extremities
C. Bowel and bladder, lower extremities, proximal upper extremities, distal upper extremities
D. Proximal upper extremities, lower extremities, bowel and bladder, distal upper extremities

Answer: B.

Central cord syndrome is the most common clinical spinal cord syndrome, accounting for approximately 50% of all incomplete injuries and 9% of traumatic SCI (McKinley et al. 2007). This syndrome is characterized by greater motor weakness in the upper extremities compared to the lower extremities and the presence of sacral sparing (Schneider et al. 1973). This clinical syndrome most commonly occurs in older individuals with cervical spondylosis who experience a hyperextension injury, usually in the setting of a fall. In central cord syndrome, recovery typically occurs the earliest and to the greatest extent in the lower extremities, followed by bowel and bladder, followed by the proximal upper extremities, followed by the distal upper extremities including intrinsic hand function.

McKinley W, Santos K, Meade M, Brooke K. Incidence and outcomes of spinal cord injury clinical syndromes. J Spinal Cord Med. 2007;30(3):215–24. https://doi.org/10.1080/10790268.2007.11753929.
Schneider RC, Crosby EC, Russo RH, Gosch HH. Chapter 32. Traumatic spinal cord syndromes and their management. Clin Neurosurg. 1973;20:424–92. https://doi.org/10.1093/neurosurgery/20.cn_suppl_1.424.

The following clinical scenario applies to questions 9 and 10. You are consulted on a patient who is admitted to the hospital with a spinal cord injury after sustaining a stab wound to the neck. Your exam reveals patchy impairments of light touch sensation below the C5 dermatome on the right side with relatively spared pin prick sensation in the same distribution. On the left, the patient has patchy impairments in pin prick sensation below the C4 dermatome. The motor exam reveals the following:

	Right	Left
C5	3	4
C6	2	4
C7	1	5
C8	0	4
T1	1	3
L2	2	3
L3	1	4
L4	2	4
L5	2	4
S1	2	5

9. Which incomplete spinal cord syndrome is characterized by the patient's neurological exam findings:

    A. Anterior cord syndrome
    B. Posterior cord syndrome
    C. Central cord syndrome
    D. Brown-Séquard-Plus syndrome

Answer: D.

This case describes physical exam findings consistent with Brown-Sequard syndrome. In the classic presentation of Brown Sequard, there is ipsilateral loss of all sensation at the level of the lesion, ipsilateral flaccid paralysis at the level of the lesion, ipsilateral loss of proprioception and vibration below the lesion, contralateral loss of pain and temperature below the lesion, and ipsilateral UMN pattern weakness below the level of the lesion. This syndrome accounts for 2–4% of all traumatic SCI (Bohlman 1979; Bosch et al. 1971; Brown-Séquard 1868; Pappas et al. 1991).

The spinothalamic tracts decussate resulting in contralateral pain and temperature loss while the corticospinal tracts and the dorsal columns decussate in the medulla in the brainstem, resulting in ipsilateral paralysis and proprioception and vibratory sensation loss with injuries at the level of the spinal cord. The syndrome is classically associated with hemisection injuries to the spinal cord resulting from knife or gunshot wounds, however a variety of other etiologies have been described. It is rare in clinical practice to see "pure" Brown-Sequard syndrome. More commonly, patients present with a combination of features of Brown-Séquard and central cord syndrome, with varying degrees of ipsilateral hemiplegia and contralateral hemianalgesia, which has been termed Brown-Séquard-Plus syndrome (Roth et al. 1991).

Bohlman HH. Acute fractures and dislocations of the cervical spine. An analysis of three hundred hospitalized patients and review of the literature. J Bone Joint Surg Am. 1979;61(8):1119–42.

Bosch A, Stauffer ES, Nickel VL. Incomplete traumatic quadriplegia. A ten-year review. JAMA. 1971;216(3):473–8.

Brown-Séquard, CE. Lectures on the physiology and pathology of the nervous system; and on the treatment of organic nervous affections. Lancet. 1868;92(2358): 593–6. https://doi.org/10.1016/S0140-6736(02)72108-9

Pappas CT, Gibson AR, Sonntag VK. Decussation of hind-limb and fore-limb fibers in the monkey corticospinal tract: relevance to cruciate paralysis. J Neurosurg. 1991;75(6):935–40. https://doi.org/10.3171/jns.1991.75.6.0935.

Roth EJ, Park T, Pang T, Yarkony GM, Lee MY. Traumatic cervical brown-sequard and brown-sequard-plus syndromes: the spectrum of presentations and outcomes. Paraplegia. 1991;29(9):582–9. https://doi.org/10.1038/sc.1991.86.

10. What percentage of individuals who have the incomplete spinal cord syndrome described above ambulate independently at the time of discharge from rehabilitation?

    A. <10%
    B. 20–50%
    C. 50–75%
    D. 75–90%

Answer: D.

The prognosis in Brown-Sequard syndrome is favorable. Nearly 75–90% of patients ambulate independently at the time of discharge from rehabilitation, and 70% are independent with activities of daily living (Koehler and Endtz 1986). Recovery of bowel and bladder function is also favorable, with continence achieved in over 80% of individuals in one study.

Koehler PJ, Endtz LJ. The Brown-Séquard syndrome. True or false? Arch Neurol. 1986;43(9):921–4. https://doi.org/10.1001/archneur.1986.00520090051015.

11. You are evaluating a patient who is newly admitted to your rehabilitation unit after a traumatic spinal cord injury from a fall. The patient has intact pinprick and light touch sensation superior to the acromioclavicular joint bilaterally with patchy impairments in sensation below this level through S4–S5. The motor exam reveals the following:

	Right	Left
C5	2	1
C6	1	1
C7	0	2
C8	2	3
T1	3	2
L2	3	3
L3	4	4
L4	3	4
L5	3	4
S1	4	5

What is the ISNSCI classification of this patient's spinal cord injury?

A. C4 AIS C
B. C4 AIS D
C. C5 AIS C
D. C5 AIS D

Answer: B.

The ISNSCI classification in this case is C4 AIS D. The sensory level is determined by the most caudal level at which light touch and pin prick sensory modalities are intact. The acromioclavicular joint corresponds with the C4 dermatome. The motor level is the same as the sensory level in this case as the first testable muscle group at C5 does not have at least 3/5 strength. The patient has motor function preserved >3 levels below the motor level on each side in the setting of sacral sparing, indicating at least AIS C (motor incomplete) classification. Furthermore, more than half of the testable muscles below the neurologic level of injury are at least 3/5 strength, which makes confers AIS D status.

American Spinal Injury Association. International standards for neurological classification of spinal cord injury. Richmond, VA: American Spinal Injury Association; 2019.

12. A construction worker is admitted to the hospital after falling from a roof and landing on his feet. He sustained bilateral calcaneal fractures and a L3 burst fracture. Which type of clinical spinal cord syndrome is he most likely to have?

A. Cauda equina syndrome
B. Conus medullaris syndrome
C. Anterior cord syndrome
D. Posterior cord syndrome

Answer: A.

The spinal cord terminates in the conus medullaris, which typically occurs at the T10–L2 vertebral level. Injuries caudal to the L1 vertebral level therefore do not typically result in injury to the spinal cord but rather to the cauda equina. Cauda equina syndrome is a lower motor neuron syndrome that results in patchy and often asymmetric findings of lumbosacral impairment, which can range from profound flaccid weakness to relatively preserved strength with loss of sensation in radicular patterns to loss of deep tendon reflexes and bowel/bladder control (Kirshblum and Solinsky 2018).

Kirshblum S, Solinsky R. Neurological assessment and classification of spinal cord injury. In: Kirshblum S, Lin VS, editors. Spinal cord medicine: 3rd ed. New York City: Springer Publishing Company. 2019. pp. 63–76. https://doi.org/10.1891/9780826137753.0005

13. How does one distinguish between ASIA Impairment Scale B and C?

    A. Presence of preserved pin prick sensation in the S4–5 dermatome
    B. Presence of bulbocavernosus reflex (BCR)
    C. Presence of motor function >3 levels below the motor level on either side of the body
    D. Presence of motor function >3 levels below the neurologic level of injury

Answer: C.

Motor incomplete status is defined by the presence of voluntary anal contraction or by preservation of motor function >3 levels below the motor level on either side of the body. This can be assessed either in key muscle groups or non-key muscle groups. Note that the motor level is the reference point for distinguishing AIS B vs C, but neurological level of injury is the reference point for determining AIS C vs D (Answer D). Preserved sensation in the S4–S5 dermatome (Answer A) would help determine between classification of AIS A vs B. Presence of BCR (Answer B) is not directly used for the ASIA Impairment scale but can be a clinically useful indicator of upper vs lower motor neuron patterns for bowel program and/or the presence of spinal shock.

American Spinal Injury Association. International standards for neurological classification of spinal cord injury. Richmond, VA: American Spinal Injury Association; 2019.

14. Which of the following is the most important prognostic factor for the recovery of functional ambulation, independence with dressing, and bowel and bladder function in individuals with central cord syndrome?

    A. Neurologic level of injury
    B. Age
    C. Extent of spinal cord edema on neuroimaging
    D. Degree of sensory impairment in sacral dermatomes

Answer: B.

In central cord syndrome, prognosis for functional recovery of ambulation, independence with dressing, and bowel and bladder function is dependent on age. Patients <50 years old are more likely to achieve functional ambulation (87–97% vs. 31–41%), dressing (77% vs. 12%), independent bladder function (83% vs. 29%), and independent bowel function (63% vs. 24%) compared to those ≥50-years-old. For those with AIS D classification with initial neurological examination (<72 h), prognosis for functional ambulation was favorable, even for those ≥50-years-old (Burns et al. 1997).

Burns SP, Golding DG, Rolle WA Jr, Graziani V, Ditunno JF Jr. Recovery of ambulation in motor-incomplete tetraplegia. Arch Phys Med Rehabil. 1997;78(11):1169–72. https://doi.org/10.1016/s0003-9993(97)90326-9.

15. You are consulted to evaluate a patient who sustained a thoracic spinal cord injury after a motor vehicle accident. The patient has intact sensation to the level of the nipple line bilaterally with patchy impairments in sensation below. Deep anal pressure is intact; voluntary anal contraction is absent. The motor exam reveals the following:

	Right	Left
C5	5	5
C6	5	5
C7	5	5
C8	5	5
T1	5	5
L2	0	0
L3	0	0
L4	0	0
L5	0	0
S1	0	0

What is the ISNCSCI classification of this patient's spinal cord injury?

A. T4 AIS A
B. T4 AIS B
C. T4 AIS C
D. T4 AIS D

Answer: B.

This patient's ISNSCI classification is T4 AIS B. Sensory function is intact to the level of the nipple, which corresponds to a sensory level of T4. The motor level corresponds with the sensory level in this case as this is a region without testable muscles. The patient is sensory incomplete as evidenced by the presence of deep anal pressure. There is no sparing of motor function >3 levels below the motor level on each side of the body. As a result, the AIS classification is B.

American Spinal Injury Association. International standards for neurological classification of spinal cord injury. Richmond, VA: American Spinal Injury Association; 2019.

16. When present within the first 2 days after initial injury, the following can lead to an inaccurate initial ISNCSCI evaluation EXCEPT:

    A. Language barrier, severe pain, cerebral palsy
    B. Closed head injury, psychiatric illness
    C. Mechanical ventilation, intoxication, sedation, or paralysis
    D. Cervical level of injury

Answer: D.

Burns et al. (2003) examined 103 patients in the first 2 days after their injury. They reexamined 101 of these subjects after 1 week and 68 of them after 1 year. Those with the concerns listed in answers choices A, B, and C had a higher conversion rate from complete to incomplete than those without such concerns, implying that those examined with the above issues likely did not have an accurate initial exam. Cervical level of injury did not lead to inaccurate initial ISNCSCI evaluations.

Burns AS, Lee BS, Ditunno JF Jr, Tessler A. Patient selection for clinical trials: the reliability of the early spinal cord injury examination. J Neurotrauma. 2003;20(5):477–82. https://doi.org/10.1089/089771503765355540.

17. What percent of those with initial AIS A spinal cord injuries are expected to convert to having motor or sensory incomplete injuries after 1 year?

    A. 10%
    B. 20%
    C. 50%
    D. 100%

Answer: B.

The guidelines for the conduct of clinical trials for spinal cord injury reviewed multiple studies and concluded that 80% of individuals with AIS A SCI on exam between 3 and 28 days following their injury continued to be classified as AIS A after 1 year, 10% became sensory incomplete/AIS B, and 10% improved to motor incomplete/AIS C or AIS D. It should be noted that the studies reviewed were both pre- and post-2000, when sacral sparing became required to be considered incomplete.

Fawcett JW, Curt A, Steeves JD, Coleman WP, Tuszynski MH, Lammertse D, Bartlett PF, Blight AR, Dietz V, Ditunno J, Dobkin BH, Havton LA, Ellaway PH, Fehlings MG, Privat A, Grossman R, Guest JD, Kleitman N, Nakamura M, Gaviria M, Short D. Guidelines for the conduct of clinical trials for spinal cord injury as developed by the ICCP panel: spontaneous recovery after spinal cord injury and statistical power needed for therapeutic clinical trials. Spinal Cord. 2007;45(3):190–205. https://doi.org/10.1038/sj.sc.3102007. Epub 2006 Dec 19.

18. You have recently completed an ISNCSCI examination on a person with complete tetraplegia and you have the following results:

	Right	Left
C5	5	5
C6	4	4
C7	2	2
C8	1	1
T1	0	0
L2	0	0
L3	0	0
L4	0	0
L5	0	0
S1	0	0

They do not have sacral sparing.

After completing the exam, your very astute resident asks you what are the chances that your patient recovers antigravity strength at the C7, C8 and T1 myotomes. Based on the study by Waters et al (1993), how do you respond? C7, C8, T1

A. 50%, 20%, 10%
B. 95%, 50%, 30%
C. 100%, 90%, 10%
D. 100%, 90%, 50%

Answer: C.

Waters et al. (1993) examined a group of 45 people with complete tetraplegia at 1 month and 1 year, representing 450 muscles and found an improvement of Motor Score on average from 8.6 ± 4.7. They also found of the 266 muscles with 0/5 strength (one level below the most caudal voluntary muscle) at 1 month, 27 of them improved greater than equal to 3/5 strength after 1 year. Of the 51 muscles with 1/5 strength at 1 month, 46 of them improved to antigravity strength at 1 year. Of the 43 muscles with 2/5 strength at 1 month all 43 of them had strength of 3/5 or better at 1 year.

Waters RL, Adkins RH, Yakura JS, Sie I. Motor and sensory recovery following complete tetraplegia. Arch Phys Med Rehabil. 1993;74(3):242–7.

19. How does advanced age impact recovery after a spinal cord injury?

A. Similar AIS score conversion rate and motor recovery compared to their younger counterparts, but decreased functional recovery
B. Worse AIS score conversion rate and motor recovery compared to their younger counterparts as well as decreased functional recovery

C. Improved AIS score conversion rate and motor recovery, compared to their younger counterparts, but decreased functional recovery
D. Similar AIS score conversion rate and motor recovery compared to their younger counterparts, as well as similar functional recovery

Answer: A.

In a study of 376 patients, Wilson et al. (2014) found no difference in AIS motor score or AIS grade conversion rate between those greater than or equal to 65 years of age and those younger than 65 years old. However, they did find that FIM motor scores were on average lower for the group that was greater than or equal to 65 years of age after 1 year.

Wilson JR, Davis AM, Kulkarni AV, Kiss A, Frankowski RF, Grossman RG, Fehlings MG. Defining age-related differences in outcome after traumatic spinal cord injury: analysis of a combined, multicenter dataset. Spine J. 2014;14(7):1192–8. https://doi.org/10.1016/j.spinee.2013.08.005.

20. When is the ideal time to perform decompressive surgery after spinal cord injury?

A. Within 12 h
B. Between 12 and 24 h
C. Between 24–48 h
D. Between 48–72 h

Answer: C.

In a review of 22 articles, pooled relative risk (RR) for 14 studies comparing early vs late decompression was 0.77 (95% CI: 0.68–0.89) and 0.84 (95% CI: 0.77–0.92) for neurological improvement of at least 1 grade and at least two grades on AIS/Frankel scales. When looking at pooled RR for various time points for spinal decompression surgery, there is noted improvement in neurological outcomes with shorter time periods preceding surgery with pooled RR being 0.26 (95% CI: 0.13–0.52; $p < 0.001$) at 12 h post-injury, 0.75 (95% CI: 0.63–0.90; $p = 0.002$) within 24 h post-injury, and 0.93 (95% CI: 0.76–1.14; $p = 0.48$) within 72 h post-injury. Finally, when decompression is performed within 24 h of injury, a significant lower risk of post-op complications was noted (RR = 0.77; 95% CI: 0.68–0.86; $p < 0.001$).

Yousefifard M, Rahimi-Movaghar V, Baikpour M, Ghelichkhani P, Hosseini M, Jafari A, Aziznejad H, Tafakhori A. Early versus late spinal decompression surgery in treatment of traumatic spinal cord injuries; a systematic review and meta-analysis. Emerg (Tehran). 2017;5(1):e37. Epub 2017 Jan 11.

21. You are completing a discharge ISNSCI examination on a patient over 4 months after his post-injury examination showed T12 AIS A paraplegia, and you excitedly note that he now has an incomplete injury. According to a study by Waters et al. (1992), how common is late conversion from complete to incomplete?

    A. 1%
    B. 4%
    C. 20%
    D. 50%

Answer: B.

In a study of 148 people with complete paraplegia on admission, Waters et al. noted that six out 148 converted to incomplete paraplegia after greater than 4 months.

Waters RL, Yakura JS, Adkins RH, Sie I. Recovery following complete paraplegia. Arch Phys Med Rehabil. 1992;73(9):784–9.

22. What percentage of patients with late conversion (as described in question 20) regain voluntary voiding and bowel function?

    A. 10%
    B. 30%
    C. 50%
    D. 75%

Answer: C.

In a study of 148 people with complete paraplegia on admission, Waters et al. (1992) noted that six out 148 converted to incomplete paraplegia after greater than 4 months. Of these six, three regained voluntary voiding and bowel function.

Waters RL, Yakura JS, Adkins RH, Sie I. Recovery following complete paraplegia. Arch Phys Med Rehabil. 1992;73(9):784–9.

23. In the four-phase model of reflex recovery after spinal cord injury, what is the correct order of the phases listed below?

    A. Initial reflex return (0–1 days), Areflexia/hyporeflexia (1–3 days), Early hyperreflexia (4–30 days), Spasticity and hyperreflexia (1–12 months)
    B. Areflexia/hyporeflexia (0–1 days), Initial reflex return (1–3 days), Early hyperreflexia (4–30 days), Spasticity and hyperreflexia (1–12 months)

   C. Early hyperreflexia (0–1 days), Initial reflex return (1–3 days), Areflexia/
      hyporeflexia (4–30 days), Spasticity and hyperreflexia (1–12 months)

   D. Spasticity and hyperreflexia (0–1 days), Initial reflex return (1–3 days),
      Early hyperreflexia (4–30 days), Areflexia/hyporeflexia (1–12 months)

Answer: B.

Ditunno et al. (2004) described a new four-phase model of reflex recovery which consisted of the following: Phase 1—Areflexia/hyporeflexia (0–1 days), which was characterized by lack of reflexes and flaccid muscles. Phase 2—Initial return of reflexes (1–3 days) with strengthening of cutaneous reflexes such as anal wink, bulbocavernosus and cremasteric reflexes, with continued lack of deep tendon reflexes. Phase 3—Early hyperflexia (4–30 days), having noted return of deep tendon reflexes. Phase 4—spasticity and hyperreflexia (1–12 months), noted elevation and hyperresponse of all reflexes.

Ditunno JF, Little JW, Tessler A, Burns AS. Spinal shock revisited: a four-phase model. Spinal Cord. 2004;42(7):383–95. https://doi.org/10.1038/sj.sc.3101603.

24. You have been consulted on a patient currently admitted to the intensive care unit who has a new spinal cord injury. Your resident brings up the MRI of their cervical spine and notes there is hemorrhage in the cord. Your resident asks you how the hemorrhage will impact prognosis. How do you respond?

   A. The prognosis of recovering strength in his upper extremities is equivalent compared to individuals without hemorrhage on their initial MRI.

   B. The prognosis of recovering strength in his upper extremities is more likely compared to individuals without hemorrhage on their initial MRI.

   C. The prognosis of recovering strength in his upper extremities is less likely compared to individuals without hemorrhage on their initial MRI.

   D. You tell your resident that you do not know and he should look it up on the internet

Answer: C.

In a study of 24 individuals, Marciello et al. (1993) found that all 15 of the individuals who had hemorrhage on their MRIs had motor complete injuries, while 8 of the 9 subjects without hemorrhage had a motor incomplete injury. 16% of upper extremity muscles and 3% of the lower extremity muscles in the hemorrhage group improved to at least anti-gravity strength, while the non-hemorrhage group had 73% in the upper extremities and 74% in the lower extremities improving.

Marciello MA, Flanders AE, Herbison GJ, Schaefer DM, Friedman DP, Lane JI. Magnetic resonance imaging related to neurologic outcome in cervical spinal cord injury. Arch Phys Med Rehabil. 1993;74(9):940–6.

25. It is a week later, and you are now seeing another patient admitted to the ICU with a spinal cord injury. The same resident brings up the MRI of the patient's cervical spine and sees no hemorrhage but notes that there is edema. What do you tell him about how edema will impact recovery?

    A. The amount of edema on the cord is not helpful to predict amount of motor recovery
    B. No additional information can be gleaned from assessing the length of the edema in relation to the spinal cord
    C. Edema and hemorrhage have equivalent prognostic value regarding motor recovery
    D. The greater the length of edema on the spinal cord, the less motor recovery is likely

Answer: D.

In a study comparing motor recovery following spinal cord injury, it was found that those with hemorrhage had the worse motor outcomes (median percentage of motor score recovery of 9%), followed by edema across more than one level of the spinal cord (41%), and edema over a single level of the spinal cord (72%).

Schaefer DM, Flanders AE, Osterholm JL, Northrup BE. Prognostic significance of magnetic resonance imaging in the acute phase of cervical spine injury. J Neurosurg. 1992;76(2):218–23. https://doi.org/10.3171/jns.1992.76.2.0218.

26. What percentage of people with complete paraplegia will become community ambulators 1 year after injury?

    A. 5%
    B. 15%
    C. 50%
    D. 75%

Answer: A.

Waters et al. (1992) found that 7 out of 148 (5%) of people with complete paraplegia were able to become community ambulators after 1 year.

Waters RL, Yakura JS, Adkins RH, Sie I. Recovery following complete paraplegia. Arch Phys Med Rehabil. 1992;73(9):784–9.

27. What percentage of people with incomplete paraplegia and incomplete tetraplegia will become community ambulators (respectively)?

    A. 96%, 76%
    B. 76%, 46%

C. 56%, 26%
D. 26%, 6%

Answer: B.

76% of individuals with incomplete paraplegia and 46% of those with incomplete tetraplegia will return to community ambulation, however it is cautioned that these percentages are dependent on AIS grade and type of sensory of sparing.

Kirshblum S, Lin VS, editors. Spinal cord medicine: 3rd ed. New York City: Springer Publishing Company. 2019. https://doi.org/10.1891/9780826137753.0005

28. What level of strength is needed in which muscles to allow for a reciprocal gait pattern?

A. Antigravity strength in one quadriceps and both ankle dorsiflexors
B. Antigravity strength in one hip flexor and both quadriceps
C. Antigravity strength in both hip flexors and one quadriceps
D. Antigravity strength in both hip flexors and both quadriceps

Answer: C.

Hussey and Staffer (1973) conducted a study of 164 individuals that regained ambulation following a spinal cord injury. They found that 95% of those in the community ambulator group and 92% of those in the household ambulator group had proprioception in the hips. They also noted that those in the community and household group had much better strength in their hip flexor muscles compared to non-ambulatory groups. Finally, similar data was found for strength in quadriceps muscles in one leg for community and household ambulators compared to the non-ambulatory groups.

Hussey RW, Stauffer ES. Spinal cord injury: requirements for ambulation. Arch Phys Med Rehabil. 1973;54(12):544–7.

29. What can be inferred from the lower extremity motor scores (LEMS) regarding overall energy expenditure?

A. LEMS is not relevant to overall energy expenditure
B. Decreased LEMS is associated with lower overall energy expenditure compared to having higher LEMS
C. Decreased LEMS is associated with equivalent overall energy expenditure compared to having higher LEMS
D. Increased LEMS is associated with lower overall energy expenditure compared to having lower LEMS

Answer: D.

In a study of 36 patients, Waters et al. (1994) found that those with LEMS of ≤20 had greater energy expenditure compared to individuals with LEMS ≥ 30.

Waters RL, Adkins R, Yakura J, Vigil D. Prediction of ambulatory performance based on motor scores derived from standards of the American Spinal Injury Association. Arch Phys Med Rehabil. 1994;75(7):756–60.

30. How do people with spinal cord injury compare to the general population on scales of life satisfaction?

    A. People with spinal cord injury have significantly higher satisfaction with life
    B. People with spinal cord injury have significantly lower satisfaction with life
    C. People with spinal cord injury have life satisfaction that is not significantly different than the general population
    D. There is no data on the life satisfaction of people with spinal cord injury

Answer: C.

The Diener Satisfaction with Life Scale has an average score of 23.5 ± 6.43. Those with high tetraplegia have a Diener score of 17.6, those with low tetraplegia of a score 19.1, those with paraplegia have a score of 20.1 and those with a AIS score of D have a score of 21.1. While lower, these values are within the standard deviation of the normative values listed above.

Diener E, Emmons RA, Larsen RJ, Griffin S. The satisfaction with life scale. J Pers Assess. 1985;49(1):71–5. https://doi.org/10.1207/s15327752jpa4901_13.
Consortium for Spinal Cord Medicine. Outcomes following traumatic spinal cord injury: clinical practice guidelines for health-care professionals. J Spinal Cord Med. 2000;23(4):289–316. https://doi.org/10.1080/10790268.2000.11753539.

31. You are consulted to evaluate a 16-year-old male who presented with paraplegia after a motor vehicle accident 3 weeks ago. Upon your encounter at bedside, you note that his sensation to light touch and pinprick is normal from head to the xiphisternal joint and absent below that region. His rectal exam shows loose rectal tone with absent deep anal pressure sensation. With regards to predicting his needed bowel program, what other physical examination would provide the most information in his functional assessment?

    A. Testing for plantarflexion at his ankles
    B. Testing for proprioception at his great toe
    C. Testing for a bulbocavernosus reflex
    D. Testing for patellar reflex

Answer: C.

With sensation intact to light touch and pinprick at and above the xiphisternal region in a paraplegic, his overall neurological level is T6. Usually with regards to bowel function, one would expect an upper motor neuron neurogenic bowel with a neurological level above T10; however, his rectal exam displayed loose rectal tone (a lower motor neuron neurogenic bowel picture) instead of the expected spastic or tight rectal tone. Therefore, testing for the bulbocavernosus reflex would provide more information with regards to if the patient is still in spinal shock; if the bulbocavernosus reflex is absent, then he would likely still be in spinal shock which would also explain his loose rectal tone; as time progresses and he is no longer in spinal shock, then an upper motor neuron neurogenic bowel would likely present. Of note, spinal shock can at times remain after an acute spinal cord injury for up to 4 weeks to 12 weeks, depending on the individual. A person who has exited spinal shock and has a bulbocavernosus reflex would likely be more appropriate for an upper motor bowel program.

Ko HY. Revisit spinal shock: pattern of reflex evolution during spinal shock. Korean J Neurotrauma. 2018;14(2):47–54. https://doi.org/10.13004/kjnt.2018.14.2.47. Epub 2018 Oct 31.

Chen D, Anschel AS. Gastrointestinal Disorders. In: Kirshblum S, Campagnolo DI, editors. Spinal cord medicine. 2nd ed. Philadelphia: Lipincott Williams & Wilkins; 2011.

Doherty JG, Burns AS, O'Ferrall DM, Ditunno JF Jr. Prevalence of upper motor neuron vs lower motor neuron lesions in complete lower thoracic and lumbar spinal cord injuries. J Spinal Cord Med. 2002;25(4):289–92. https://doi.org/10.1080/10790268.2002.11753630.

32. A 72-year-old male with intense mid back pain particularly while lying supine at night comes into clinic for further evaluation after he also started having urinary accidents overnight and has been wetting his pants more frequently. He mentions falling a week ago because his legs gave out. When asking about his medical history, he mentions having a prostate cancer diagnosed 2 years ago although he had completed radiation therapy. If the patient had electrodiagnostic studies for further assessment, what would you expect to see with regards to the motor-evoked potentials (MEPs) of his legs?

A. Normal MEPs
B. Increased amplitude of MEPs
C. Prolonged latency of MEPs
D. Absent MEPs

Answer: D.

The patient comes into clinic with symptoms correlating to a neoplastic lesion as very high in the differential, particularly with a history of prostate cancer that was treated with radiation therapy only, there is a possibility of a metastatic lesion to the thoracic spine now, which would likely be blastic in nature if the primary lesion is from the prostate. While likely not the first step in evaluation, motor-evoked potentials (MEPs) can be evaluated. There is a good correlation between MEP findings and motor function. For neoplastic lesions, there is most often decreased MEP amplitudes or absent MEP responses. Neoplastic lesions tend to have decreased latencies compared to inflammatory lesions. Other diagnostic studies include MRI (ideally with contrast if looking for neoplastic lesions). Another diagnostic imaging that could be performed is a bone scan, which may be able to identify blastic bone lesions.

Kawaguchi Y, Kitagawa H, Nakamura H, Gejo R, Kimura T. Neurophysiological tests of respiratory function by compound muscle action potentials from the diaphragm. Detection of lesions in the higher cervical cord. J Bone Joint Surg Br. 2000;82(5):695–701. https://doi.org/10.1302/0301-620x.82b5.10390.

Tegenthoff M. Clinical applications of magnetic transcranial stimulation in acute spinal cord injury. In: Lissens MA, editor. Clinical applications of magnetic transcranial stimulation. Leuven, Belgium: Peeters Press; 1992. pp. 33–41.

Dimitrijević MR, Kofler M, McKay WB, Sherwood AM, Van der Linden C, Lissens MA. Early and late lower limb motor evoked potentials elicited by transcranial magnetic motor cortex stimulation. Electroencephalogr Clin Neurophysiol. 1992;85(6):365–73. https://doi.org/10.1016/0168-5597(92)90049-h.

Meyer B, Zentner J. Do motor evoked potentials allow quantitative assessment of motor function in patients with spinal cord lesions? Eur Arch Psychiatry Clin Neurosci. 1992;241(4):201–4. https://doi.org/10.1007/BF02190253.

Linden D, Berlit P. Magnetic motor evoked potentials (MEP) in diseases of the spinal cord. Acta Neurol Scand. 1994;90(5):348–53. https://doi.org/10.1111/j.1600-0404.1994. tb02736.x.

33. A 47-year-old female with a history of multiple sclerosis comes into your clinic for a follow-up visit after having a recent MRI lumbar spine with new findings of a demyelinating lesion. If electrodiagnostic studies were performed, what would you expect to see with regards to motor-evoked potentials (MEPs)?

    A. Increased amplitudes and increased latencies of MEPs
    B. Increased amplitudes and decreased latencies of MEPs
    C. Decreased amplitudes and increased latencies of MEPs
    D. Decreased amplitudes and decreased latencies of MEPs

Answer: C.

The patient has history of multiple sclerosis with new findings of demyelinating lesion of the lumbar spine on MRI. Given the medical history, the patient has an inflammatory lesion of the spinal cord. For inflammatory lesions, usually the motor-evoked potential (MEP) has a decreased amplitude and the MEP for inflammatory lesions often demonstrate increased or prolonged latencies. This is in contrast to neoplastic lesions which have decreased latencies.

Linden D, Berlit P. Magnetic motor evoked potentials (MEP) in diseases of the spinal cord. Acta Neurol Scand. 1994;90(5):348–53. https://doi.org/10.1111/j.1600-0404.1994. tb02736.x.

34. A 25-year-old male presents to the emergency room after a motor vehicle accident, and he is not moving his arms or his legs. Imaging of his spine shows translation of the vertebral body C5 on C6 with cord compression. He is brought emergently into the operating room with the neurosurgical team. During the surgery, electrodes were placed for monitoring of somatosensory-evoked potentials (SEPs) and motor-evoked potentials (MEPs). Which of the following would be most suggestive of a poor prognosis?

A. Normal SEPs and decreased amplitude of MEPs
B. Absent SEPs and decreased amplitudes of MEPs
C. Normal SEPs and normal MEPs
D. Reduced SEPs and normal MEPs

Answer: B.

Patients will often have monitoring of SEPs and MEPs during neurosurgical procedures. In the acute stages of spinal cord injury, having absent SEPs are very sensitive for a poor prognosis when predicting outcome, though less specific. However, when combining SEPs with MEPs the specificity of the assessment increases. Therefore, having the combination of absent SEPs and either decreased amplitude MEPs or absent MEPs would be the most suggestive of a poor prognosis. Of the answer choices, normal SEPs and normal MEPs would have the best prognosis.

Maugière F. Clinical utility of somatosensory evoked potentials (SEPs): present debates and future trends. Electroencephalogr Clin Neurophysiol Suppl. 1996;46:27–33.
Spielholz NI, Sell GH, Goodgold J, Rusk HA, Greens SK. Electrophysiological studies in patients with spinal cord lesions. Arch Phys Med Rehabil. 1972;53(12):558–62.
Curt A, Dietz V. Electrophysiological recordings in patients with spinal cord injury: significance for predicting outcome. Spinal Cord. 1999;37(3):157–65. https://doi.org/10.1038/sj.sc.3100809.
Boakye M, Harkema S, Ellaway PH, Skelly AC. Quantitative testing in spinal cord injury: overview of reliability and predictive validity. J Neurosurg Spine. 2012;17(Suppl. 1):141–50. https://doi.org/10.3171/2012.5.AOSPINE1296.

35. Which of the following functional assessment measures may be used to assess the capacity of individuals with spinal cord injury to perform daily tasks covering three domains?

A. Physical Activity Recall Assessment for People with SCI (PARA-SCI)
B. Spinal Cord Independence Measure (SCIM)
C. Functional Independence Measure (FIM)
D. Barthel Index or Modified Barthel Index (BI)

Answer: B.

The Spinal Cord Independence Measure (SCIM) assesses the capacity of individuals with SCI to perform daily tasks using 19 items covering 3 domains: self-care (feeding, grooming, bathing, and dressing), respiration and sphincter management, and mobility (bed, transfers, indoor/outdoor). Observation or self- or proxy-report may be utilized to collect the information; the items are weighted to reflect assumed clinical relevance.

The Physical Activity Recall Assessment for People with SCI (PARA-SCI) was developed to measure the physical activity of individuals with spinal cord injury who use wheelchairs at their primary means of mobility. The Functional Independence Measure (FIM) is a measure of the level of assistance individuals need to carry out daily activities.

The Barthel Index (BI) consists of 10 self-care items which may be completed based on observation or self or proxy reported; the original Barthel index has 3 score options for most items (0 = inability; 5 = assistance required; 10 = total independence), but the modified Barthel index utilizes a 5 point scale and weighing of the items to increase the sensitivity.

Anderson K, Aito S, Atkins M, Biering-Sørensen F, Charlifue S, Curt A, Ditunno J, Glass C, Marino R, Marshall R, Mulcahey MJ, Post M, Savic G, Scivoletto G, Catz A; Functional Recovery Outcome Measures Work Group. Functional recovery measures for spinal cord injury: an evidence-based review for clinical practice and research. J Spinal Cord Med. 2008;31(2):133–44. https://doi.org/10.1080/10790268.2008.11760704.

Dawson J, Shamley D, Jamous MA. A structured review of outcome measures used for the assessment of rehabilitation interventions for spinal cord injury. Spinal Cord. 2008;46(12):768–80. https://doi.org/10.1038/sc.2008.50. Epub 2008 Jun 3.

Furlan JC, Noonan V, Singh A, Fehlings MG. Assessment of disability in patients with acute traumatic spinal cord injury: a systematic review of the literature. J Neurotrauma. 2011;28(8):1413–30. https://doi.org/10.1089/neu.2009.1148. Epub 2010 Aug 28.

36. A 45-year-old male with central cord syndrome who recently transferred to the spinal cord unit begins mobilizing in bed, attempting to transfer over to the wheelchair, and trial standing in place with the therapist. There is noticeable wobbling and instability with these activities. In order to assess his risk of falling, which if the following functional assessment measures would be useful?

    A. Berg Balance Scale (BBS)
    B. Spinal Cord Ability Ruler (SCAR)
    C. International Standards of Neurological Classification of SCI (ISNCSCI)
    D. 6-minute Walk Test (6MWT)

    Answer: A.

    The Berg Balance Scale (BBS) is a 14-item measure to assess risk of falling based on ability to perform balance-challenging tasks, such as standing with eyes closed or on one foot. The scale was originally developed for older individuals and usually best suited for incomplete SCI with some ability to stand and walk. The Spinal Cord Ability Ruler (SCAR) combines aspects of function with strength in order to address challenges with "volitional performance." The International Standards of Neurological Classification of SCI (ISNCSCI) tests motor and sensory components in order to determine a level of injury and the severity of the injury. The 6-Minute Walk Test (6MWT) measures the distance that a patient can walk at their own pace on a flat surface that is hard over the timespan of 6 min.

Kahn JH, Tappan R, Newman CP, Palma P, Romney W, Tseng Stultz E, Tefertiller C, Weisbach CL. Outcome measure recommendations from the spinal cord injury EDGE Task Force. Phys Ther. 2016;96(11):1832–42. https://doi.org/10.2522/ptj.20150453. Epub 2016 May 26.

Reed R, Mehra M, Kirshblum S, Maier D, Lammertse D, Blight A, Rupp R, Jones L, Abel R, Weidner N; EMSCI Study Group; SCOPE, Curt A, Steeves J. Spinal cord ability ruler: an interval scale to measure volitional performance after spinal cord injury. Spinal Cord. 2017;55(8):730–8. https://doi.org/10.1038/sc.2017.1. Epub 2017 Mar 21.

37. A 33-year-old female with C6 AIS B SCI has been working with the occupational therapist on feeding and grooming and utilizing a universal cuff for utensils. She has also been working on picking up large and small objects and stacking items. Which of the following functional tests would be helpful to evaluate her use of her upper extremities?

   A. Assessment of Life Habits (LIFE-H)
   B. Reintegration to Normal Living Index (RNL)
   C. Needs Assessment Checklist. (NAC)
   D. Jebsen-Taylor Hand Function Test (JHFT)

Answer: D.

The Jebsen-Taylor Hand Function Test (JHFT) is a standardized performance-based measure that tests fine and gross motor hand function using simulated ADLs, such as writing, turning over cards, picking up small common objects, simulated feeding, stacking checkers, and picking up large heavy objects.

The Needs Assessment Checklist (NAC) comprehensively operationalizes functioning of those with SCI during inpatient rehabilitation in 9 domains, including ADLs (29 items), skin management (14 items), bladder management (10 items), bowel management (7 items), mobility (17 items), wheelchair and equipment (33 items), community preparation (24 items), discharge coordination (32 items) and psychological issues (19 items); usually a 4 point scale is utilized with 0 = completely dependent to 3 = completely independent. The Reintegration to Normal Living Index (RNL) functional measure is a self-report questionnaire that looks at satisfaction with performance in life activities (e.g. mobility, self-care, daily activity, reaction all activity, and family roles) by utilizing 11 items, with one of the three alternate scoring systems: 10 point visual analogue scale, 3 point scale, or 4 point scale.

The Assessment of Life Habits (LIFE-H) functional measure defines life habits as "those habits that ensure the survival and development of a person in society throughout their life" to include activities ranging from ADLs to social roles; it utilizes 242 items or 77 items to assess functioning in 12 domains (from nutrition to recreation) by separating rating levels of difficulty (5 point scale) and type of assistance necessary (4 point scale); satisfaction is usually measured separately.

Noonan VK, Miller WC, Noreau L; SCIRE Research Team. A review of instruments assessing participation in persons with spinal cord injury. Spinal Cord. 2009;47(6):435–46. https://doi.org/10.1038/sc.2008.171. Epub 2009 Feb 24.

Spinal Cord Injury Research Evidence Project. Outcome Measures. 2016. Available at: https://scireproject.com/outcome-measures

Rehabilitation Institute of Chicago. Rehabilitation Measures Database. 2010. Available at: www.rehabmeasures.org

38. A 69-year-old male with C5 AIS A SCI was transferred over to the SCI unit and is undergoing initial evaluations. You notice that he has severe spasticity of the bilateral lower extremities with Modified Ashworth Score (MAS) of 3 in the bilateral adductors, knee extensors, and ankle plantarflexors. He has been having bowel incontinence overnight per nursing staff, and a Foley was placed due to frequent urinary incontinence. In the last few days, his appetite has decreased, and he occasionally refuses position turns and changing his hospital gown. What functional assessment would be most appropriate to evaluate his risk of developing a pressure injury?

A. Spinal Cord Injury-Functional Index Self-care Domain (SCI-FI Self-Care)
B. Spinal cord injury-Functional Index Basic Mobility Domain (SCI-FI Basic Mobility)
C. Braden Scale (BS)
D. Barthel Index (BI)

Answer: C.

The Braden Scale (BS) assess the likelihood of developing a pressure injury; it consists of 6 subscales with total scores ranging from 6 to 23 points with lower scores indicating a higher risk of pressure injuries. The 6 subscales include: (1) Sensory—to measure the ability to feel and relieve discomfort, (2) Moisture - to assess the degree to which skin is exposed to moisture, (3) Mobility—to assess the individual's ability to relieve pressure, (4) Activity—to assess the ability to get out of bed and or ambulate, (5) Nutrition—to assess amount of food intake, (6) Friction and shear—to measure the individual's ability to assist with movement or be able to move in a way that keeps the skin free of contact with underlying surfaces.

The Barthel Index (BI) consists of 10 self-care items which may be completed based on observation or self or proxy reported; the original Barthel index has 3 score options for most items (0 = inability; 5 = assistance required; 10 = total independence), but the modified Barthel index utilizes a 5 point scale and weighing of the items to increase the sensitivity.

The Spinal Cord Injury- Functional Index Self-care Domain (SCI-FI Self-Care) includes 9- items that cover bathing, grooming, bladder and bowel management, upper and lower body dressing and feeding; it may also be administered as a 9-item short form with separate versions for those with tetraplegia or paraplegia.

The Spinal Cord Injury- Functional Index Basic Mobility Domain (SCI-FI Basic Mobility) includes 54 items referring to body positioning, transfers, carrying objects, and moving around in different locations.

Jette AM, Tulsky DS, Ni P, Kisala PA, Slavin MD, Dijkers MP, Heinemann AW, Tate DG, Whiteneck G, Charlifue S, Houlihan B, Williams S, Kirshblum S, Dyson-Hudson T, Zanca J, Fyffe D. Development and initial evaluation of the spinal cord injury-functional index. Arch Phys Med Rehabil. 2012;93(10):1733–50. https://doi.org/10.1016/j.apmr.2012.05.008. Epub 2012 May 17.
Tulsky DS, Jette AM, Kisala PA, Kalpakjian C, Dijkers MP, Whiteneck G, Ni P, Kirshblum S, Charlifue S, Heinemann AW, Forchheimer M, Slavin MD, Houlihan B, Tate DG, Dyson-Hudson T, Fyffe DG, Williams S, Zanca J. Spinal cord injury-functional index: item banks to measure physical functioning in individuals with spinal cord injury. Arch Phys Med Rehabil. 2012;93(10):1722–32. https://doi.org/10.1016/j.apmr.2012.05.007. Epub 2012 May 16.
Rehabilitation Institute of Chicago. Rehabilitation Measures Database. 2010. Available at: www.rehabmeasures.org

39. A 35-year-old male with a history of L4 AIS D SCI comes into your clinic as a 3-month follow-up visit after discharge from inpatient rehabilitation. He has been working with PT/OT as an outpatient and recently had an assessment with the Walking Index for Spinal Cord Injury (WISCI) in order to determine his ambulation status. Which of the following best describes this functional test?

A. Self-reported gait performance measure for those who can ambulate independently, based on assistive device use and walking ability
B. Measuring the time required to walk 10 m at a self-selected walking speed
C. Walking ability is characterized by a score from 0 to 20 based on distance walked and use of assistive devices, bracing, and physical assistance
D. Measuring walking performance by having the individual stand up from an armchair, walk 3 m at a self-selected speed, turn, return to the chair, and sit down.

Answer: C.

The Walking Index for Spinal Cord Injury (WISCI) is best described in answer choice C. Answer choice A refers to the SCI Functional Ambulation Inventory (SCI-FAI) functional assessment. Answer choice B refers to the 10-Meter Walk Test (10MWT). Answer choice D refers to the Timed Up and Go Test (TUG).

Furlan JC, Noonan V, Singh A, Fehlings MG. Assessment of disability in patients with acute traumatic spinal cord injury: a systematic review of the literature. J Neurotrauma. 2011;28(8):1413–30. https://doi.org/10.1089/neu.2009.1148. Epub 2010 Aug 28.

Spinal Cord Injury Research Evidence Project. Outcome Measures. 2016. Available at: https://scireproject.com/outcome-measures

Rehabilitation Institute of Chicago. Rehabilitation Measures Database. 2010. Available at: www.rehabmeasures.org

40. A 19-year-old male with C5 AIS B SCI is working with the occupational therapist on picking up objects with a neuroprosthesis. The therapist mentions performing the Grasp Release Test earlier in the week to determine his hand function. Which of the following best describes this functional assessment?

 A. Assesses hand function in those with tetraplegia based on ability to manipu- late 6 objects (peg, paperweight, fork, block, can, and videotape) using one hand.
 B. Standardized performance-based measure testing and gross motor hand function using simulated ADLs.
 C. Consists of 153 items referring to 9 classes of activities (self-care, dressing, continence, mobility, eating/drinking, work, leisure, household tasks, and miscellaneous)
 D. Consists of 35 items referring to ability to perform tasks requiring fine motor control like turning pages and opening mail.

Answer: A.

Choice A describes the Grasp Release Test (GRT). Choice B describes the Jeb- sen-Taylor Hand Function Test (JHFT). Choice C refers to the Tetraplegia Hand Activity Questionnaire (THAQ). Choice D describes the Spinal Cord Injury- Functional Index (SCI-FI)-Fine motor domain.

Sinnott KA, Dunn JA, Wangdell J, Johanson ME, Hall AS, Post MW. measurement of out- comes of upper limb reconstructive surgery for tetraplegia. Arch Phys Med Rehabil. 2016;97(Suppl. 6):S169–81. https://doi.org/10.1016/j.apmr.2015.10.110.

Kahn JH, Tappan R, Newman CP, Palma P, Romney W, Tseng Stultz E, Tefertiller C, Weis- bach CL. Outcome Measure Recommendations From the Spinal Cord Injury EDGE Task Force. Phys Ther. 2016;96(11):1832–42. https://doi.org/10.2522/ptj.20150453. Epub 2016 May 26.

Jette AM, Tulsky DS, Ni P, Kisala PA, Slavin MD, Dijkers MP, Heinemann AW, Tate DG, Whiteneck G, Charlifue S, Houlihan B, Williams S, Kirshblum S, Dyson-Hudson T, Zanca J, Fyffe D. Development and initial evaluation of the spinal cord injury-func- tional index. Arch Phys Med Rehabil. 2012;93(10):1733–50. https://doi.org/10.1016/j. apmr.2012.05.008. Epub 2012 May 17.

41. A 36-year-old male with T6 AIS B SCI is currently performing intermittent catheterization by himself without any issues reported. When attempting to transfer from the bed to his wheelchair with a slide board, he performs about 75% of the maneuver and needs one person assist. Which of the following

correctly pairs the tasks described with the appropriate Functional Independence Measure (FIM) score?

A. Bladder management – FIM 5 and Wheelchair transfers – FIM 1
B. Bladder management – FIM 4 and Wheelchair transfers – FIM 6
C. Bladder management – FIM 2 and Wheelchair transfers – FIM 5
D. Bladder management – FIM 6 and Wheelchair transfers – FIM 4

Answer: D.

The Functional Independence Measure (FIM) assesses the burden of care based on 2 domains: motor and cognitive/communication. All the items are measured on a 7-point scale as follows:
  1 = Total Assistance or not testable (Subject performs less than 25%)
  2 = Maximal Assistance (Subject performs 25% or more)
  3 = Moderate Assistance (Subject performs 50% or more)
  4 = Minimal Assistance (Subject performs 75% or more)
  5 = Supervision (Subject performs 100%)
  6 = Modified Independence (device)
  7 = Complete Independence (timely, safely)
This patient would have a FIM 6 (Modified Independence) with bladder management and FIM 4 (Minimal Assistance) with Wheelchair Transfers.

Velstra IM, Ballert CS, Cieza A. A systematic literature review of outcome measures for upper extremity function using the international classification of functioning, disability, and health as reference. PM R. 2011;3(9):846–60. https://doi.org/10.1016/j.pmrj.2011.03.014.
Anderson K, Aito S, Atkins M, Biering-Sørensen F, Charlifue S, Curt A, Ditunno J, Glass C, Marino R, Marshall R, Mulcahey MJ, Post M, Savic G, Scivoletto G, Catz A; Functional Recovery Outcome Measures Work Group. Functional recovery measures for spinal cord injury: an evidence-based review for clinical practice and research. J Spinal Cord Med. 2008;31(2):133–44. https://doi.org/10.1080/10790268.2008.11760704.
Kidd D, Stewart G, Baldry J, Johnson J, Rossiter D, Petruckevitch A, Thompson AJ. The Functional independence measure: a comparative validity and reliability study. Disabil Rehabil. 1995;17(1):10–4. https://doi.org/10.3109/09638289509166622.

42. A 75-year-old male presents to the hospital after falling off a ladder while placing Christmas lights on the roof of his house. He is found to have a neurological level of C8 AIS C on examination. When speaking with his therapist and nursing staff, he is only able to perform about 50% of the task when transferring onto the mobile shower commode chair. He can feed himself with a universal cuff to hold the utensils. He is not able to insert the suppository for his bowel care (nursing is performing). Which of the following correctly pairs the tasks described with the appropriate Functional Independence Measure (FIM) score?

A. Shower transfers – FIM 6, Feeding – FIM 2, Bowel management – FIM 5
B. Shower transfers – FIM 3, Feeding – FIM 6, Bowel management – FIM 1

C. Shower transfers – FIM 2, Feeding – FIM 5, Bowel management – FIM 2
D. Shower transfers – FIM 4, Feeding – FIM 3, Bowel management – FIM 3

Answer: B.

The Functional Independence Measure (FIM) assesses the burden of care based on 2 domains: motor and cognitive/communication (see Question 40). This patient would score FIM 3 on shower transfers (Moderate Assistance), FIM 6 (Modified Independence) on feeding, and FIM 1 (Complete Dependence) on Bowel Management.

Velstra IM, Ballert CS, Cieza A. A systematic literature review of outcome measures for upper extremity function using the international classification of functioning, disability, and health as reference. PM R. 2011;3(9):846–60. https://doi.org/10.1016/j.pmrj.2011.03.014.
Anderson K, Aito S, Atkins M, Biering-Sørensen F, Charlifue S, Curt A, Ditunno J, Glass C, Marino R, Marshall R, Mulcahey MJ, Post M, Savic G, Scivoletto G, Catz A; Functional Recovery Outcome Measures Work Group. Functional recovery measures for spinal cord injury: an evidence-based review for clinical practice and research. J Spinal Cord Med. 2008;31(2):133–44. https://doi.org/10.1080/10790268.2008.11760704.

43. A 45-year-old female with AIS T5 AIS B spinal cord injury after a motor vehicle accident was admitted to your SCI unit. She has been participating with the therapists and making progress in her mobility, ADLs, and iADLs. Which of the following functional assessments would review the patient's participation or any participation restrictions?

    A. Continuity Assessment Record and Evaluation (CARE Tool)
    B. Craig Handicap and Reporting Technique (CHART)
    C. Quadriplegia Index of Function (QIF)
    D. Functional Independence Measure Locomotion Item (FIM-L)

Answer: B.

The Craig Handicap and Reporting Technique (CHART) operationalizes participation and participation restrictions in 5 domains (physical independence, mobility, occupation, social integration, and economic self-sufficiency) using 27 items that may be completed by the individual with a disability or a proxy.

The Continuity Assessment Record and Evaluation (CARE Tool) consists of items covering self-care, functional mobility, supplemental functional ability, and iADLs.

The Quadriplegia Index of Function (QIF) was developed since the Barthel index was deemed too insensitive to document small functional gains made by tetraplegics during rehabilitation; the short form QIF utilizes 6 items to replace the 37 QIF items covering 10 domains; the modified QIF utilizes 14 items to cover 3 domains such as grooming, bathing, and feeding.

The Functional Independence Measure Locomotion item (FIM-L) assesses the burden of care with respect to primary mode of locomotion (walking or using wheelchair); scores are given by a trained observer and are based on a combination of assistive device use, distance traveled, and assistance provided by others.

Magasi SR, Heinemann AW, Whiteneck GG; Quality of Life/Participation Committee. Participation following traumatic spinal cord injury: an evidence-based review for research. J Spinal Cord Med. 2008;31(2):145–56. https://doi.org/10.1080/10790268.2008.11760705.

Noonan VK, Miller WC, Noreau L; SCIRE Research Team. A review of instruments assessing participation in persons with spinal cord injury. Spinal Cord. 2009;47(6):435–46. https://doi.org/10.1038/sc.2008.171. Epub 2009 Feb 24.

Centers for Medicare & Medicaid Services. CARE Item Set and B-CARE. 2015. Available at: https://www.cms.gov/Medicare/Quality-Initiatives-Patient-Assessment-Instruments/Post-Acute-Care-Quality-Initiatives/CARE-Item-Set-and-B-CARE.html

Sinnott KA, Dunn JA, Wangdell J, Johanson ME, Hall AS, Post MW. Measurement of outcomes of upper limb reconstructive surgery for tetraplegia. Arch Phys Med Rehabil. 2016;97(Suppl. 6):S169–81. https://doi.org/10.1016/j.apmr.2015.10.110.

Velstra IM, Ballert CS, Cieza A. A systematic literature review of outcome measures for upper extremity function using the international classification of functioning, disability, and health as reference. PM R. 2011;3(9):846–60. https://doi.org/10.1016/j.pmrj.2011.03.014.

44. A 23-year-old male presented to the hospital after a diving accident resulting in C5 AIS B spinal cord injury. He is now transferring to the SCI unit for comprehensive inpatient rehabilitation. During his initial evaluation, the Spinal Cord Independence Measure (SCIM) is utilized. Which of the following is NOT part of the domains covered in this functional assessment?

A. Feeding
B. Bathing
C. Sphincter management
D. Pressure relief

Answer: D.

The Spinal Cord Independence Measure (SCIM) assesses the capacity of individuals with SCI to perform daily tasks using 19 items covering 3 domains: self-care (that includes feeding, grooming, bathing, and dressing), respiration and sphincter management, and mobility (that includes bed, transfers, indoor/outdoor).

Anderson K, Aito S, Atkins M, Biering-Sørensen F, Charlifue S, Curt A, Ditunno J, Glass C, Marino R, Marshall R, Mulcahey MJ, Post M, Savic G, Scivoletto G, Catz A; Functional Recovery Outcome Measures Work Group. Functional recovery measures for spinal cord injury: an evidence-based review for clinical practice and research. J Spinal Cord Med. 2008;31(2):133–44. https://doi.org/10.1080/10790268.2008.11760704.

Dawson J, Shamley D, Jamous MA. A structured review of outcome measures used for the assessment of rehabilitation interventions for spinal cord injury. Spinal Cord. 2008;46(12):768–80. https://doi.org/10.1038/sc.2008.50. Epub 2008 Jun 3.

Acute Evaluation and Management of Spinal Cord Injuries

Beverly Hon and Michelle M. Didesch

Questions

1. Emergency medical services (EMS) are called to a scene where a middle-aged man has been found unconscious outside of his home. He is minimally moving his arms and legs. There is alcohol beside him. The exact mechanism of his injury is unclear. Clinical decision is made to stabilize his cervical spine in preparation for transport to the nearest hospital. All of the following are key clinical criteria that raise suspicion for cervical spine injury EXCEPT?

   A. Possible intoxication
   B. Altered mental status
   C. Age
   D. Possible neurologic deficit

   Answer: C.

   When EMS are assessing a patient, there are critical criteria that raise red flags for possible cervical spine injury. These include alteration in mental status, concern for being under the influence of substances, spine pain, neurologic deficit, or another injury such as a painful fracture that is distracting from possible

B. Hon (✉)
Veteran Affairs New Jersey Health Care System, Spinal Cord Injury and Disorders Service, East Orange, NJ, USA
e-mail: Beverly.hon@va.gov

M. M. Didesch
Department of Neuro Rehab Physiatry, Confluence Health—Wenatchee Valley Medical Group, Wenatchee, WA, USA
e-mail: michelle.didesch@confluencehealth.org

spine injury. If any of these criteria are met, standard of care is to stabilize the cervical spine until further evaluation can be completed. Age itself is not considered a criterion for cervical stabilization, making "C" an incorrect answer. Older age could be associated with cervical spine degenerative changes; however, this patient is middle aged and there is no specific suspicion of underlying cervical spine disease at baseline.

Consortium for Spinal Cord Medicine. Early acute management in adults with spinal cord injury: a clinical practice guideline for health-care professionals. J Spinal Cord Med. 2008;31(4):403–79. https://doi.org/10.1043/1079-0268-31.4.408.

Domeier RM. Indications for prehospital spinal immobilization. National Association of EMS Physicians Standards and Clinical Practice Committee. Prehosp Emerg Care. 1999;3(3):251–3. https://doi.org/10.1080/10903129908958946.

2. A patient is being treated in the Emergency Department after suffering a severe motor vehicle accident with resultant cervical spine injury. On physical examination, he is able to flex his elbows but not fully against gravity. He has no other volitional movement noted. While being evaluated for his injuries, it is noted that he is becoming increasingly somnolent with respirations becoming more labored. What is the most appropriate next step?

A. Check complete blood count, metabolic panel and urine drug screen to help determine differential for altered mental status.
B. Transport patient for stat head computed tomography (CT) to rule out intracranial bleed.
C. Call for additional respiratory assistance for possible intubation and obtain stat arterial blood gas.
D. Obtain urinalysis to rule out urinary tract infection.

Answer: C.

This patient has a neurologic spinal cord injury that is affecting the C5 level. He has potential compromise of his diaphragm and has compromise of his accessory respiratory muscles. While patients may initially seem to be stable from a respiratory standpoint, there must be close monitoring of respiratory status because of neurologic involvement of the diaphragm and accessory muscles and potential to fatigue over time. It is appropriate to call for additional respiratory assistance and obtain a stat arterial blood gas with onset of respiratory distress. If the patient continues to decline, intubation should be performed. Checking additional lab work such as urinalysis, complete blood count, metabolic panel, and urine drug screen may be important but do not take precedent to the key components of resuscitation of airway and breathing. Attempts should be made to first stabilize the patient before additional imaging.

Berlly M, Shem K. Respiratory management during the first five days after spinal cord injury. J Spinal Cord Med. 2007;30(4):309–18. https://doi.org/10.1080/10790268.2007.11753946.

3. A patient is hospitalized in the intensive care unit after suffering a cervical spinal cord injury. He has been afebrile with normal complete blood count. He is persistently having low blood pressures and bradycardia. He is on a dopamine drip. What is the most likely cause for his abnormal vital signs?

   A. Neurogenic shock
   B. Septic shock
   C. Effect of pressor medication
   D. Autonomic dysreflexia

Answer: A.

Patients with tetraplegia may demonstrate neurogenic shock which is a loss of sympathetic input below the level of injury. This will often manifest as low blood pressure due to peripheral vasodilation and bradycardia due to lack of sympathetic outflow to compensate for ongoing vagal nerve input. Septic shock is less likely in this case as patient is afebrile with a normal white blood cell count. Dopamine would result in improvement in blood pressure and heart rate, not hypotension and bradycardia. Autonomic dysreflexia leads to elevated blood pressures.

Hachem LD, Ahuja CS, Fehlings MG. Assessment and management of acute spinal cord injury: from point of injury to rehabilitation. J Spinal Cord Med. 2017;40(6):665–75. https://doi.org/10.1080/10790268.2017.1329076. Epub 2017 Jun 1.

Bilello JF, Davis JW, Cunningham MA, Groom TF, Lemaster D, Sue LP. Cervical spinal cord injury and the need for cardiovascular intervention. Arch Surg. 2003;138(10):1127–9. https://doi.org/10.1001/archsurg.138.10.1127.

4. A patient with tetraplegia is being monitored in the intensive care unit. She has not required intubation, but nursing staff has been concerned about possibility of respiratory failure given her tetraplegia. Which of the following parameters does NOT help to predict the need for intubation?

   A. Vital capacity
   B. Negative inspiratory force
   C. Arterial blood gas
   D. Diaphragm fluoroscopy

Answer: D.

Vital capacity or negative inspiratory force can help monitor patients for impending need for intubation. An individual with a vital capacity less than 15 ml/Kg of ideal body weight (particularly if decreasing or below 10 ml/Kg) requires close monitoring and potentially consideration of intubation. Similarly, individuals with negative inspiratory force <20 cm H_2O also require close monitoring. Arterial blood gas assesses pO2 and pCO2 levels for hypoxemia and hypercapnia which should be monitored if concerning changes in respiratory status. Continuous pulse oximetry, chest x-ray, FEV1 may also be used to help assess for respiratory risk and compromise. It is not recommended to rely on any given number, as the entire clinical context and often a combination of parameters requires assessment. While diaphragm fluoroscopy can be used to assess phrenic nerve and diaphragmatic function, it is not typically used to assess for need for intubation.

Berlly M, Shem K. Respiratory management during the first five days after spinal cord injury. J Spinal Cord Med. 2007;30(4):309–18. https://doi.org/10.1080/10790268.2007.11753946.
Consortium for Spinal Cord Medicine. Respiratory management following spinal cord injury: a clinical practice guideline for health-care professionals. J Spinal Cord Med. 2005;28(3):259–93. https://doi.org/10.1080/10790268.2005.11753821.

5. Which of the following is NOT a key risk factor for respiratory complications after spinal cord injury?

   A. Completeness of injury
   B. Neurologic level of injury
   C. Younger age
   D. Concurrent severe traumatic brain injuries

Answer: C.

Higher neurologic level of injury and more complete injuries are correlated with higher risk for developing respiratory complications. Older age is also considered a risk factor, but not younger age. Concurrent severe traumatic brain injuries increase the risk of respiratory complications.

Berlly M, Shem K. Respiratory management during the first five days after spinal cord injury. J Spinal Cord Med. 2007;30(4):309–18. https://doi.org/10.1080/10790268.2007.11753946.
Jensen MP, Truitt AR, Schomer KG, Yorkston KM, Baylor C, Molton IR. Frequency and age effects of secondary health conditions in individuals with spinal cord injury: a scoping review. Spinal Cord. 2013;51(12):882–92. https://doi.org/10.1038/sc.2013.112. Epub 2013 Oct 15.

6. Head cervical orthoses such as Miami J, Aspen, or Philadelphia collars primarily provide what type of restriction?

   A. Restriction of flexion and extension
   B. Restriction of lateral bending
   C. Restriction of rotation
   D. Restriction of incision dressing removal

Answer: A.

Head cervical orthoses such as Miami J, Aspen, or Philadelphia collars mostly restrict flexion and extension movement but are not effective for adequate restriction of lateral bending or rotation in the cervical spine. Head cervical thoracic orthosis such as Halo orthosis provides further restriction for lateral bending and rotation of the cervical spine. They are not designed to restrict dressing removal and can all be easily taken off.

Holla M, Huisman JM, Verdonschot N, Goosen J, Hosman AJ, Hannink G. The ability of external immobilizers to restrict movement of the cervical spine: a systematic review. Eur Spine J. 2016;25(7):2023–36. https://doi.org/10.1007/s00586-016-4379-6. Epub 2016 Mar 31.
Harrington AL, Cleveland C. Spinal orthoses. In: Kirshblum S, Lin V, editors. Spinal cord medicine. 3rd ed. New York, NY: Springer; 2019, pp. 744–53.

7. A patient is involved in a severe motor vehicle accident with subsequent thoracic burst fracture resulting in spinal cord injury. The orthotist is requested to make the most restrictive thoracolumbosacral (TLSO) option for the patient. What of the following is most restrictive?

   A. Crusiform Anterior Spinal Hyperextension (CASH) brace
   B. Jewett brace
   C. Custom TLSO
   D. Knight-Taylor Orthosis

Answer: C.

Custom TLSO is the most restrictive thoracolumbar spinal orthosis. CASH and Jewett braces primarily limit spinal forward flexion. Knight-Taylor orthosis provides restriction at flexion, extension, and lateral bending but custom TLSO provides more restriction.

Harrington AL, Cleveland C. Spinal orthoses. In: Kirshblum S, Lin V, editors. Spinal cord medicine. 3rd ed. New York, NY: Springer; 2019, pp. 744–53.

8. A patient has been diagnosed with a thoracic spine fracture and spinal cord injury. As a consultant, you are being asked if further imaging of the cervical or lumbar spine is needed as diagnosis has been established?

   A. Yes; CT imaging of the entire spine should be obtained after spinal cord injury to rule out other areas of spine injury.
   B. Yes; MRI imaging of the entire spine should be obtained after spinal cord injury to rule out other areas of spine injury.
   C. No; diagnosis has already been established. It is not cost effective to image further areas of the spine at this time.
   D. No; physical exam should be sufficient to rule out other injury.

Answer: A.

For a patient with spinal cord injury, the entire spine should be imaged to rule out other regions of spine injury. Assuming that a preliminary diagnosis rules out other injuries may save cost but is not a clinically appropriate decision. Physical exam is insufficient to completely rule out other injuries as a distracting injury can limit quality of the physical exam. CT imaging is ideal to rule out other bony injuries. Magnetic resonance imaging (MRI) can be helpful to further evaluate spinal cord and ligamentous injuries but is not always needed for the entire spine.

Consortium for Spinal Cord Medicine. Early acute management in adults with spinal cord injury: a clinical practice guideline for health-care professionals. J Spinal Cord Med. 2008;31(4):403–79. https://doi.org/10.1043/1079-0268-31.4.408.

9. Generally, how long should gastrointestinal ulcer prophylaxis be utilized after acute spinal cord injury?

   A. Gastrointestinal prophylaxis is not recommended
   B. 4 weeks
   C. 3 months
   D. 6 months

Answer: B.

Gastrointestinal ulcer prophylaxis is recommended for 4 weeks after acute spinal cord injury. This can be continued on an individual basis if there are other risk factors for ulcer development.

Consortium for Spinal Cord Medicine. Early acute management in adults with spinal cord injury: a clinical practice guideline for health-care professionals. J Spinal Cord Med. 2008;31(4):403–79. https://doi.org/10.1043/1079-0268-31.4.408.

10. A patient with acute tetraplegia is recovering in the hospital. A family member requests to bring the patient outside for a few hours on a warm summer day. When she returns, it is noted that her temperature is 100 °F. She has no leukocytosis, normal urinalysis, and no new pain, skin issues, or swelling. What is the most likely diagnosis?

    A. Autonomic dysreflexia
    B. Venous thrombosis
    C. Urinary tract infection
    D. Poikilothermia

Answer: D.

Patients with tetraplegia are at increased risk for poikolthermia, which is the inability to regulate body temperature resulting in changes in body temperature depending on environmental temperature. For example, being outside during a warm day or wearing excessive blankets can result in elevated temperatures.

Incorrect temperature reading is less likely diagnosis. Given lack of leukocytosis, normal urinalysis, and no other concerns for skin breakdown or increased pain, infection is low on the differential. Although a possible cause of fever, the patient does not have any findings to suggest venous thrombosis. Fever is not a common symptom of autonomic dysreflexia.

Consortium for Spinal Cord Medicine. Early acute management in adults with spinal cord injury: a clinical practice guideline for health-care professionals. J Spinal Cord Med. 2008;31(4):403–79. https://doi.org/10.1043/1079-0268-31.4.408.

11. When is the earliest time that a comprehensive International Standards for Neurological and Functional Classification provides reliable information on prognosis after acute spinal cord injury?

    A. First six hours
    B. 3–7 days after initial injury
    C. 2 weeks after initial injury
    D. 1 month after initial injury

Answer: B.

3–7 days after initial injury is generally considered the earliest time that a comprehensive exam provides information of prognosis for neurologic recovery. An exam conducted in the first six hours may not be reliable for information on neurologic recovery.

Brown PJ, Marino RJ, Herbison GJ, Ditunno JF Jr. The 72-hour examination as a predictor of recovery in motor complete quadriplegia. Arch Phys Med Rehabil. 1991;72(8):546–8.
Consortium for Spinal Cord Medicine. Outcomes following traumatic spinal cord injury: clinical practice guidelines for health-care professionals. J Spinal Cord Med. 2000;23(4):289–316. https://doi.org/10.1080/10790268.2000.11753539.

12. A patient is hospitalized after an acute spinal cord injury. When attempting to elicit a Babinski sign on exam, there is a delayed, slow toe flexion and then relaxation. What is the likely reason for this finding?

    A. Early neurologic recovery
    B. Incorrect examination technique
    C. Spinal shock with delayed plantar reflex
    D. Development of spasticity

Answer: C.

This finding is called a delayed plantar reflex. This is one of the first reflexes that returns after spinal shock. Prolonged presence of delayed plantar reflex is associated with worse neurologic outcomes. Therefore, this is not a sign of neurologic recovery. This should also not be mistaken for volitional movement.

Ko HY. Revisit spinal shock: pattern of reflex evolution during spinal shock. Korean J Neurotrauma. 2018;14(2):47–54. https://doi.org/10.13004/kjnt.2018.14.2.47. Epub 2018 Oct 31.

Weinstein DE, Ko HY, Graziani V, Ditunno JF Jr. Prognostic significance of the delayed plantar reflex following spinal cord injury. J Spinal Cord Med. 1997;20(2):207–11. https://doi.org/10.1080/10790268.1997.11719470.

Ditunno JF, Little JW, Tessler A, Burns AS. Spinal shock revisited: a four-phase model. Spinal Cord. 2004;42(7):383–95. https://doi.org/10.1038/sj.sc.3101603.

13. Which of the following is the least likely to indicate a poor prognosis on MRI imaging?

A. Intramedullary hemorrhage
B. Intramedullary edema <36mm
C. Cord transection
D. Bilateral facet dislocation

Answer: B.

Spinal cord hemorrhage is considered a poor prognostic indicator for acute spinal cord injury and associated more often with complete injuries. Cord transection is also associated with poor prognosis and more likely to result in a complete injury. Edema itself is not a poor prognostic indicator and in fact may be considered a positive prognostic indicator in incomplete injuries. Bilateral facet dislocation is associated with worse outcomes.

Marciello MA, Flanders AE, Herbison GJ, Schaefer DM, Friedman DP, Lane JI. Magnetic resonance imaging related to neurologic outcome in cervical spinal cord injury. Arch Phys Med Rehabil. 1993;74(9):940–6.

Ramón S, Domínguez R, Ramírez L, Paraira M, Olona M, Castelló T, García Fernández L. Clinical and magnetic resonance imaging correlation in acute spinal cord injury. Spinal Cord. 1997;35(10):664–73. https://doi.org/10.1038/sj.sc.3100490.

Wilson JR, Vaccaro A, Harrop JS, Aarabi B, Shaffrey C, Dvorak M, Fisher C, Arnold P, Massicotte EM, Lewis S, Rampersaud R, Okonkwo DO, Fehlings MG. The impact of facet dislocation on clinical outcomes after cervical spinal cord injury: results of a multicenter North American prospective cohort study. Spine (Phila Pa 1976). 2013;38(2):97–103. https://doi.org/10.1097/BRS.0b013e31826e2b91.

14. What is NOT a common complication of halo fixation?

A. Dysphagia
B. Pin loosening
C. Pin infection
D. Intracranial penetration of pins

Answer: D.

Complications from halo fixation include pin loosening, pin infection, as well as dysphagia. Care must be taken to monitor for these complications with halo placement. Brain injury from pin insertion is not common. While intracranial penetration of pins has been reported, it is extremely rare.

Lee D, Adeoye AL, Dahdaleh NS. Indications and complications of crown halo vest placement: a review. J Clin Neurosci. 2017;40:27–33. https://doi.org/10.1016/j.jocn.2017.01.002. Epub 2017 Feb 10.

15. Which pharmacological treatment is recommended for orthostatic hypotension in individuals with acute spinal cord injury?

    A. Amitriptyline
    B. Gabapentin
    C. Midodrine
    D. Baclofen

Answer: C.

Midodrine is an alpha$_1$ agonist that can be used to help augment blood pressure in individuals with hypotension due to spinal cord injuries. The other medications are not used to increase blood pressure.

Claydon VE, Steeves JD, Krassioukov A. Orthostatic hypotension following spinal cord injury: understanding clinical pathophysiology. Spinal Cord. 2006;44(6):341–51. https://doi.org/10.1038/sj.sc.3101855. Epub 2005 Nov 22.
Consortium for Spinal Cord Medicine. Early acute management in adults with spinal cord injury: a clinical practice guideline for health-care professionals. J Spinal Cord Med. 2008;31(4):403–79. https://doi.org/10.1043/1079-0268-31.4.408.
Evans LT, Lollis SS, Ball PA. Management of acute spinal cord injury in the neurocritical care unit. Neurosurg Clin N Am. 2013;24(3):339–47. https://doi.org/10.1016/j.nec.2013.02.007. Epub 2013 Apr 17.

16. Which is a typical presentation of autonomic dysreflexia?

    A. A sudden decrease in blood pressure, headache, bradycardia, and profuse sweating below the level of injury.
    B. A sudden increase in blood pressure, headache, tachycardia, and profuse sweating above the level of injury.
    C. A sudden decrease in blood pressure, headache, tachycardia, and profuse sweating below the level of injury.
    D. A sudden increase in blood pressure, headache, bradycardia, and profuse sweating above the level of injury.

Answer: D.

The typical presentation of autonomic dysreflexia is a sudden increase in blood pressure, decrease in heart rate, and profuse sweating above the level of injury. Headache and a flushed face are also common seen in individuals suffering from an autonomic dysreflexia.

Consortium for Spinal Cord Medicine. Acute management of autonomic dysreflexia: individuals with spinal cord injury presenting to health-care facilities. J Spinal Cord Med. 2002;25(Suppl. 1):S67–88.

17. For individuals with severe acute bradycardia following SCI, treatment options include:

    A. Atropine
    B. Fludrocortisone
    C. Midodrine
    D. No treatment is needed as acute symptomatic bradycardia will not lead to any issues.

Answer: A.

Atropine is recommended for treatment of acute severe or symptomatic bradycardia. Midodrine is used for pharmacological treatment of orthostatic hypotension. Fludrocortisone is also used for pharmacological treatment of orthostatic hypotension. In the acute stages, bradycardia can lead to asystole if severe. In patients with recurrent episodes of bradycardia, temporary pacing may be needed. Implantation of a permanent pacemaker is rarely needed.

Consortium for Spinal Cord Medicine. Early acute management in adults with spinal cord injury: a clinical practice guideline for health-care professionals. J Spinal Cord Med. 2008;31(4):403–79. https://doi.org/10.1043/1079-0268-31.4.408.

18. What is the pharmacological agent of choice for chemoprophylaxis in individuals with acute spinal cord injury?

    A. Heparin drip
    B. Low molecular weight heparin
    C. Inferior vena cava filter placement
    D. Aspirin

Answer: B.

The Consortium for Spinal Cord Medicine Clinical Practice Guidelines recommends low-molecular weight heparin to be started in individuals with acute spinal cord injury once there are no signs of active bleeding and there is no upcoming surgical intervention planned. Inferior vena cava filter placement is not typically placed in individuals with acute spinal cord injury as a prophylactic measurement. Heparin drip is considered for therapeutic anti-coagulation.

Prevention of Venous Thromboembolism in Individuals with Spinal Cord Injury: Clinical Practice Guidelines for Health Care Providers, 3rd ed.: Consortium for spinal cord medicine. Top Spinal Cord Inj Rehabil. 2016;22(3):209–240. https://doi.org/10.1310/sci2203-209.

Geerts WH, Heit JA, Clagett GP, Pineo GF, Colwell CW, Anderson FA Jr, Wheeler HB. Prevention of venous thromboembolism. Chest. 2001;119(Suppl. 1):132S–175S. https://doi.org/10.1378/chest.119.1_suppl.132s.

19. A 28-year-old male with T6 AIS A paraplegia is one-week post-injury due to a motor vehicle accident. He required two surgical procedures and remained under anesthesia for a total of 16 hours. He is complaining of nausea and had two episodes of emesis. On examination, his abdomen is distended and bowel sounds are minimal. He has not had a bowel movement since his initial injury. What is your diagnosis?

   A. Peptic ulcer perforation
   B. Ileus
   C. Pancreatitis
   D. Constipation

   Answer: B.

   Impairment of colonic motility occurs early after an acute spinal cord injury. During ileus, bowel sound may be absent to hypoactive. Proposed mechanism of ileus is thought to be due to loss of both sympathetic and parasympathetic innervation from spinal shock. Individuals may experience bowel distension, inadequate elimination with resultant nausea and emesis, as well as poor appetite. Peptic ulceration perforation with resultant gastrointestinal bleeding occurs most often during the first month post injury. Pancreatitis is another complication that may occur during the first month post injury and should be monitored for. While neurogenic bowel and constipation are common, it is unlikely to lead to absence of bowel sounds. Abdominal imaging may be useful to distinguish between colonic obstruction, constipation, and ileus.

   Chen DA, Anschel A. Gastrointestinal disorders. In: Kirshblum S, Campagnolo DI, editors. Spinal cord medicine. 2nd ed. Philadelphia: Lipincott Williams & Wilkins; 2011. pp. 6–30.
   Consortium for Spinal Cord Medicine. Early acute management in adults with spinal cord injury: a clinical practice guideline for health-care professionals. J Spinal Cord Med. 2008;31(4):403–79. https://doi.org/10.1043/1079-0268-31.4.408.

20. A 40-year-old male suffered a spinal cord injury 3 weeks ago and is found with C6 AIS B tetraplegia. He is currently in acute rehabilitation. He has been having episodes of bowel incontinence throughout the day. He is interested in establishing a bowel program. What would you recommend?

   A. It is recommended to wait at least 6 weeks post injury to start a bowel program due to increased risk of autonomic dysreflexia with a bowel program.
   B. Insert a rectal tube to minimize incontinence and possible skin break down.

C. Start a daily bowel program in the morning about 30 min after breakfast.
D. Bowel program should be started as an outpatient as the main focus of acute rehabilitation is ambulation.

Answer: C.

Daily bowel program should be institute about 30 min after a meal at approximately the same time each day. The goal of a bowel program is to minimize episodes of incontinence. Bowel program training should be initiated in the acute care hospital to help decrease complication of impaction, obstruction, or colorectal distention. It would be improper to wait until the outpatient setting to start a formal bowel program. A regular bowel program may decrease the risk of autonomic dysreflexia.

Clinical practice guidelines: Neurogenic bowel management in adults with spinal cord injury. Spinal Cord Medicine Consortium. J Spinal Cord Med. 1998;21(3):248–93. https://doi.org/10.1080/10790268.1998.11719536.

21. In the initial acute phase after injury, what is the recommendation for neurogenic bladder management?

A. Texas catheter to preserve skin integrity
B. Intermittent catheterization program to decrease risk of urinary tract infection
C. Indwelling catheter in case fluid resuscitation or intravenous (IV) medications are required
D. Insertion of suprapubic catheter as soon as possible to prevent urethral trauma

Answer: C.

In the initial acute phase after spinal cord injury, an indwelling catheter is recommended while a patient is being medically stabilized as urgent fluid resuscitation or intravenous medications may be required. However, when a patient no longer requires significant amounts of IV administration, an indwelling catheter can be discontinued. At that time, when medically stable, initiation of intermittent catheterization program is recommended for a patient that can perform or has the potential to perform catheterizations independently. Intermittent catheterization volumes should be maintained below 500 ml. While a Texas catheter (aka condom catheter) and other external catheter devices can help to minimize leakage from urinary incontinence, they do not adequately address issues of urinary retention. Suprapubic catheter placement may be beneficial for individuals with neurogenic bladders who are unable to independently perform intermittent catheterizations to help maximize independence and quality of life.

Consortium for Spinal Cord Medicine. Early acute management in adults with spinal cord injury: a clinical practice guideline for health-care professionals. J Spinal Cord Med. 2008;31(4):403–79. https://doi.org/10.1043/1079-0268-31.4.408.

22. Which factor has been determined to decrease likelihood of pressure injuries during the acute care hospitalization?

    A. admission to a specialized spinal cord injury trauma center
    B. increased family involvement
    C. higher educational status
    D. higher socioeconomic status

Answer: A.

Patients who were admitted to an inpatient rehabilitation facility from a specialized spinal cord injury trauma center were found to have significantly shorter acute care length of stay as well as total length of stay when compared with patients transferred from a non-specialized acute care hospital. In addition, a statistically significant higher incidence of patients from a non-specialized acute care hospital had pressure injuries when compared to patients from an organized spinal cord injury trauma center.

Ploumis A, Kolli S, Patrick M, Owens M, Beris A, Marino RJ. Length of stay and medical stability for spinal cord-injured patients on admission to an inpatient rehabilitation hospital: a comparison between a model SCI trauma center and non-SCI trauma center. Spinal Cord. 2011;49(3):411–5. https://doi.org/10.1038/sc.2010.132. Epub 2010 Oct 5.

23. Which factor is associated with increased risk of pressure injury in individuals with acute traumatic spinal cord injury?

    A. Age
    B. Complete neurological injury
    C. Body mass index
    D. Skin color

Answer: B.

Factors associated with the development of pressure injuries in persons with acute traumatic spinal cord injury include pneumonia, requirement of mechanical ventilation, and complete neurological injury.

Brienza D, Krishnan S, Karg P, Sowa G, Allegretti AL. Predictors of pressure ulcer incidence following traumatic spinal cord injury: a secondary analysis of a prospective longitudinal study. Spinal Cord. 2018 Jan;56(1):28–34. https://doi.org/10.1038/sc.2017.96. Epub 2017 Sep 12.

24. Which is NOT a risk factor associated with the development of venous thromboembolism in individuals with acute spinal cord injury

    A. Injury resulting from ground level falls
    B. Complete neurological injury
    C. Older age
    D. Concurrent long bone fracture

Answer: A.

Individuals with acute spinal cord injury are at increased risk of venous thromboembolism, including both deep vein thrombosis (DVT) as well as pulmonary embolism. Duplex ultrasound is the preferred method for detection of DVTs in the clinical setting. Risk factors associated with venous thromboembolism include complete neurological injury, absent or delayed chemoprophylaxis, concurrent lower extremity fractures, and older age.

Prevention of Venous Thromboembolism in Individuals with Spinal Cord Injury: Clinical Practice Guidelines for Health Care Providers, 3rd ed. Consortium for spinal cord medicine. Top Spinal Cord Inj Rehabil. 2016;22(3):209–40. https://doi.org/10.1310/sci2203-209.

25. Which of the following is true regarding bradycardia in those with acute spinal cord injury?

    A. Bradycardia is more common in those with paraplegia than tetraplegia.
    B. Bradycardia usually requires placement of permanent pacemaker.
    C. Bradycardia usually improves within 2–6 weeks post injury.
    D. Bradycardia is usually improved by endotracheal suctioning.

Answer: C.

Bradycardia usually occurs in individuals with a cervical spinal cord injury with an incidence of 17–77%. In contrast, individuals with thoracolumbar injuries experienced a 0–3% incidence of bradycardia. Noxious stimuli, such as endotracheal suctioning, can elicit episodes of bradycardia. In most cases, bradycardia is self-limiting and will improve between 2 and 6 weeks post injury. Persistent or life-threatening episodes of bradycardia may require implantation of a permanent pacemaker. Severe bradycardia can lead to asystole.

Hector SM, Biering-Sørensen T, Krassioukov A, Biering-Sørensen F. Cardiac arrhythmias associated with spinal cord injury. J Spinal Cord Med. 2013;36(6):591–9. https://doi.org/10.1179/2045772313Y.0000000114. Epub 2013 Apr 11.

26. Which of the following medications used to prevent hypotension following spinal cord injury is NOT matched with the appropriate mechanism of action?

    A. Fludrocortisone—Mineralocorticoid that promotes reabsorption of sodium from the distal tubules.
    B. Midodrine—Alpha$_2$ Agonist that leads to increased arteriolar and venous tone
    C. Epinephrine—Leads to release of norepinephrine and vasoconstriction
    D. Norepinephrine—Stimulates beta$_1$-adrenergic receptors and alpha-adrenergic receptors leading to vasoconstriction

Answer: B.

All of the following are correct except that midodrine is an Alpha$_1$ Agonist. Alpha$_2$ Agonists, such as clonidine, generally reduce blood pressure.

Claydon VE, Steeves JD, Krassioukov A. Orthostatic hypotension following spinal cord injury: understanding clinical pathophysiology. Spinal Cord. 2006;44(6):341–51. https://doi.org/10.1038/sj.sc.3101855. Epub 2005 Nov 22.
Consortium for Spinal Cord Medicine. Early acute management in adults with spinal cord injury: a clinical practice guideline for health-care professionals. J Spinal Cord Med. 2008;31(4):403–79. https://doi.org/10.1043/1079-0268-31.4.408.
Evans LT, Lollis SS, Ball PA. Management of acute spinal cord injury in the neurocritical care unit. Neurosurg Clin N Am. 2013;24(3):339–47. https://doi.org/10.1016/j.nec.2013.02.007. Epub 2013 Apr 17.

27. What is the major risk of indwelling catheters for individuals in the intensive care unit following spinal cord injury?

    A. Increased risk of bladder dependency
    B. Decrease in therapy time due to presence of the catheter
    C. Increased risk of renal injury
    D. Increased risk for catheter associated urinary tract infection

Answer: D.

Indwelling catheters are associated with a higher risk of a catheter associated urinary tract infections than intermittent catheterization. Although removal of indwelling catheters is recommended, other factors including patient quality of life, upper extremity function, urine output, and family support need to be considered prior to removal.

Zermann D, Wunderlich H, Derry F, Schröder S, Schubert J. Audit of early bladder management complications after spinal cord injury in first-treating hospitals. Eur Urol. 2000;37(2):156–60. https://doi.org/10.1159/000020133.
Markandaya M, Stein DM, Menaker J. Acute treatment options for spinal cord injury. Curr Treat Options Neurol. 2012. https://doi.org/10.1007/s11940-011-0162-5. Epub ahead of print.

Cardiovascular Issues in Spinal Cord Injury

6

Chloe McCloskey, D. Frank Distel, and Benjamin A. Abramoff

Questions

1. All of the following are causes of disrupted cardiovascular control following spinal cord injury (SCI) EXCEPT:

   A. Generalized reduction in sympathetic activity
   B. Loss of supraspinal sympathetic control
   C. Peripheral alpha-adrenoreceptor hypo-responsiveness
   D. Morphologic changes in sympathetic neurons

   Answer: C.

   Following SCI, there has been found to be peripheral alpha-adrenoreceptor hyper-responsiveness, which may play a significant role in the development of autonomic dysreflexia. The remainder of the answer options are correct. There is a generalized reduction in sympathetic activity associated with low plasma adrenaline and noradrenaline levels, with this effect more pronounced in higher cervical lesions. There is also a loss of descending supraspinal excitatory and inhibitory control; the extent to which this disrupts sympathetic control is directly related to the level at which the injury occurred. Finally, there is evidence of morphologic changes in the sympathetic preganglionic neurons (SPN). Initially following injury there is atrophy of the SPN which is followed by axonal sprouting and new (often inappropriate) synaptic connections.

C. McCloskey · D. F. Distel · B. A. Abramoff (✉)
Department of Physical Medicine & Rehabilitation, University of Pennsylvania, Philadelphia, PA, USA
e-mail: Benjamin.abramoff@pennmedicine.upenn.edu

© The Author(s), under exclusive license to Springer Nature Switzerland AG 2022
B. A. Abramoff et al. (eds.), *The Essential Spinal Cord Injury Medicine Question Bank*, https://doi.org/10.1007/978-3-031-07796-8_6

Claydon VE, Steeves JD, Krassioukov A. Orthostatic hypotension following spinal cord injury: understanding clinical pathophysiology. Spinal Cord. 2006;44(6):341–51. https://doi.org/10.1038/sj.sc.3101855. Epub 2005 Nov 22.

2. Which of the following patients is most likely to experience orthostatic hypotension?

   A. A 44-year-old male with a non-traumatic T12 American Spinal Injury Association (ASIA) C SCI
   B. A 30-year-old female with a traumatic C7 ASIA A SCI
   C. A 87-year-old male with a traumatic L2 ASIA A SCI
   D. A 70-year-old female with a non-traumatic C7 ASIA C SCI

Answer: B.

Orthostatic hypotension is defined as a decrease in systolic blood pressure of 20 mmHg or more, or in diastolic blood pressure of 10 mmHg or more, upon the assumption of an upright posture from a supine position, regardless of whether symptoms occur. The level and severity of the spinal cord injury correlates to the likelihood of developing orthostatic hypotension. Spinal cord injury patients with tetraplegia and complete injuries have been noted to have larger falls in blood pressure than those with paraplegia. There is also increased risk of orthostatic hypotension in those that suffer a traumatic injury in comparison to those with nontraumatic injury. Lastly, there is little evidence that orthostatic hypotension occurs more in elderly patients with SCI.

Claydon VE, Steeves JD, Krassioukov A. Orthostatic hypotension following spinal cord injury: understanding clinical pathophysiology. Spinal Cord. 2006;44(6):341–51. https://doi.org/10.1038/sj.sc.3101855. Epub 2005 Nov 22.

3. A 57-year-old male with history of a C7 ASIA B SCI, congestive heart failure, diabetes mellitus type 2, and hyperlipidemia is experiencing light-headedness, nausea, and blurred vision while working on transfers with therapy. The patient's vitals include temperature of 98.6, heart rate of 105, blood pressure of 92/65, oxygen saturation of 98% during transfers compared to his baseline of temperature of 98.6, heart rate of 94, blood pressure of 118/85, and oxygen saturation of 98%. The patient's symptoms resolve with return to bed. Your first step in managing this patient is to:

   A. Discontinue the patient's furosemide
   B. Encourage the patient to eat a large meal each morning
   C. Recommend compression stockings & abdominal binder for the patient to use when he is out of bed
   D. Start the patient on an alpha-1 adrenoreceptor agonist

Answer: C.

This patient is suffering from orthostatic hypotension. The first step in managing this condition in SCI is to try non-pharmacologic measures. Compression stockings and abdominal binders restrict venous pooling (which is due to the loss of sympathetic innervation). Other non-pharmacologic measures include ensuring adequate fluid intake, avoiding large meals (which can lead to postprandial hypotension), sleeping in a semi-upright position (10–20° head-up) and avoiding heat stress. If these supportive measures are not effective, the next step would be to hold the patient's diuretic if safe from a cardiac perspective. If these measures continued to be ineffective, further pharmacologic management may be needed, including possibly volume expansion with fludrocortisone or increasing vascular tone with the alpha-1 adrenoreceptor agonist midodrine.

Phillips AA, Krassioukov AV. Contemporary cardiovascular concerns after spinal cord injury: mechanisms, maladaptations, and management. J Neurotrauma. 2015;32(24):1927–42. https://doi.org/10.1089/neu.2015.3903. Epub 2015 Sep 1.

Claydon VE, Steeves JD, Krassioukov A. Orthostatic hypotension following spinal cord injury: understanding clinical pathophysiology. Spinal Cord. 2006;44(6):341–51. https://doi.org/10.1038/sj.sc.3101855. Epub 2005 Nov 22.

4. A patient with a C5 ASIA B traumatic spinal cord injury has had significant limitations in therapy and upright tolerance due to orthostatic hypotension despite numerous non-pharmacologic measures. You have initiated the patient on midodrine, with dose titrated up to 5 mg three times per day (TID) (6 AM, 2 PM, 10 PM) with significant improvement. The patient is now able to tolerate eating his meals upright in his wheelchair and transfer training. However, the patient's evening blood pressure prior to bed is noted to be 162/88. Your next step is to:

A. Stop the midodrine immediately and initiate the patient on fludrocortisone
B. Decrease the dose of midodrine to 2.5 mg TID
C. Adjust the timing of midodrine to 6 AM, 10 AM and 2 PM
D. Make no changes to medication and continue to monitor

Answer: C.

This patient has had excellent response to the initiation of midodrine to support his blood pressure, however he has now developed supine hypertension as a medication side-effect. Since the patient has had an excellent response to the therapy, the first step would be to adjust the time of the medication to avoid any dose within 4 h of bedtime. It can also be beneficial to have the patient sleep in a semi-upright position. Midodrine acts as an alpha-1 adrenoreceptor agonist with well-established evidence for treating neurogenic orthostatic hypotension. Midodrine is 93% absorbed following oral administration with bio-availability not effected by food. It is typically initiated at a dose of 2.5–5 mg at breakfast and lunch with rapid titration to a maximum daily dose of 30 mg.

Sabharwal S. Cardiovascular dysfunction in spinal cord injury. In: Kirshblum S, Lin VS, editors. Spinal cord medicine: 3rd ed. New York City: Springer Publishing Company. 2019. pp. 63–76. https://doi.org/10.1891/9780826137753.0005

5. A patient with paraplegia follows up outpatient requesting recommendations on what exercise program they should enter to improve their cardiovascular health. Based on the US Department of Health and Human Services Physical Activity Guidelines, you advise them to initiate an exercise regimen of:

   A. 150–300 min a week of moderate-intensity aerobic exercise
   B. 150–300 min a week of high-intensity aerobic exercise
   C. 75–150 min a week of moderate-intensity aerobic exercise
   D. 75–150 min a week of high- intensity resistance exercise

   Answer: A.

   The United States Department of Health and Human Services Physical Activity Guidelines recommends that adults with disabilities should do at least 150–300 min a week of moderate-intensity aerobic exercise or 75–150 min of high-intensity aerobic exercise per week. They also advise muscle strengthening (resistance) exercise of moderate or greater intensity of all major muscle groups 2 or more days a week. Aerobic exercise in persons with SCI can be achieved by arm ergometry, bodyweight supported treadmill training and functional electrical stimulation.

US Department of Health and Human Services Physical Activity Guidelines for Americans. 2019. Available at: https://www.hhs.gov/fitness/be-active/physical-activity-guidelines-for-americans/index.html.
Warburton DE, Eng JJ, Krassioukov A, Sproule S; the SCIRE Research Team. Cardiovascular health and exercise rehabilitation in spinal cord injury. Top Spinal Cord Inj Rehabil. 2007;13(1):98–122. https://doi.org/10.1310/sci1301-98.

6. The most common precipitant for an episode of autonomic dysreflexia (AD) is:

   A. Rectal distention
   B. Bladder distention
   C. Pressure injury
   D. Musculoskeletal injury

   Answer: B.

   Bladder distension accounts for up to 85% of episodes of AD. This can be due to a blocked or kinked indwelling catheter or a delay in intermittent catheterization. For some patients, catheterization itself can trigger an episode of AD, as well as other GU procedures such as urodynamic studies, cystoscopy, percutaneous lithotripsy, or assisted ejaculation. The second most common precipitant are gastrointestinal issues such as fecal impaction, rectal distention, hemorrhoids, or anal fissures. Other precipitants include skin ulceration, fractures, heterotopic ossification or ingrown toenails.

Bycroft J, Shergill IS, Chung EA, Arya N, Shah PJ. Autonomic dysreflexia: a medical emergency. Postgrad Med J. 2005;81(954):232–5. https://doi.org/10.1136/pgmj.2004.024463.

7. Common symptoms of autonomic dysreflexia include all the following EXCEPT:

   A. Nausea
   B. Nasal congestion
   C. Flushing below the level of injury
   D. Sweating above the level of Injury

Answer: C.

It common to see flushing ABOVE the level of injury, rather than below in cases of AD. This is due to the predominant parasympathetic excitation above the level of injury and sympathetic excitation below the level of injury. Nasal congestion occurs secondary to vasodilation from parasympathetic excitation. Patients can additionally experience headache, hypertension, and bradycardia (although it is not uncommon to also see tachycardia). Untreated episodes can result in intracranial hemorrhage, retinal detachment, seizures and death.

Bycroft J, Shergill IS, Chung EA, Arya N, Shah PJ. Autonomic dysreflexia: a medical emergency. Postgrad Med J. 2005 ;81(954):232–5. https://doi.org/10.1136/pgmj.2004.024463.

8. You are taking care of a patient with baseline hypotension, who is also suffering from frequent episodes of autonomic dysreflexia (4–5 times per day) that have been resistant to nonpharmacologic management. Given these concerns, you decide to start the patient on a daily medication. Which of the following should you choose?

   A. Prazosin
   B. Nifedipine
   C. Captopril
   D. Nitroglycerine

Answer: A.

While all of these agents have pharmacologic roles in the management of AD, only prazosin (dosed 0.5–1 mg three times daily) has shown to be effective as a prophylactic medicine to prevent episodes of AD. In randomized controlled trials, prazosin did not excessively lower baseline blood pressure while reducing AD episodes. The other options are used for acute management of episodes of

AD and can significantly lower blood pressures, thus patients should be monitored very closely following their administration.

Krassioukov A, Warburton DE, Teasell R, Eng JJ; Spinal Cord Injury Rehabilitation Evidence Research Team. A systematic review of the management of autonomic dysreflexia after spinal cord injury. Arch Phys Med Rehabil. 2009;90(4):682–95. https://doi.org/10.1016/j.apmr.2008.10.017.

9. Following spinal cord injury, patients have a _____ resting stroke volume, and _____ cardiac output response to exercise.

   A. Reduced, normal
   B. Increased, normal
   C. Normal, attenuated
   D. Reduced, attenuated

Answer: D.

At all levels of injury, SCI patients demonstrate lower stroke volumes at rest and an attenuated response in cardiac output to exercise. This is true even of patients with level of injury below T6. Chronically, these changes may result in myocardial atrophy, although not universally.

Myers J, Lee M, Kiratli J. Cardiovascular disease in spinal cord injury: an overview of prevalence, risk, evaluation, and management. Am J Phys Med Rehabil. 2007;86(2):142–52. https://doi.org/10.1097/PHM.0b013e31802f0247.

10. According to the 2016 International Paralympic Committee guidelines, what criteria is used to remove a Paralympian from play due to concern of "boosting"?

    A. Systolic blood pressure (SBP) >160, with continued elevation of SBP >160 on re-check 10 min later
    B. SBP >140, with continued elevation of SBP >140 on re-check 10 min later
    C. An SBP 20 mmHg greater than athlete's baseline that persists on re-check 10 min later
    D. A single reading of SBP >160

Answer: A.

According to the 2016 IPC guidelines, a hazardous dysreflexic state is considered to be present when SBP is >160. An athlete with an SBP >160 mmHg is to be re-examined 10 min later. If the second examination remains with SBP >160, the person examining the athlete is to inform the technical delegate to withdraw the athlete from the event.

International Paralymic Committee Handbook. Chapter 4.2 Position Statement on Autonomic Dysreflexia and Boosting. 2016. Available at: https://www.paralympic.org/ipc-handbook

11. You are taking care of a patient who has been suffering from orthostatic hypotension. You recommend initiation of fludrocortisone. The patient asks what side effects to expect on the medication. You counsel them on all of the following common side effects except:

    A. Fluid retention
    B. Electrolyte abnormalities
    C. Headaches
    D. Palpitations

    Answer: D.

    Fludrocortisone is a mineralocorticoid with vasopressor activity resulting from sodium retention and by increasing sensitivity of arterioles to norepinephrine. Fludrocortisone is typically started at a dose of 0.1 mg daily, with titration over intervals of 1–2 weeks. Patients should be advised to expect 5–8 pounds of weight gain from fluid retention. Electrolyte abnormalities also occur, primarily hypokalemia and hypomagnesemia requiring supplementation. Headaches are also common particularly in younger patients. Palpitations are not a common side effect of fludrocortisone but can be a side effect of ephedrine which is also used for management of orthostatic hypotension.

    Sabharwal S. Cardiovascular Dysfunction in Spinal Cord Injury. In: Kirshblum S, Lin VS, editors. Spinal cord medicine. 3rd ed. New York City: Springer Publishing Company; 2019. pp. 63–76. https://doi.org/10.1891/9780826137753.0005

12. What is the most frequent cardiac dysrhythmia in the acute phase following spinal cord injury?

    A. Atrial fibrillation
    B. Sinus tachycardia
    C. Bradycardia
    D. Supraventricular tachycardia

    Answer: C.

    The risk of cardiac dysrhythmia is higher in the acute phase and diminishes with time from injury. In the first few weeks, this can be life-threatening and patients should be monitored closely due to risk of cardiac arrest. In both the acute and chronic phase, ventricular bradyarrhythmias remain the most frequent cardiac arrhythmia, although atrial fibrillation can occur in the setting of autonomic dysreflexia. The frequency of bradycardia peaks at day 4 following injury, and gradually decreases thereafter. These events can be further triggered by vagal endotracheal suctioning, laryngoscopy, or even bowel movements due to unopposed vagal response.

    Grigorean VT, Sandu AM, Popescu M, Iacobini MA, Stoian R, Neascu C, Strambu V, Popa F. Cardiac dysfunctions following spinal cord injury. J Med Life. 2009;2(2):133–45.

13. Following an episode of autonomic dysreflexia, how long is it recommended that the patient's symptoms and blood pressure continue to be monitored?

A. 30 min
B. 1 h
C. 2 h
D. 4 h

Answer: C.

According to expert opinion, patients should be monitored for recurrent symptoms for at least 2 h following an episode of AD. Patients should be advised to seek medical attention if the symptoms recur, and admission for close monitoring should be considered, particularly if the patient is pregnant or if the cause of the episode is unclear. It is advised that all episodes of AD be documented in the patient's medical record.

Consortium for Spinal Cord Medicine. Acute management of autonomic dysreflexia: individuals with spinal cord injury presenting to health-care facilities. J Spinal Cord Med. 2002;25(Suppl. 1):S67–88.

14. In children 6–12 years old, at what systolic blood pressure should you consider pharmacologic intervention in an episode of autonomic dysreflexia?

A. 110
B. 120
C. 130
D. 140

Answer: C.

According to expert opinion, at age 6–12 pharmacologic intervention should be considered at a systolic blood pressure above 130 mmHg. For under 5 years old, it should be considered for SBP > 120 mmHg and for adolescents it should be considered >140 mmHg. It is always optimal to have the patient's baseline blood pressure as a point of comparison, however these guidelines can be used if that information is unavailable. It is very important to ensure that you are using an appropriate size BP cuff when assessing for AD in a child, particularly because their ability to communicate symptoms accurately can be limited depending on their age.

Consortium for Spinal Cord Medicine. Acute management of autonomic dysreflexia: individuals with spinal cord injury presenting to health-care facilities. J Spinal Cord Med. 2002;25(Suppl. 1):S67–88.

15. For pregnant patients with SCIs, what is recommended to prevent episodes of autonomic dysreflexia during labor?

    A. Vaginal delivery with epidural anesthesia
    B. Cesarean section under general anesthesia
    C. Vaginal delivery without anesthesia
    D. Vaginal delivery with intravenous analgesia

Answer: A.

Although studies are limited, epidural or spinal anesthesia is the recommended prevention of episodes of AD during labor for either vaginal or Cesarean delivery. Although some patients, depending on their level of injury, may not experience labor pains, they continue to be at risk for development of AD. AD or increased spasticity can sometimes be a prominent sign that a patient is in labor. It is essential that the patient has adequate analgesia through epidural or spinal anesthetic to prevent serious complications from uncontrolled hypertension in the setting of AD.

Krassioukov A, Warburton DE, Teasell R, Eng JJ; Spinal Cord Injury Rehabilitation Evidence Research Team. A systematic review of the management of autonomic dysreflexia after spinal cord injury. Arch Phys Med Rehabil. 2009;90(4):682–95. https://doi.org/10.1016/j.apmr.2008.10.017.

16. Initiation of anti-hypertensive medications should be considered in most individuals with SCI and no other past medical history who have consistent blood pressure readings above what threshold?

    A. 130/80 mmHg
    B. 140/90 mmHg
    C. 160/80 mmHg
    D. 160/100 mmHg

Answer B.

There is insufficient evidence that individuals with SCI should have a different threshold for treating hypertension than the general population. Current guidelines by most organizations recommend the initiation of pharmacologic agents when blood pressure is consistently above 140/90 in individuals with no other significant past medical history. Making the diagnosis of hypertension in individuals with SCI can be challenging as blood pressure can be highly variable as a result of postural influences and autonomic dysfunction. Blood pressure should be checked at every routine visit and at least annually. Elevated blood pressure should be confirmed on a subsequent visit prior to diagnosing hypertension.

Nash MS, Groah SL, Gater DR Jr, Dyson-Hudson TA, Lieberman JA, Myers J, Sabharwal S, Taylor AJ; Consortium for Spinal Cord Medicine. Identification and management of cardio-metabolic risk after spinal cord injury: clinical practice guideline for health care providers. Top Spinal Cord Inj Rehabil. 2018;24(4):379–423. https://doi.org/10.1310/sci2404-379.

17. A patient with T4 AISA D SCI with a past medical history of diabetes mellitus should be initiated on anti-hypertensive medications when blood pressure readings are consistently above what threshold, despite lifestyle interventions?

    A. 120/80 mmHg
    B. 130/80 mmHg
    C. 140/90 mmHg
    D. 160/100 mmHg

Answer B.

There is insufficient evidence that individuals with SCI should have a different threshold for treating hypertension than the general population. The Joint National Commission guidelines recommend a goal blood pressure of less than 130/80 mmHg for individuals with chronic kidney disease or diabetes mellitus. Current guidelines by most organizations recommend the initiation of pharmacologic agents when blood pressure is consistently above 140/90 in individuals with no past medical history.

Armstrong C; Joint National Committee. JNC8 guidelines for the management of hypertension in adults. Am Fam Physician. 20141;90(7):503–4.
Nash MS, Groah SL, Gater DR Jr, Dyson-Hudson TA, Lieberman JA, Myers J, Sabharwal S, Taylor AJ; Consortium for Spinal Cord Medicine. Identification and management of cardiometabolic risk after spinal cord injury: clinical practice guideline for health care providers. Top Spinal Cord Inj Rehabil. 2018;24(4):379–423. https://doi.org/10.1310/sci2404-379.

18. Which of the following would NOT be recommend as first line pharmacologic intervention for treatment of hypertension in a 40-year-old male with history of a traumatic C5 ASIA D SCI and no other past medical history?

    A. Calcium channel blocker
    B. Beta blocker
    C. Thiazide diuretic
    D. Angiotensin-converting enzyme inhibitor

Answer B.

There is insufficient data investigating antihypertensive agents in the SCI population. Recommendations for blood pressure management are based on guidelines for the general population. First line agents include calcium channel blockers, angiotensin-converting enzyme inhibitors, angiotensin receptor blockers, and thiazide diuretics. Beta blockers are recommended as first line in individuals who have suffered a myocardial infarction but are not recommended as first line in this patient with no other significant past medical history. Individual factors must also be taken into account for each patient and the use of diuretics should be carefully considered in individuals with SCI who require intermittent bladder catheterization as these may change bladder volumes.

Nash MS, Groah SL, Gater DR Jr, Dyson-Hudson TA, Lieberman JA, Myers J, Sabharwal S, Taylor AJ; Consortium for Spinal Cord Medicine. Identification and management of cardiometabolic risk after spinal cord injury: clinical practice guideline for health care providers. Top Spinal Cord Inj Rehabil. 2018;24(4):379–423. https://doi.org/10.1310/sci2404-379.

19. How often should an adult with SCI and no other past medical history, who's initial post-injury lipid panel was normal, be screened for hyperlipidemia?

    A. Annually
    B. Every 6 months for the 1st year, and then if normal, annually
    C. Every 3 years
    D. Every 2 years

Answer C.

A patient with a normal post-injury lipid panel without other risk factors should be screened for hyperlipidemia every 3 years. If the patient has multiple risk factors for dyslipidemia, such as smoking, diabetes or obesity, a lipid panel should be checked annually. The decision to screen should always be based on clinical judgement.

Nash MS, Groah SL, Gater DR Jr, Dyson-Hudson TA, Lieberman JA, Myers J, Sabharwal S, Taylor AJ; Consortium for Spinal Cord Medicine. Identification and management of cardiometabolic risk after spinal cord injury: clinical practice guideline for health care providers. Top Spinal Cord Inj Rehabil. 2018;24(4):379–423. https://doi.org/10.1310/sci2404-379.

20. Clinicians should recommend their patients with SCI participate in at least how many minutes of physical exercise per week?

    A. 200 min
    B. 150 min
    C. 120 min
    D. 60 min

Answer B.

Individuals with SCI should participate in at least 150 min of physical exercise per week in order to lower their risk of cardiometabolic disease and improve their general fitness. Exercise should begin as soon as possible following injury. Exercise can be broken up into 30–60 min sessions, 3–5 days per week. Exercise can also occur in three 10-min sessions, 5 days per week, in those unable to tolerate longer exercise durations. Anything above this (A) would be beneficial, but 150 min is the recommended minimum.

Nash MS, Groah SL, Gater DR Jr, Dyson-Hudson TA, Lieberman JA, Myers J, Sabharwal S, Taylor AJ; Consortium for Spinal Cord Medicine. Identification and management of cardiometabolic risk after spinal cord injury: clinical practice guideline for health care providers. Top Spinal Cord Inj Rehabil. 2018;24(4):379–423. https://doi.org/10.1310/sci2404-379.

21. At what level (and above) is transmission of angina less likely to be perceived by a patient with a SCI?

    A. T5
    B. T6
    C. T7
    D. T8

Answer A.

Cardiac pain is transmitted in afferent sympathetic nerves through the first five thoracic segments. It is then carried through the spinal cord through the spino-thalamic tract, to the thalamus, and then to the cortex. Individuals with injuries to T5 and above may fail to perceive cardiac chest pain due to interruption of this pathway.

Malliani A, Lombardi F. Consideration of the fundamental mechanisms eliciting cardiac pain. Am Heart J. 1982;103(4 Pt 1):575–8. https://doi.org/10.1016/0002-8703(82)90352-0.
Malliani A, Lombardi F, Pagani M. Sensory innervation of the heart. Prog Brain Res. 1986;67:39–48. https://doi.org/10.1016/s0079-6123(08)62755-7.

22. Which anesthetic should be avoided for individuals with thoracolumbar SCI undergoing general anesthesia?

    A. Rocuronium
    B. Propofol
    C. Vecuronium
    D. Succinylcholine

Answer D.

Rapid development of hyperkalemia in succinylcholine induced cardiac arrest in individuals with thoracolumbar SCI has been described in the literature. The presumed mechanism is that a larger potassium efflux will occur following depolarization due to changes in acetylcholine and succinylcholine sensitivity following denervation. Specifically, following denervation there is spread of the acetylcholine and succinylcholine sensitive area of the myoneural junction to a larger area of the muscle membrane, upregulation of acetylcholine receptors with spread of these receptors throughout the muscle membrane, and expression of acetylcholine receptor isomers. Patients with a thoracolumbar injury should receive alternatives to succinylcholine when undergoing anesthesia for surgical procedures.

Brooke MM, Donovon WH, Stolov WC. Paraplegia: succinylcholine-induced hyperkalemia and cardiac arrest. Arch Phys Med Rehabil. 1978;59(7):306–9.
Martyn JA, Richtsfeld M. Succinylcholine-induced hyperkalemia in acquired pathologic states: etiologic factors and molecular mechanisms. Anesthesiology. 2006;104(1):158–69. https://doi.org/10.1097/00000542-200601000-00022.

23. A 24-year-old male with a traumatic T4 ASIA B SCI presents to your clinic seeking advice regarding sexual function. He reports that he has been having trouble achieving an erection and is requesting a prescription for sildenafil. Which of the following comorbidities must this patient be screened for prior to prescribing this medication due to concerns related to polypharmacy?

A. Heterotopic ossification
B. Autonomic dysreflexia
C. Urinary retention
D. Osteoporosis

Answer B.

Concomitant use of topical or intravenous nitrates with a phosphodiesterase-5 inhibitor, such as sildenafil, can cause severe hypotension which could result in death. The two agents should not be prescribed together because of this serious interaction. Topical nitrates are often prescribed for individuals who suffer from autonomic dysreflexia. Individuals with injury at or above T6 are predisposed to autonomic dysreflexia and thus, should be screened for AD prior to prescribing a phosphodiesterase-5 inhibitor. Patients should be counseled about the serious risk of using these agents together. The other choices are not contraindications to the use of sildenafil.

Sabharwal S. Cardiovascular Dysfunction in Spinal Cord Injury. In: Kirshblum S, Lin VS, editors. Spinal cord medicine. 3rd ed. New York City: Springer Publishing Company; 2019. pp. 63–76. https://doi.org/10.1891/9780826137753.0005.

24. Which of the following diagnostic components of cardiometabolic disease has not been validated in the SCI population?

    A. Elevated blood pressure ≥ 130/80 mmHg
    B. Fasting glucose ≥ 100 mg/dL
    C. Waist circumference greater than 40" in men and 35" in women
    D. Reduced high-density lipoprotein (HDL)

Answer C.

All of the above are components of establishing the diagnosis of cardiometabolic disease. However, waist circumference has not been validated in the SCI population. It is instead recommended to use a BMI ≥ 22 kg/m² or >22% body fat when using 3 or 4 compartment modeling to assess body composition.

Nash MS, Groah SL, Gater DR Jr, Dyson-Hudson TA, Lieberman JA, Myers J, Sabharwal S, Taylor AJ; Consortium for Spinal Cord Medicine. Identification and management of cardiometabolic risk after spinal cord injury: clinical practice guideline for health care providers. Top Spinal Cord Inj Rehabil. 2018;24(4):379–423. https://doi.org/10.1310/sci2404-379.
Grundy SM, Brewer HB Jr, Cleeman JI, Smith SC Jr, Lenfant C; National Heart, Lung, and Blood Institute; American Heart Association. Definition of metabolic syndrome: report of the National Heart, Lung, and Blood Institute/American Heart Association conference on scientific issues related to definition. Arterioscler Thromb Vasc Biol. 2004;24(2):e13–8. https://doi.org/10.1161/01.ATV.0000111245.75752.C6.

25. Which of the following statements regarding nutritional counseling in patients with SCI is FALSE?

    A. Patients should undergo a caloric assessment using indirect calorimetry to estimate energy expenditure and establish caloric goals
    B. The Mediterranean or Dietary Approach to Stop Hypertension (DASH) diets should be adopted by individuals with SCI and cardiometabolic risk factors
    C. Saturated fats should be limited to 5–6% of total caloric intake
    D. Daily sodium intake should be limited to <3000 mg for individuals with hypertension

Answer D.

The daily sodium intake in individuals with SCI and hypertension should be ≤ 2400 mg. The other answer options are accurate recommendations.

Nash MS, Groah SL, Gater DR Jr, Dyson-Hudson TA, Lieberman JA, Myers J, Sabharwal S, Taylor AJ; Consortium for Spinal Cord Medicine. Identification and management of cardiometabolic risk after spinal cord injury: clinical practice guideline for health care providers. Top Spinal Cord Inj Rehabil. 2018;24(4):379–423. https://doi.org/10.1310/sci2404-379.

26. An 80-year-old woman presents to your rehabilitation unit after sustaining a C7 ASIA B Spinal Cord Injury along with bilateral femur fractures. Which of the following is the preferred venous thromboembolism (VTE) prophylaxis?

A. Heparin 5000 units subcutaneous TID for 6 weeks
B. Enoxaparin 40 mg daily for 6 weeks
C. Rivaroxaban 10 mg daily for 12 weeks
D. Enoxaparin 20 mg daily for 12 weeks

Answer: C.

According to PVA guidelines, anticoagulation in patients at increased risk for VTE following SCI should be continued for at least 8 weeks. Longer duration of thromboprophylaxis may be appropriate for individuals with increased risk factors for VTE. Risk factors in this patient include the bilateral femoral fractures and older age. Other risk factors include motor complete injuries, previous VTE and coexisting cancer. Preferred anticoagulants include LMWH, DOAC, oral vitamin K antagonists.

Prevention of Venous Thromboembolism in Individuals with Spinal Cord Injury: Clinical Practice Guidelines for Health Care Providers, 3rd ed.: Consortium for spinal cord medicine. Top Spinal Cord Inj Rehabil. 2016;22(3):209–40. https://doi.org/10.1310/sci2203-209.

27. What is the sensitivity/specificity of the following tests in screening for deep vein thromboses (DVT):

A. Duplex Ultrasound: Good/Good D-Dimer: Good/Poor
B. Duplex Ultrasound: Good/Good D-Dimer: Poor/Poor
C. Duplex Ultrasound: Poor/Good D-Dimer: Good/Poor
D. Duplex Ultrasound: Good/Good D-Dimer: Poor/Poor"

Answer: A.

Duplex ultrasound has good sensitivity (94.2% for proximal DVTs) and specificity (94%). D-Dimer has good sensitivity (mid 90%s) but poor specificity (mid 40%s).

Goodacre S, Sampson F, Thomas S, van Beek E, Sutton A. Systematic review and meta-analysis of the diagnostic accuracy of ultrasonography for deep vein thrombosis. BMC Med Imaging. 2005;5:6. https://doi.org/10.1186/1471-2342-5-6.
Wells P, Anderson D. The diagnosis and treatment of venous thromboembolism. Hematology Am Soc Hematol Educ Program. 2013;2013:457–63. https://doi.org/10.1182/asheducation-2013.1.457.

28. After a patients sustains an acute spinal cord injury, which of the following would be your first choice to prevent venous thromboembolism once there is no evidence of active bleeding?

    A. Low molecular weight heparin
    B. Low dose unfractionated heparin
    C. Oral vitamin K antagonist
    D. Direct thrombin inhibitor

Answer: A.

According to PVA guidelines [level 1B recommendation], low molecular weight heparin (LMWH) should be initiated as soon as there is no evidence of active bleeding as LMWH has been shown to be superior to low dose unfractionated heparin in prevention of pulmonary embolism with a trend towards decreased DVT and no major differences in bleeding risk.

Prevention of Venous Thromboembolism in Individuals with Spinal Cord Injury: Clinical Practice Guidelines for Health Care Providers, 3rd ed.: Consortium for Spinal Cord Medicine. Top Spinal Cord Inj Rehabil. 2016;22(3):209–40. https://doi.org/10.1310/sci2203-209.

Paciaroni M, Ageno W, Agnelli G. Prevention of venous thromboembolism after acute spinal cord injury with low-dose heparin or low-molecular-weight heparin. Thromb Haemost. 2008;99(5):978–80. https://doi.org/10.1160/TH07-09-0540.

29. Which of the following increases the risk of VTE after SCI?

    A. Female gender
    B. Obesity
    C. Surgical intervention for spine stabilization
    D. Complete injury

Answer: D.

Factors which have been shown to increase the risk of VTE after SCI in many studies include tetraplegia, older age, complete injuries, delayed or absent thromboprophylaxis, thrombophilia, time from injury, and concomitant lower-extremity fractures. Other factors including gender, obesity, non-orthopedic injuries and surgical management have not consistently been shown to increase VTE risk after spinal cord injury.

Matsumoto S, Suda K, Iimoto S, Yasui K, Komatsu M, Ushiku C, Takahata M, Kobayashi Y, Tojo Y, Fujita K, Minami A. Prospective study of deep vein thrombosis in patients with spinal cord injury not receiving anticoagulant therapy. Spinal Cord. 2015;53(4):306–9. https://doi.org/10.1038/sc.2015.4. Epub 2015 Feb 3.

Prevention of Venous Thromboembolism in Individuals with Spinal Cord Injury: Clinical Practice Guidelines for Health Care Providers, 3rd ed.: Consortium for spinal cord medicine. Top Spinal Cord Inj Rehabil. 2016;22(3):209–40. https://doi.org/10.1310/sci2203-209.

30. Which of the following is true regarding children under the age of 13 with acute spinal cord injuries in regards to the prevention of venous thromboembolism?

    A. Children with acquired SCI should have an IVC filter placed
    B. Children should be started on mechanical prophylaxis if appropriate sizing is available
    C. Children should be started on chemoprophylaxis as soon as possible
    D. Children with acquired SCI are not at high risk venous thromboembolism and therefore no VTE prophylaxis should be used

Answer: B.

DVTs are uncommon in children with acquired spinal cord injuries when sustained under the age of 12. In one retrospective analysis of all patients with newly acquired spinal cord injury in California between 1991–2001 only 1.1% of patients aged 8–13 years old and 4.8% of those 14–19 years old were found to have DVTs. There are no widely publicized prospective studies looking at the use of mechanical or chemoprophylaxis for children with SCI. Mechanical prophylaxis should be used if the appropriate size is available.

Vogel L, Betz R, Mulcahey M. 2011. Pediatric spinal cord disorders. In: Kirshblum S, Campagnolo DI, editors. Spinal cord medicine. 2nd ed. Philadelphia: Lipincott Williams & Wilkins; 2011. pp. 533–64.
Schottler J, Vogel LC, Sturm P. Spinal cord injuries in young children: a review of children injured at 5 years of age and younger. Dev Med Child Neurol. 2012;54(12):1138–43. https://doi.org/10.1111/j.1469-8749.2012.04411.x. Epub 2012 Sep 23.

31. You are the director on an inpatient spinal cord injury unit. Which of the following measures should you undertake in order to prevent venous thromboembolism on your unit?

    A. Allow all of your spinal cord injury physicians who are fellowship trained to use the method of VTE prevention they used during their fellowship training.
    B. Educate all new hires to your SCI unit on the standard thromboembolism prophylaxis policy.
    C. Discuss with your pharmacist a standard thromboprophylaxis policy and have them remind all physicians of the policy after patients have been admitted.
    D. Create a written thromboprophylaxis policy and incorporate two additional implementation strategies including a standard admission documentation template and chemoprophylaxis order set.

Answer: D.

Publication of clinical practice guidelines alone has not been shown to significantly change clinical practice. Use of structured implementation practices after publication of guidelines, including measures such as standard templates and order sets as well as marketing and outreach, have been shown to increase rates of adherence in the clinical setting.

Burns SP, Nelson AL, Bosshart HT, Goetz LL, Harrow JJ, Gerhart KD, Bowers H, Krasnicka B, Guihan M. Implementation of clinical practice guidelines for prevention of thromboembolism in spinal cord injury. J Spinal Cord Med. 2005;28(1):33–42. https://doi.org/10.1080/10790268.2005.11753796. PMID: 15832902.

Pulmonary Changes After Spinal Cord Injury

7

Ellia Ciammaichella, Darby Cruz, and Christine Krull

Questions

1. People with cervical spinal cord injury are more at risk for sleep disorders than the general population due to all the following EXCEPT:

    A. Existence of neuromuscular respiratory weakness
    B. Disproportionate male representation
    C. Reduced nighttime circulation levels of melatonin
    D. Higher use of indwelling catheters

    Answer: D.

    Use of indwelling catheters would likely reduce nighttime awakenings if present due to less need to wake to catheterize. On the other hand, neuromuscular respiratory weakness, especially in the intercostal muscles, may be a cause of hypoventilation during sleep possibly due to the rib cage contribution to tidal volume during non-REM sleep relative to wakefulness. Male sex is a risk factor

E. Ciammaichella (✉)
Department of Physical Medicine and Rehabilitation, Renown Regional Medical Center, Reno, NV, USA
e-mail: el@ciammaichella.com

D. Cruz
Department of Respiratory Therapy, TIRR Memorial Hermann, Houston, TX, USA
e-mail: darby.cruz@memorialhermann.org

C. Krull
Spinal Cord Injury/Dysfunction Service, VA St. Louis Health Care System, St. Louis, MO, USA

Department of Physical Medicine and Rehabilitation, Baylor College of Medicine, TIRR Memorial Hermann, Houston, TX, USA
e-mail: Christine.krull@va.gov

© The Author(s), under exclusive license to Springer Nature Switzerland AG 2022
B. A. Abramoff et al. (eds.), *The Essential Spinal Cord Injury Medicine Question Bank*, https://doi.org/10.1007/978-3-031-07796-8_7

109

for sleep-disordered breathing and there is a disproportionate representation of male sex in spinal cord injury compared to the general population. In addition, because the sympathetic nerves below the level of injury are affected, the pathway between the suprachiasmatic nuclei to the superior cervical ganglion is interrupted, resulting in disruption of the circadian melatonin rhythmicity.

Bascom AT, Sankari A, Goshgarian HG, Badr MS. Sleep onset hypoventilation in chronic spinal cord injury. Physiol Rep. 2015;3(8):e12490.
Sankari A, Badr MS, Martin JL, Ayas NT, Berlowitz DJ. Impact of spinal cord injury on sleep: current perspectives. Nat Sci Sleep. 2019;11:219–29.

2. Which tracheostomy management strategy is accurate regarding the ability to talk and eat with a tracheostomy tube?

   A. Increasing the diameter of the tracheostomy tube may be helpful.
   B. Deflation of the cuff, or changing to a cuffless tracheostomy may be helpful.
   C. Stopping use of a one-way valves may be helpful.
   D. It is never safe to eat with a tracheostomy but speech may be possible with appropriate therapy.

Answer: B.

The following strategies may be employed to improve the ability to talk and/ or eat when a tracheostomy is present: downsizing of the tracheostomy tube; deflating the cuff (it is recommended to suction before deflating to prevent aspiration of pooled pharyngeal contents); changing to a cuffless tracheostomy; utilizing a one-way speaking valve (such as a Passy Muir speaking valve); occluding the tracheostomy with a finger when the cuff is deflated; and utilizing a fenestrated tracheostomy tube (although these tubes pose an increased risk of forming granulation tissue).

   These measures help the pharyngeal structures move more unencumbered and generate the appropriate pressure differentials for swallowing and speech movements. It is important to note that capping the tracheostomy, using a one speaking valve and finger occlusion should not be used in the setting of an inflated cuff.

Hess DR. Tracheostomy tubes and related appliances. Respiratory Care. 2005;50(4):497–510.
Hess DR, Altobelli NP. Tracheostomy tubes discussion. Respiratory Care. 2014;59(6):956–73.

3. Complications of sleep disordered breathing include all of the following EXCEPT:

   A. Sexual dysfunction
   B. Poor attention and information processing
   C. Daytime sleepiness
   D. Nocturnal hypertension

Answer: A.

Common complications of sleep-disordered breathing include poor attention and information processing, daytime sleepiness, and nocturnal hypertension.

Sankari A, Badr MS, Martin JL, Ayas NT, Berlowitz DJ. Impact of spinal cord injury on sleep: current perspectives. Nat Sci Sleep. 2019;11:219–29.
Sankari A, Vaughan S, Bascom A, Martin JL, Badr MS. Sleep-disordered breathing and spinal cord injury: a state-of-the-art review. Chest. 2019;155(2):438–45.

4. Compromise in which system is the most common cause of death after spinal cord injury in the United States?

   A. Cardiac
   B. Renal
   C. Gastrointestinal
   D. Respiratory

   Answer: D.

   According to the National Spinal Cord Injury Statistical Center, over the past 45 years, pneumonia and septicemia have had the greatest impact on reducing life expectancy in the SCI population. Prior to that, the renal and urinary system compromise were the primary causes of death in this population.

Frankel HL, Coll JR, Charlifue SW, Whiteneck GG, Gardner BP, Jamous MA, et al. Long-term survival in spinal cord injury: a fifty year investigation. Spinal Cord. 1998;36(4):266–74.
University of Alabama at Birmingham. National Spinal Cord Injury Statistical Center, Facts and Figures at a Glance [Internet]. 2020. Available from: https://www.nscisc.uab.edu/Public/Facts%20and%20Figures%202020.pdf
van den Berg MEL, Castellote JM, de Pedro-Cuesta J, Mahillo-Fernandez I. Survival after spinal cord injury: a systematic review. J Neurotrauma. 2010;27(8):1517–28.

5. Which of the following is true about access to high quality care for sleep-disordered breathing for individuals with spinal cord injury?

   A. Sleep-disordered breathing in the spinal cord injury (SCI) population is recognized early and often.
   B. Diagnostic services for sleep-disordered breathing is generally accessible for those with mobility impairment.
   C. Diagnostic criteria for sleep-disordered breathing is based on studies done with people with SCI.
   D. People with SCI often do not tolerate the standard treatment options offered for sleep-disordered breathing.

   Answer: D.

   Studies note that people with spinal cord injury have a higher rate of discontinuation of positive airway pressure (PAP) use compared to the general population. This is related to weakness of the upper limbs, mask claustrophobia, increased awakenings, nasal congestion, lack of education and inconvenience. Using a nasal interface and extensive education can alleviate some of these issues. Further studies of alternative treatments, as well as alternative modes of PAP, should be pursued. Despite a high prevalence, a diagnosis of sleep-disordered breathing in the SCI population is often missed or significantly delayed due to inaccessible diagnostic services and inadvertent missed symptoms. For this reason, the American Academy of Sleep Medicine recommends that clinicians carefully assess all people with SCI for sleep disordered breathing. Interestingly, the diagnostic criteria for sleep-disordered breathing is not based on studies that included people with SCI so the diagnostic criteria may not accurately reflect the needs of the SCI population.

Patients with spinal cord injuries should be assessed for sleep apnea [Internet]. Aasm.org. 2014 [cited 2021 Apr 26]. Available from: https://aasm.org/patients-with-spinal-cord-injuries-should-be-assessed-for-sleep-apnea
Sankari A, Martin JL, Safwan Badr M. Sleep-disordered breathing and spinal cord injury: Challenges and opportunities. Curr Sleep Med Rep. 2017;3(4):272–8.

6. Which of the following is NOT a sign of readiness for decannulation of a tracheostomy tube?

   A. Peak cough flow >160 mL/min
   B. Successful capping trials for at least 24 h with no stridor
   C. No sign of respiratory compromise with a size 8 tracheostomy in place and 5 L of oxygen via trach collar
   D. Endoscopic/fiberoptic evaluation with no signs of tracheal stenosis or other abnormalities in the upper airway

   Answer: C.

   When evaluating a patient for decannulation, there are several considerations to determine if a patient is ready. Ultimately, the patient needs to have a good prognosis for not needing to go back on respiratory support. Before decannulation, a patient needs to demonstrate an ability to keep respiratory secretions under control without tracheal suctioning and be able to cough effectively to remove secretions/mucus. A peak cough flow of >160 mL/min has been found to be a good predictor of success with decannulation. Success with capping trials with no stridor and ability to cough up secretions are favorable signs as well. Decannulation should not be pursued in the presence of an upper airway obstruction such as significant tracheal stenosis. A tracheostomy tube should be downsized before removal, as higher sizes (such as size 8 mm) may have an increased chance of a large soft tissue defect with prolonged healing/closure of the stoma, which would be accompanied by a prolonged air leak. Before decannulation it is preferred to downsize at least to a size 6mm tube, or potentially further to a 4mm tube. Level of consciousness is another consideration in decannulation readiness. If a patient has upcoming plans for surgery, it may be worth waiting until after the procedure is done to pursue decannulation so any respiratory needs in the operating room or in the postoperative period may be met effectively without risk of repeat intubation or tracheostomy.

Bach JR, Saporito LR. Criteria for extubation and tracheostomy tube removal for patients with ventilatory failure: a different approach to weaning. Chest. 1996;110(6):1566–71.
Hess DR, Altobelli NP. Tracheostomy tubes discussion. Respiratory Care. 2014;59(6):956–73.

7. A 35-year-old woman is admitted to acute inpatient rehabilitation after polytrauma and a complicated hospital course including tracheostomy. She was noted to have undergone decannulation recently. However, she is observed to have an odd high-pitched musical sound when she breathes. She also feels short of breath on exertion. Her oxygen saturations at rest are 94–97% on room air, and she appears to be breathing comfortably at rest. What is the next best step?

A. Bedside replacement of a tracheostomy tube should be attempted immediately.
B. Otolaryngology should be consulted.
C. She should be sent emergently to a higher level of care (i.e. emergency department).
D. A chest tube should be inserted emergently.

Answer: B.

After tracheostomy procedures, early complications may include obstruction (such as by the posterior membranous trachea), subcutaneous emphysema, and pneumothorax. Other potential complications after tracheostomy include infection of the stoma, tracheitis, tracheal stenosis, tracheomalacia, tracheoesophageal fistula, tracheo-arterial fistula, hemorrhage, aspiration, swallowing dysfunction, and reduced phonation.

The presented case describes the sound of stridor, which is often caused by tracheal stenosis. Other clinical manifestations of tracheal stenosis include inability to tolerate a one-way speaking valve or capping, dysphonia, exertional dyspnea which may progress to dyspnea at rest, increased cough, difficulty clearing secretions, and high peak airway pressures. Tracheal stenosis can make both vent weaning and decannulation more difficult. Significant stenosis is estimated to occur in 8% of patients following tracheostomy. The risk is higher in those with an overly large tracheal stoma, oversized cannula, overdistention of the cuff, excessive tube motion causing mechanical irritation, and fenestrated tracheostomy tubes. Definitive diagnosis can be made by bronchoscopy or laryngotracheoscopy. Patients with tracheal stenosis should not be decannulated without otolaryngology evaluation, as surgical strategies are often necessary.

In the case presented, the patient is not showing immediate signs of decompensation although she is at high risk of decompensating if the tracheal stenosis is not addressed. It is appropriate to proceed with a timely otolaryngology consultation and close monitoring of her respiratory status, with a low threshold to transfer her promptly to a higher level of care should any signs of decompensation occur. A bedside attempt to replace the tracheostomy tube is not indicated and would likely be unsuccessful depending how long ago the tube was removed, as the stoma tends to close quickly. Such an attempt may also risk introducing a false passage.

Epstein SK. Late complications of tracheostomy. Respiratory Care. 2005;50(4):542–9.
Wood DE, Mathisen DJ. Late complications of tracheostomy. Clin Chest Med. 1991;12(3):597–609.

8. A 21-year-old male suffered a C5 American Spinal Injury Association Impairment Scale (AIS) A spinal cord injury after a high-speed motor vehicle collision about 6 months ago. While in acute inpatient rehabilitation, he had significant difficulty with worsening orthostatic hypotension. He also had asymptomatic spikes in blood pressure at night. He was evaluated for autonomic dysreflexia but no inciting noxious stimuli was discovered. Nursing noted some apneic-like events at night. He underwent a sleep study and was found to have an apnea-hypopnea index (AHI) of 6 per hour. Which of the following is true?

A. He does not have sleep-disordered breathing.
B. He has mild sleep-disordered breathing.
C. He has moderate sleep-disordered breathing.
D. He has severe sleep-disordered breathing.

Answer: B.

Based on studies on able bodied persons, he has mild sleep apnea as defined by an AHI between 5–14 per hour. (Moderate sleep apnea: 15–29; severe sleep apnea >29.) Some studies have shown a correlation between sleep-disordered breathing and nocturnal hypertension resulting in nighttime diuresis and daytime orthostatic hypotension with improvement of all three conditions with the use of positive air pressure.

Berry RB, Brooks R, Gamaldo CE, Harding SM, Lloyd RM, Cl M, et al. The AASM manual for the scoring of sleep and associated events: rules, terminology and technical specifications, Version 2.6. www.aasmnet.org. Darien, IL: American Academy of Sleep Medicine; 2020.
Brown JP, Bauman KA, Kurili A, Rodriguez GM, Chiodo AE, Sitrin RG, et al. Positive airway pressure therapy for sleep-disordered breathing confers short-term benefits to patients with spinal cord injury despite widely ranging patterns of use. Spinal Cord. 2018;56(8):777–89.

9. Paradoxical breathing is seen on physical examination when:

   A. On inhalation, chest wall rises and diaphragm descends
   B. On inhalation, chest wall depresses and diaphragm descends
   C. On inhalation, chest wall rises and diaphragm ascends
   D. On inhalation, chest wall depresses and diaphragm ascends

Answer: B.

In the able-bodied population, when breathing is initiated, the diaphragm descends and the chest wall rises to provide negative pressure for inhalation. However, when the accessory muscles of respiration are weak and flaccid as in spinal shock, paradoxical breathing may be seen. During paradoxical breathing, the diaphragm is activated which creates negative pressure in the lungs to suck air into the lungs. Because of chest wall weakness and flaccidity, the negative pressure causes the chest wall to depress. Sometimes, a rise in the abdomen will be seen.

Berlly M, Shem K. Respiratory management during the first five days after spinal cord injury. J Spinal Cord Med. 2007;30(4):309–18.

10. Which of the following is NOT a contraindication to manual assisted cough:

   A. Unstable spine
   B. Recently placed vena cava filter
   C. Pneumonia
   D. Pregnancy

Answer: C.

A manual assisted cough, colloquially called a "quad cough," is a maneuver that can be performed by the patient or a caretaker to assist with expectoration. In the seated position, patients can splint the abdomen below the xiphoid with the use of their hands or by flexing forward and grabbing their legs, using the pressure of their knees in their abdomen. Similarly, a caretaker can provide a gentle abdominal thrust that is coordinated with the patient's breath. Pneumonia is not a contraindication to a manual assisted cough. Contraindications of a quad cough include: an unstable spine, a recently placed vena cava filter, chest trauma, abdominal complications, and pregnancy.

Berlly M, Shem K. Respiratory management during the first five days after spinal cord injury. J Spinal Cord Med. 2007;30(4):309–18.

11. Which of the following is unlikely related to the development of acute respiratory distress syndrome (ARDS) in a patient with spinal cord injury?

    A. Sepsis
    B. Dysphagia
    C. Pancreatitis
    D. Pulmonary embolism

Answer: D.

Although the SCI population is predisposed to developing a pulmonary embolism, it is rarely related to ARDS. On the other hand, studies have shown a relationship between ARDS and lung injuries such as aspiration pneumonia as well as sepsis and pancreatitis. Furthermore, studies have shown that respiratory complications are not only more prevalent in the SCI population but are more severe. Because of this, a high index of suspicion should be maintained for dysphagia and pneumonia.

Veeravagu A, Jiang B, Rincon F, Maltenfort M, Jallo J, Ratliff JK. Acute respiratory distress syndrome and acute lung injury in patients with vertebral column fracture(s) and spinal cord injury: a nationwide inpatient sample study. Spinal Cord. 2013;51(6):461–5.

12. Secondary respiratory muscles are innervated by the following levels:

    A. C1–C4
    B. C2–T12
    C. T2–T12
    D. L1–S5

Answer: B.

The primary muscle of respiration is the diaphragm which is innervated by C3, C4, and C5 via the phrenic nerve. The secondary respiratory muscles include: sternocleidomastoid (spinal accessory nerve and C2/C3), scalenes (C3–C8), upper trapezius (spinal accessory nerve and C3/C4), external intercostals (T1–T11), internal intercostals (T1–T11), and abdominal muscles (T6–T12).

Terson de Paleville DG, McKay WB, Folz RJ, Ovechkin AV. Respiratory motor control disrupted by spinal cord injury: mechanisms, evaluation, and restoration. Transl Stroke Res. 2011;2(4):463–73. https://doi.org/10.1007/s12975-011-0114-0.

13. Which of the following strategies is employed to prevent pneumonia in individuals with subacute spinal cord injury?

A. Minimize tidal volume to very low levels
B. Use of a mechanical insufflator-exsufflator
C. Avoiding noninvasive ventilation
D. Encourage patient to minimize activity

Answer: B.

Aggressive secretion management is key to pneumonia prevention. One key method is the use of a mechanical insufflator-exsufflator (also known as a coughalator or cough assist). For a ventilated patient in the subacute period, increasing tidal volume to a minimum of 10 cc per kg of ideal body weight (while maintaining plateau pressure below 30 cm H_2O) may reduce the instances of atelectasis and encourage surfactant production. Invasive or noninvasive ventilation may be necessary, particularly when patients are fatiguing. Finally, good pulmonary toilet and maximizing (not minimizing) the patient's activity are essential.

Consortium for Spinal Cord Medicine. Respiratory management following spinal cord injury: a clinical practice guideline for health-care professionals. J Spinal Cord Med. 2005;28(3):259–93.

14. Increased secretion production after cervical spinal cord injury is due to:

A. Unopposed parasympathetic activity
B. Unopposed sympathetic activity
C. Hyperactive parasympathetic activity
D. Hyperactive sympathetic activity

Answer: A.

After a cervical spinal cord injury, the cranial parasympathetic connections are generally unaffected (through the Vagus nerve). However, the sympathetic neurons originate in the intermediolateral nuclei from spinal cord segments of T1 through L2, which are impaired in a cervical spinal cord injury. For this reason, there is unopposed parasympathetic activity or vagal tone. This causes increased secretions and changes in secretion consistency. Impaired clearance of secretions is also a likely contributor but this is affected by the somatic system.

Berlowitz DJ, Wadsworth B, Ross J. Respiratory problems and management in people with spinal cord injury. Breathe (Sheff). 2016;12(4):328–40.

15. Which of the following scenarios would best be treated with the initiation of noninvasive ventilation?

    A. Patient with a new (s/p 5 days) C3 SCI with bibasilar atelectasis on chest radiograph, ABG results of pH 7.25, pCO_2 58 mmHg, PO_2 77 mmHg on 40% oxygen via venturi-mask
    B. Patient with C7 SCI with shortness of breath, respiratory rate 34 per minute, mild intercostal retractions, ABG results pH 7.49, pCO_2 31 mmHg, PO_2 65 mmHg on 45% oxygen mask
    C. Patient with C6 SCI who has been requiring nasotracheal suctioning Q2hrs for excessive secretions
    D. Patient with an acute T2 SCI unresponsive to sternal rub

Answer: B.

The ABG results and the clinical presentation of this patient suggest impending respiratory failure with tachypnea and respiratory alkalosis with decreased oxygenation on supplemental O_2. Since the SCI level is at C7, the functioning of the diaphragm is likely intact.

    Patients with excessive secretions are not candidates for noninvasive ventilation as maintenance of the airway may be compromised (Answer C). Interventions would include aggressive pulmonary toilet and eventual intubation if respiratory compromise ensued.

    Patients with severely decreased levels of consciousness are not candidates for noninvasive ventilation (Answer D). Patients with high level spinal cord injuries (C1–C4) in the acute period are generally not candidates for noninvasive ventilation due to the high risk of failure with non-invasive ventilation and likely need for intubation. This is particularly true in cases of impending respiratory failure. (Answer A).

Rabinstein AA. Noninvasive ventilation for neuromuscular respiratory failure. Curr Opin Crit Care. 2016; 1.

16. All of the following should be considered when deciding to place patients with chronic high level SCI on noninvasive ventilation (NIV) EXCEPT:

    A. Cognition
    B. Swallowing status
    C. Urine output
    D. Ability to cough

Answer: C.

The indications for NIV are the absence of swallowing disorders, good comprehension and cooperation, ability to cough and ability to ventilate. While urine output may play a role in conditions like congestive heart failure, it does not factor in to determining whether a SCI patient is a candidate for NIV.

Toki A, Nakamura T, Nishimura Y, Sumida M, Tajima F. Clinical introduction and benefits of non-invasive ventilation for above C3 cervical spinal cord injury. J Spinal Cord Med. 2019;44(1):70–6.

17. The following methods can be used to improve secretion management EXCEPT:

    A. Mucolytics
    B. Mechanical insufflation and exsufflation
    C. Bed rest to reserve energy
    D. Bronchoscopy

Answer: C.

Aggressive secretion management can include the use of: mucolytics and expectorants, suctioning, muscarinic antagonist, hydration, chest physiotherapy and postural drainage, mechanical insufflation and exsufflation, manual assisted cough, intrapulmonary percussive ventilation, and bronchoscopy. On the other hand, relative rest or bed rest will limit aggressive pulmonary hygiene and is not a treatment for improving secretion management.

Berlly M, Shem K. Respiratory management during the first five days after spinal cord injury. J Spinal Cord Med. 2007;30(4):309–18.

18. The theory behind the neurogenic restrictive lung includes all of the following EXCEPT:

    A. Weak inspiratory muscles resulting in hypoventilation
    B. Lack of stretch of the alveoli resulting in reduced surfactant production
    C. Reduced surfactant availability causing alveolar collapse
    D. Collapsed alveoli leading neighboring alveoli to absorb more oxygen

Answer: D.

Collapsed alveoli do not recruit neighboring alveoli to absorb more oxygen. Rather, collapsed alveoli will create a negative pressure differential on the inter-alveolar septum, making the neighboring alveoli more susceptible to collapse as well.

The following cascade of events is thought to occur. First, weak inspiratory muscles result in hypoventilation of the alveoli. This results in less mechanical stretching of the Type II alveolar epithelial cells, also called pneumocytes. Mechanical stretch plays an important role to stimulate the production of surfactant, which reduces the surface tension and stabilizes the phospholipid molecules in the alveoli to prevent the collapse of the alveoli. On the other hand, with less surfactant, the alveoli tend to collapse, making the neighboring alveoli prone to collapsing as well. These changes result in a cascade of restrictive lung disease. Thus, care should be taken to avoid hypoventilation.

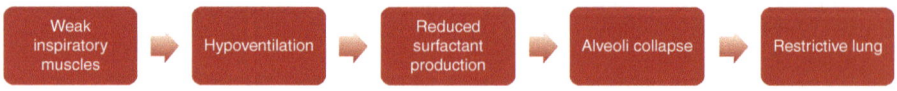

Consortium for Spinal Cord Medicine. Respiratory management following spinal cord injury: a clinical practice guideline for health-care professionals. J Spinal Cord Med. 2005;28(3):259–93.

Ihalainen T, Rinta-Kiikka I, Luoto TM, Helminen M, Thesleff T, Korpijaakko-Huuhka A-M, et al. Reply to Saeid Safiri's Letter to the Editor: Risk factors for laryngeal penetration-aspiration in patients with acute traumatic cervical spinal cord injury. Spine J 2017;17(12):1956–7.

19. Which of the following modalities is described as applying positive airway pressure to obtain a large volume of air within the lungs and then quickly reversing the air flow by shifting to negative air pressure, resulting in high expiratory flow that helps mobilize secretions out of the airway?

    A. Incentive spirometry
    B. Chest percussion and drainage
    C. Intrapulmonary percussive ventilation
    D. Mechanical insufflation-exsufflation

    Answer: D.

    Mechanical insufflation-exsufflation (MIE), also known as cough assist or Coughalator, is designed to noninvasively clear secretions from the lungs by simulating a natural cough for those persons who have a weak or ineffective cough. It is the rapid shift in the pressure that allows for the glottis to close and move secretions up and out of the airway. It is also used to improve recruitment of the lungs for patients with neurogenic restrictive respiratory disease to prevent atelectasis and pneumonia.

    Philips. CoughAssist T70 Airway clearance device: Philips Healthcare [Internet]. CoughAssist T70 Mechanical Insufflator-Exsufflator. [cited 2021Apr14]. Available from: https://www.usa.philips.com/healthcare/product/HC0066000/coughassist-t70-airway-clearance-device

20. Which of the following patients would be the most appropriate candidate for implantation of a diaphragmatic pacer to assist with ventilator weaning?

    A. History of C4 AIS A SCI, 14 months post injury, ventilator dependent with avulsed phrenic nerve
    B. History of C2 AIS A SCI, 12 weeks post injury, ventilator dependent, with intact phrenic nerve on nerve conduction testing

C. History of C7 AIS A SCI, 3 weeks post injury, ventilator dependent, with intact phrenic nerve on nerve conduction testing and recurrent respiratory infections and acute respiratory distress syndrome (ARDS)
D. History of T2 AIS A SCI, 12 weeks post injury, ventilator dependent, with intact phrenic nerve on nerve conduction testing

Answer: B.

Implantation of a diaphragm pacer requires an intact phrenic nerve. The phrenic nerve is initially tested by cutaneous electromyography (EMG) but EMG often results in a false negative. For this reason, even if the phrenic nerve testing by EMG is negative, patients often undergo intraoperative EMG testing.

Patients generally also have a high cervical spinal cord injury level. Lower spinal cord injuries like those at the thoracic level do not have loss of innervation to their diaphragm as the diaphragm is innervated at the cervical levels of C3–C5.

Posluszny JA, Onders R, Kerwin AJ, Weinstein MS, Stein DM, Knight J, et al. Multi-center review of diaphragm pacing in spinal cord injury. J Trauma Acute Care Surg. 2014;76(2):303–10.

21. The following factors may indicate spinal cord injury-related pharyngeal dysfunction EXCEPT for:

A. Coughing and throat clearing
B. Status post anterior cervical discectomy and fusion
C. Stomach pain
D. Watery eyes during or following meals

Answer: C.

Penetration aspiration is common among patients with acute cervical SCI. Signs of laryngeal penetration and aspiration include: wet vocal quality, coughing/choking, watery eyes or runny nose during or following meals, decreased excursion of the larynx, uncoordinated laryngeal movement, audible swallowing sounds, clearing of the throat after swallowing, drooling, weight loss (due to fear of eating), or recurrent respiratory infections. Stomach pain is not a direct symptom of aspiration.

Chaw E, Shem K, Castillo K, Wong SL, Chang J. Dysphagia and associated respiratory considerations in cervical spinal cord injury. Top Spinal Cord Inj Rehabil. 2012;18(4):291–9. https://doi.org/10.1310/sci1804-291.

22. Cervical spinal cord injuries are sometimes irreversible and many patients cannot sustain their own effective ventilation. Options like diaphragmatic and phrenic nerve pacing exist that can facilitate long term ventilation in these patients. In what way does pacing diminish the incidence of respiratory infections and atelectasis versus traditional mechanical ventilation?

A. Pacing improves swallowing.
B. Pacing provides intrathoracic pressures similar to physiologic processes in non-spinal cord injured individuals.
C. Pacing facilitates verbal communication.
D. Pacing provides larger volumes to the lungs.

Answer: B.

Since pacing works by stimulating the phrenic nerve to contract the diaphragm, there are no "positive pressure" breaths applied to the airway and lungs therefore providing a more physiologic breath for the patient. This allows the diaphragm to descend and creates a negative pressure by which to draw air into the lungs.

Romero FJ, Gambarrutta C, Garcia-Forcada A, Marín MA, Diaz de la Lastra E, Paz F, et al. Long-term evaluation of phrenic nerve pacing for respiratory failure due to high cervical spinal cord injury. Spinal Cord. 2012;50(12):895–8.

23. First-line treatment for sleep-related hypoventilation in individuals with spinal cord injuries is:

A. Supplemental oxygen
B. Continuous positive airway pressure
C. Bi-level positive airway pressure
D. D. Tracheostomy

Answer: C.

Bi-level positive airway pressure is the first line treatment for sleep-related hypoventilation (and possibly a back-up rate as well). On the other hand, obstructive sleep apnea is often treated with continuous positive airway pressure. Central sleep apnea also requires a back-up rate.

The American Academy of Sleep Medicine (AASM) defines sleep-related hypoventilation as elevated $PaCO_2$ levels by either an increase in CO_2 levels ($ETCO_2$ or $TCCO_2$) to > 55 mmHg for greater than or equal to 10 min or increase in CO_2 levels ($ETCO_2$ or $TCCO_2$) by at least 10 mmHg (from awake supine value) to >50 mmHg for greater than or equal to 10 min.

Sleep-related hypoventilation is more common in cervical SCI compared to lower-level injuries, possibly due to weakness in intercostal muscles.

Bascom AT, Sankari A, Goshgarian HG, Badr MS. Sleep onset hypoventilation in chronic spinal cord injury. Physiol Rep. 2015;3(8):e12490.

Berry RB, Brooks R, Gamaldo CE, Harding SM, Lloyd RM, Cl M, et al. The AASM manual for the scoring of sleep and associated events: rules, terminology and technical specifications, version 2.6. www.aasmnet.org. Darien, IL: American Academy of Sleep Medicine; 2020.

Chiodo AE, Sitrin RG, Bauman KA. Sleep disordered breathing in spinal cord injury: a systematic review. J Spinal Cord Med. 2016;39(4):374–82.

24. Which of the following is NOT an accessory muscle of inspiration?

   A. Scalenes
   B. Internal intercostals
   C. Sternocleidomastoid
   D. Upper trapezius

Answer: B.

Internal intercostals are muscles of expiration. All the other named muscles (scalenes, sternocleidomastoid, and upper trapezius) are accessory muscles of inspiration. Additional muscles of inspiration include pectoralis major and external intercostals. The diaphragm is the primary muscle of inspiration.

Terson de Paleville DG, McKay WB, Folz RJ, Ovechkin AV. Respiratory motor control disrupted by spinal cord injury: mechanisms, evaluation, and restoration. Transl Stroke Res. 2011;2(4):463–73. https://doi.org/10.1007/s12975-011-0114-0.

25. Which of the following is NOT a risk factor for pneumonia in the spinal cord injured population?

   A. Lumbar level spinal cord injury
   B. Excess pulmonary secretions
   C. History of traumatic brain injury
   D. Weak cough

Answer: A.

All the primary and accessory muscles of respiration are innervated by nerves above the lumbar level and therefore a lumbar level spinal cord injury would not be a risk factor for pneumonia. Excess pulmonary secretions, history of traumatic brain injury and weak cough are risk factors for pneumonia.

Sultan I, Lamba N, Liew A, Doung P, Tewarie I, Amamoo JJ, et al. The safety and efficacy of steroid treatment for acute spinal cord injury: a Systematic Review and meta-analysis. Heliyon. 2020;6(2):e03414.

Berlly M, Shem K. Respiratory management during the first five days after spinal cord injury. J Spinal Cord Med. 2007;30(4):309–18.

26. All of the following would be taken into consideration for determining readiness to wean a patient with C5 tetraplegia from mechanical ventilation EXCEPT for:

    A. Pulmonary function measurements
    B. Vital signs
    C. Radiologic assessments
    D. Cervical range of motion

Answer: D.

A patient's cervical range of motion does not determine whether they are ready to wean from mechanical ventilation. Measurements such as vital capacity (generally 10–15 mL/kg/IBW), maximum inflation pressure (MIP), recent chest radiographs, and vital signs (temperature, blood pressure, heart rate within normal limits for the patient) are all important to assessing a patient's readiness to wean.

Kim TW, Yang JH, Huh SC, Koo BI, Yoon JA, Lee JS, et al. Motor and sensory function as a predictor of respiratory function associated with ventilator weaning after high cervical cord injury. Ann Rehabil Med. 2018;42(3):457–64.

27. A person with spinal cord injury with neurogenic restrictive disease may have all the following EXCEPT:

    A. Hypoventilation
    B. Bronchodilation
    C. Neuromuscular weakness
    D. Secretory changes

Answer: B.

People with cervical level spinal cord injury may have alterations to their autonomic system resulting in bronchospasms (not bronchodilation) and secretory changes. Thus, they are often placed on bronchodilators to improve their respiratory status. In addition, neurogenic restrictive disease is generally caused by neuromuscular weakness, which may initially present as flaccidity and resulting paradoxical breathing. Due to weakness, the lungs may not fully recruit alveoli, resulting in hypoventilation.

Berlly M, Shem K. Respiratory management during the first five days after spinal cord injury. J Spinal Cord Med. 2007;30(4):309–18.

28. To facilitate a voice in a patient with a tracheostomy, all of the following must exist EXCEPT:

    A. The patient must be completely weaned from the ventilator.
    B. There should be no suspicion of upper airway obstruction.
    C. The patient should be able to use upper extremities to remove a speaking valve.
    D. A cuffed tracheostomy tube must be deflated.

Answer: A.

To facilitate speech, a path from the trachea to the pharynx should be clear for air to pass through the vocal cords for phonation to occur. If the patient has a cuffed tracheostomy tube, the cuff must be deflated for this to occur. The patient should have no upper airway abnormality such as tracheomalacia or stenosis that would prevent air passing through the pharynx. Speech can be facilitated while a patient is on a ventilator either through "leak speech" or an in-line one way speaking valve.

Johansson K, Seiger Å, Forsén M, Holmgren Nilsson J, Hartelius L, Schalling E. Assessment of voice, speech and communication changes associated with cervical spinal cord injury. Int J Lang Commun Disord. 2018;53(4):761–75.

29. The most used strategy for mechanical ventilation in the acute care setting is low tidal volume via a cuffed inflated tracheostomy tube, which focuses on prevention of acute lung injury. In comparison, which of the below strategies is often utilized in individuals with SCI/D in the post-acute phase, focusing on prevention of atelectasis, sensation of distress, and improving the ability to vocalize and swallow:

    A. Higher tidal volumes and higher PEEP
    B. Lower tidal volumes and higher PEEP
    C. Higher respiratory rate and lower tidal volumes
    D. Higher tidal volumes and lower respiratory rates

Answer: D.

Higher ventilator volumes are recommended to overcome leaks caused from deflated or uncuffed tracheostomy tubes and to prevent atelectasis and pneumonia. The higher tidal volumes are also better tolerated by patients in the chronic phase, relieving the sense of "air hunger". Not enough studies have been done in the post-acute phase surrounding use of PEEP in weaning strategies.

While many ventilation strategies are similar in spinal cord injury patients compared to those with respiratory dysfunction of other etiologies, there are unique considerations. Nationally recognized recommendations in the context of acute respiratory distress syndrome (ARDS) call for a low tidal volume of approximately 6 mL/kg, due to a concern for increased mortality risk thought to be related to volutrauma at higher volumes. However, many spinal cord injury patients have intrinsically healthy lungs, and the cause for impaired ventilation is more purely neuromuscular in nature. Traditionally accepted spinal cord injury guidelines describe a target tidal volume of 10–20 mL per kg of ideal body weight. However, the strength of evidence to provide definitive recommendations on ventilator settings after spinal cord injury is limited and warrants further investigation.

Acute Respiratory Distress Syndrome Network. Ventilation with lower tidal volumes as compared with traditional tidal volumes for acute lung injury and the acute respiratory distress syndrome. N Engl J Med. 2000;342(18):1301–8.
Korupolu R, Stampas A, Uhlig-Reche H, Ciammaichella E, Mollett PJ, Achilike EC, Pedroza C. Comparing outcomes of mechanical ventilation with high vs. moderate tidal volumes in tracheostomized patients with spinal cord injury in acute inpatient rehabilitation setting: a retrospective cohort study. Spinal Cord. 2020:1–8.
Toki A, Nakamura T, Nishimura Y, Sumida M, Tajima F. Clinical introduction and benefits of non-invasive ventilation for above C3 cervical spinal cord injury. J Spinal Cord Med. 2019;44(1):70–6.
Consortium for Spinal Cord Medicine. Respiratory management following spinal cord injury: a clinical practice guideline for health-care professionals. J Spinal Cord Med. 2005;28(3):259–93.

30. Hypoventilation due to neurogenic restrictive respiratory disease results in reduction of all the following EXCEPT:

A. Vital capacity
B. Tidal volume
C. Ratio of residual volume to total lung capacity
D. Ratio of vital capacity to total lung capacity

Answer: C.

The ratio of residual volume to total lung capacity (RV/TLC) is the only listed value that increases due to hypoventilation in neurogenic restrictive respiratory disease. This is a measure of relative hyperinflation or air trapping that is occurring in the lungs. All other values decrease.

Sheel AW, Welch J, Townson AF (2018). Respiratory management following spinal cord injury. In: Eng JJ, Teasell RW, Miller WC, Wolfe DL, Townson AF, Hsieh JTC, Connolly SJ, Noonan VK, Loh E, Sproule S, Querée M, McIntyre A, editors. Spinal cord injury rehabilitation evidence. Version 6.0. Vancouver: p. 1–72.

31. Strategies that have shown to reduce the rate of ventilator acquired pneumonia and the duration of mechanical ventilation include all of the following EXCEPT:

    A. Early tracheostomy
    B. Head of bed 30°
    C. Assist control ventilation mode
    D. Chest physiotherapy and secretion mobilization

Answer: C.

The most effective strategies for prevention of VAP include semirecumbent position, physiotherapy and mobilization techniques for secretion management, application of PEEP (5 or more) and early tracheostomy. Selection of a specific ventilation mode (such as assist-control) has not been shown to be a strategy to reduce the rate of ventilator acquired pneumonia, although specific modes may have other benefits for management of ventilator-dependent patients with spinal cord injury.

Roquilly A, Seguin P, Mimoz O, Feuillet F, Rosenczweig E, Chevalier F, et al. Risk factors for prolonged duration of mechanical ventilation in acute traumatic tetraplegic patients—a retrospective cohort study. J Crit Care. 2014;29(2).

Gastrointestinal Disorders in Spinal Cord Injury

8

Lisa Wenzel and Christina Draganich

Questions

1. What part of the nervous system is responsible for intestinal secretion and absorption?

   A. Myenteric plexus
   B. Auerbach's plexus
   C. Meissner's plexus
   D. Gaston's plexus

   Answer: C.

   The gastrointestinal system's innervation is complex and involves both central and local control from the intrinsic (enteric) nervous system and extrinsic (autonomic) nervous system. The enteric nervous system consists of two major plexuses, the submucosal plexus (Meissner's plexus) and the myenteric plexus (Auerbach's plexus). Meissner's plexus is located within the submucosal layer of the gastrointestinal wall and functions to control local intestinal secretion and absorption (Answer C).

   The autonomic nervous system may also influence the enteric nervous system. For example, increased parasympathetic activity potentiates the function

L. Wenzel (✉)
H. Ben Taub Department of Physical Medicine and Rehabilitation, Baylor College of Medicine, TIRR Memorial Hermann Hospital, Houston, TX, USA
e-mail: Lisa.Wenzel@memorialhermann.org

C. Draganich
Physical Medicine and Rehabilitation Department, University of Colorado, Aurora, CO, USA
e-mail: Christina.Draganich@cuanschutz.edu

© The Author(s), under exclusive license to Springer Nature Switzerland AG 2022
B. A. Abramoff et al. (eds.), *The Essential Spinal Cord Injury Medicine Question Bank*, https://doi.org/10.1007/978-3-031-07796-8_8

of both the submucosal and myenteric plexuses, whereas increased sympathetic activity decreases their functions.

(Answers A and B) The myenteric plexus (also known as Auerbach's plexus) serves to control mechanical mixing and propelling of intestinal contents. Interstitial cells of cajal are found in both Meissner's and Auerbach's plexuses where they function as electrical pacemakers to produce rhythmic bowel contractions.

(Answer D) Gaston's plexus does not exist.

Furness JB, Callaghan BP, Rivera LR, Cho H-J. The enteric nervous system and gastrointestinal innervation: integrated local and central control. In: Lyte M, Cryan JF, editors. Microbial endocrinology: the microbiota-gut-brain axis in health and disease [Internet]. New York, NY: Springer New York; 2014 [cited 2020 Dec 17]. pp. 39–71. (Advances in Experimental Medicine and Biology; vol. 817). Available from: http://link.springer.com/10.1007/978-1-4939-0897-4_3

Nezami BG, Srinivasan S. Enteric Nervous System in the Small Intestine: Pathophysiology and Clinical Implications. Curr Gastroenterol Rep. 2010;12(5):358–65.

Al-Shboul O. The importance of interstitial cells of cajal in the gastrointestinal tract. Saudi J Gastroenterol. 2013;19(1):3.

Uchida K, Kamikawa Y. Muscularis mucosae—the forgotten sibling. J Smooth Muscle Res. 2007;43(5):157–77.

2. A 63-year-old female with T2 complete paraplegia presents to your office with burning pain and nausea at night as well as new dry cough. You diagnose her with gastroesophageal reflux disease (GERD) and her symptoms improve with a trial of a proton-pump inhibitor (PPI). Dysfunction in what part of the autonomic nervous system is responsible for the patient's increased susceptibility to this disease process?

A. Parasympathetic system, vagus nerve
B. Parasympathetic system, pelvic splanchnic nerves
C. Sympathetic system, T5–T9
D. Sympathetic system, T10–T12

Answer: C.

Sympathetic innervation to the gastrointestinal system results in decreased peristalsis, inhibition of secretions, impaired absorption, and contraction of sphincters and blood vessels. The sympathetic nervous system originates within cell bodies of the intermediolateral column of the spinal cord from T5 to L2 and is therefore affected by injuries to the spinal cord. The sympathetic innervation to the esophagus, stomach, liver, gallbladder, pancreas, spleen, and adrenals travels from thoracic levels T5–T9 through preganglionic sympathetic fibers via the greater splanchnic nerve to the celiac ganglion and then by postganglionic axons. In a T2 level injury, the sympathetic system arising from T5 to T9 below the injury will be affected resulting in decreased function of the sympathetic innervation to the esophagus resulting in decreased contractility of the esophageal sphincter. Given the sympathetic dysfunction, parasympathetic effects will dominate with relative relaxation of the esophageal sphincter (Answer C)

(Answer A) The effect of the parasympathetic nervous system on the gastrointestinal (GI) tract results in increased peristalsis, increased secretions, and relaxation of sphincters. The vagus nerve originates from the medulla in the central nervous system and synapses on enteric neurons extending from the esophagus to the proximal colon. Since it is not a part of the spinal column it is not directly affected by injury to the spinal cord. Furthermore, injury to the parasympathetic nervous system would result in difficulty with sphincter relaxation whereas GERD results from difficulty with sphincter contraction. The majority of the parasympathetic nerves are excitatory and release acetylcholine, which modulates the submucosal and myenteric plexuses. The system is also modulated by other neuropeptides, such as vasoactive intestinal peptide (VIP) and nitric oxide (NO)

(Answer B) The pelvic splanchnic nerves originate from the anterior gray columns of the sacral spinal cord from S2 to S4 and provides parasympathetic innervation to the distal transverse colon to the anorectal region. Since the pelvic splanchnic nerves originate from the sacral spinal cord they could be affected by some injuries to the spinal cord, however they are below the level of innervation of the of the esophagus.

(Answer D) The sympathetic innervation to the small intestine and ascending and transverse colon travels from thoracic levels T10–T12 through preganglionic sympathetic fibers via the greater splanchnic nerve to the celiac ganglion and then by postganglionic axons. The inferior mesenteric ganglion receives sympathetic fibers from L1 through L2 and sends postganglionic fibers via the hypogastric plexus to the kidney, bladder, sex organs, colon, and rectal region. Thus, T10 to T12 does not innervate the esophagus or directly affect GERD.

Karlsson AK. Autonomic dysfunction in spinal cord injury: clinical presentation of symptoms and signs. Prog Brain Res. 2006;152:1–8. https://doi.org/10.1016/S0079-6123(05)52034-X.
Wecht JM, La Fountaine MF, Handrakis JP, West CR, Phillips A, Ditor DS, et al. Autonomic nervous system dysfunction following spinal cord injury: cardiovascular, cerebrovascular, and thermoregulatory effects. Curr Phys Med Rehabil Rep. 2015;3(3):197–205.
Buijs RM. The autonomic nervous system: a balancing act. Handb Clin Neurol. 2013;117:1–11. https://doi.org/10.1016/B978-0-444-53491-0.00001-8.

3. Which statement regarding the gastrocolic reflex is correct?

   A. It is defined by a decrease in colonic activity after ingestion of a meal.
   B. It is noradrenergic mediated.
   C. It typically increases minutes after eating, peaks within an hour, and lasts for a few hours.
   D. Carbohydrates provide the best stimulus for this reflex.

   Answer: C.

Gastrointestinal functioning relies on reflexes that assist with food transit through the GI tract lumen and are facilitated by interneuron communications. The three major colonic reflexes that assist with GI motility are the gastrocolic reflex, colo-colonic reflex, and recto-colic reflex. The gastrocolic reflex occurs when there is an increase in colonic activity after a meal and typically increases minutes after eating, peaks within an hour, and lasts for a few hours (Answer C).

(Answer A) The gastrocolic reflex occurs when there is an INCREASE in colonic activity after a meal is ingested.

(Answer B) The gastrocolic reflex a cholinergic mediated reflex.

(Answer D) Fatty foods and proteins are thought to provide the best stimulus for the gastrocolic reflex. There are likely also hormonal contributions from CCK, gastrin, and motilin, as well as involvement from the vagal pathway.

Chen DA, Anschel A. Gastrointestinal disorders. In: Kirshblum S, Campagnolo DI, editors. Spinal cord medicine. 2nd ed. Philadelphia: Lipincott Williams & Wilkins; 2011. pp. 6–30.

Callaghan B, Furness JB, Pustovit RV. Neural pathways for colorectal control, relevance to spinal cord injury and treatment: a narrative review. Spinal Cord. 2018;56(3):199–205.

4. Which of the following statements regarding the recto-colic reflex is INCORRECT?

A. It is mediated by pelvic nerves.
B. It is defined by increased colonic peristalsis in response to chemical or mechanical stimulation of the rectum or anal canal.
C. It is the basis for the use of suppositories and digital stimulation.
D. It occurs when the rectum is stimulated after a meal.

Answer: D.

The gastrocolic reflex occurs when there is an increase in peristalsis after a meal (Answer D). The recto-colic reflex results from chemical or mechanical stimulation of the rectum or anal canal and causes increased peristalsis. While the recto-colic reflex is not directly stimulated by eating, bowel programs are often timed after meals to take advantage of the gastrocolic reflex in addition to the recto-colic reflex.

(Answer A). The recto-colic reflex is mediated by pelvic nerves.

(Answer B). It occurs when a chemical or mechanical stimulation of the rectum or anal canal causes increased colonic peristalsis thereby promoting colonic transit of food.

(Answer C). The recto-colic reflex is the basis for suppositories and digital stimulation to assist patients with spinal cord injury (SCI) to have a bowel movement. Suppositories or other bowel irritants can be used to chemically stimulate the rectum or anal canal causing an increase in colonic peristalsis to facilitate evacuation. Similarly, digital stimulation with a digit or adaptive device can be used to stimulate the rectum or anal canal to increase colonic peristalsis. Suppositories and digital stimulation are often used together to facilitate bowel movements and constitute important components of an upper motor neuron bowel program.

Chen DA, Anschel A. Gastrointestinal disorders. In: Kirshblum S, Campagnolo DI, editors. Spinal cord medicine. 2nd ed. Philadelphia: Lipincott Williams & Wilkins; 2011. pp. 6–30
Callaghan B, Furness JB, Pustovit RV. Neural pathways for colorectal control, relevance to spinal cord injury and treatment: a narrative review. Spinal Cord. 2018;56(3):199–205.

5. A patient with C4 American Spinal Injury Association Impairment Scale (AIS) A SCI on your service is currently being seen by your speech language pathologist for dysphagia. He is on a dysphagia II diet and is scheduled for a fiberoptic endoscopic evaluation of swallowing (FEES) in the next few days. During your daily rounds he asks you questions regarding the etiology of his dysphagia and its prognosis. Which of the following statements is true regarding dysphagia following acute tetraplegia?

A. When a patient with acute tetraplegia presents with dysphagia it is typically bound to be a permanent impairment.
B. The incidence of dysphagia in individuals with acute tetraplegia is approximately 70%.
C. Swallowing impairments typically result from soft tissue swelling or weakness in the setting of an anterior spinal surgery or prolonged intubation and generally improves with time.
D. Dysphagia typically does not result from functional causes such as bracing.

Answer: C.

Dysphagia in the acute phase following tetraplegia may be an indirect complication of acute spinal cord injury. It may result from soft tissue swelling or weakness in the setting of anterior spinal surgery or prolonged intubation (Answer C). A bedside examination by a speech and language pathologist, a fiberoptic endoscopic examination of swallowing (FEES), or a videofluoroscopic study of swallowing (VFSS) should be performed to detect and classify dysphagia. Based on these studies, speech pathologists can provided treatment for dysphagia often leading to improvement and dietary progression.

(Answer A) Dysphagia is typically transient after spinal cord injury and may be a result of soft tissue swelling or weakness in the setting of surgery or intubation as above. Chronically, it may be related to esophageal dysmotility among other causes.

(Answer B) Dysphagia is common following traumatic spinal cord injury. A study by Shem et al. (2011), showed the incidence of dysphagia in acute tetraplegia to be approximately 41%.

(Answer D) The etiology of dysphagia may be functional. For example, dysphagia may be related to the presence of a cervical immobilizing brace or forced supine position in the acute period following injury. It is also important to keep in mind that dysphagia may become a new concern even in the chronic phase of injury if a patient has new functional limitations, such as supine program following flap surgery for non-healing pressure wound.

Chen DA, Anschel A. Gastrointestinal disorders. In: Kirshblum S, Campagnolo DI, editors. Spinal cord medicine. 2nd ed. Philadelphia: Lipincott Williams & Wilkins; 2011. pp. 6–30
Chaw E, Shem K, Castillo K, Wong S, Chang J. Dysphagia and associated respiratory considerations in cervical spinal cord injury. Top Spinal Cord Injury Rehabil. 2012;18(4):291–9.
Shem K, Castillo K, Wong S, Chang J. Dysphagia in individuals with tetraplegia: incidence and risk factors. J Spinal Cord Med. 2011;34(1):85–92. https://doi.org/10.1179/107902610X12911165974981.

6. A patient of yours with incomplete tetraplegia reports having heartburn that has been preventing her from lying flat. Which statement is INCORRECT regarding esophageal dysmotility following spinal cord injury?

   A. The esophagus may experience disrupted or weakened peristalsis resulting in GERD or spasm like chest pain.
   B. Research has shown that individuals with SCI are more likely to have abnormal esophageal manometry than individuals without SCI.
   C. Research has shown lower esophageal contraction amplitudes and esophageal contraction velocities in chronic SCI patients.
   D. Patients with paraplegia are not at greater risk of GERD compared to the general population.

Answer: D.

Potential factors leading to GERD in patients with SCI include chronic elevation of the diaphragm, reduced lower esophageal pressures, weakened or disrupted peristalsis, and greater time spent in supine or semi-upright positions. Since the esophagus and stomach receive sympathetic innervation from the thoracic region (T5–T9), individuals with paraplegia may have disruptions in peristalsis and esophageal pressures. They are also at risk to spend increase time in supine positions, particularly in the acute phase of injury, and in patients with lower thoracic SCI, frequent performance of Valsalva due to constipation may also lead to transient increases in the risk of GERD. Thus, individuals with both paraplegia and tetraplegia are at greater risk for GERD compared to individuals without SCI.

It is important to note that the typical symptom of heartburn may not be present in patients with neurologic levels above T7 which may also contribute to delayed diagnosis and treatment. Endoscopy may also be performed less frequently in individuals with SCI and therefore the disease may progress by the time it is detected.

(Answer A) Recent studies suggest that there may be a higher incidence of esophageal dysmotility in patients with spinal cord injury compared to age matched controls. The mechanism is thought to relate partially to disrupted or weakened peristalsis resulting in difficulty with gastroesophageal reflux disease (GERD), spasm like chest pain, or dysphagia. It is also thought to be related to sympathetic nervous system dysfunction causing relaxation in the lower esophageal sphincter.

(Answer B) Radulovic et al. (2015) studied the use of manometry to assess esophageal motility disorders in 25 participants with chronic SCI (13 individuals with injuries between C5 and C7 and 12 individuals with injuries between T4 and T12) compared to 14 individuals without SCI. They found that individuals with spinal cord injury had significantly higher prevalence of abnormal esophageal manometry (84%) compared to individuals without spinal cord injury (7%).

(Answer C) Stinneford et al. (1993) have reported significantly lower esophageal contraction amplitudes and esophageal contraction velocities in individuals with SCI compared to individuals without SCI.

Radulovic M, Schilero GJ, Yen C, Bauman WA, Wecht JM, Ivan A, et al. Greatly increased prevalence of esophageal dysmotility observed in persons with spinal cord injury: esophageal HRM in SCI. Dis Esophagus. 2015;28(7):699–704.
Stinneford JG, Keshavarzian A, Nemchausky BA, Doria MI, Durkin M. Esophagitis and esophageal motor abnormalities in patients with chronic spinal cord injuries. Spinal Cord. 1993;31(6):384–92.
Chen DA, Anschel A. Gastrointestinal disorders. In: Kirshblum S, Campagnolo DI, editors. Spinal cord medicine. 2nd ed. Philadelphia: Lipincott Williams & Wilkins; 2011. pp. 6–30
Karlsson AK. Autonomic dysfunction in spinal cord injury: clinical presentation of symptoms and signs. Prog Brain Res. 2006;152:1–8. https://doi.org/10.1016/S0079-6123(05)52034-X.

7. A 28-year-old male with C8 AIS B tetraplegia s/p motor vehicle accident 2 weeks ago reports nausea, vomiting, and early satiety after small meals. Workup reveals delayed gastric emptying and you start him on reglan. Which statement is INCORRECT regarding gastric emptying following spinal cord injury?

A. Impaired gastrocolic reflex may contribute to gastric-emptying impairments.
B. Impaired emptying may be a result of dissociation of antral and duodenal motility.
C. Impairment in autonomic and enteric neurons may contribute to delayed gastric emptying.
D. A study showed that gastric emptying time in individuals with SCI was on average twice as long as for individuals without SCI.

Answer: D.

A study by Williams et al. (2012) compared gastric motility times for individuals with SCI with those without SCI. They showed delayed gastric emptying time in individuals with SCI compared to age and gender matched controls (10.6 vs. 3.5 h) as well as delayed colonic transit time (52.3 vs. 14.2 h) and delayed whole gut transit time (3.3 vs. 1 days). Thus, gastric emptying was shown to be approximately three times as long for individuals with SCI compared to those without SCI.

(Answer A) The gastrocolic reflex may be impaired following injury to the spinal cord and may contribute to difficulty with gastric emptying. A study by Aaronson et al. (1985) found that this reflex was absent after SCI, however more studies are needed to elucidate the effect of SCI on this reflex.

(Answers B and C) Impaired emptying is thought to be the result of the dissociation of antral and duodenal motility as a result of autonomic and enteric dysfunction. Interstitial cells of cajal are also thought to be dysfunctional as a result of injury.

Williams RE, Bauman WA, Spungen AM, Vinnakota RR, Farid RZ, Galea M, et al. SmartPill technology provides safe and effective assessment of gastrointestinal function in persons with spinal cord injury. Spinal Cord. 2012;50(1):81–4.
Aaronson MJ, Freed MM, Burakoff R. Colonic myoelectric activity in persons with spinal cord injury. Digest Dis Sci. 1985;30(4):295–300.
Pacheco MS, Garstang SV. Gastric dysmotility after abdominal surgery in persons with cervical spinal cord injury: a case series. J Spinal Cord Med. 2007;30(4):378–84. https://doi.org/10.1080/10790268.2007.11771866.

8. You visit your 38-year-old patient with T6 paraplegia to educate her on changes in bowel patterns after spinal cord injury. How long should you tell her that it would take on average for the lunch she just ate to make it all the way through her system as compared to an able bodied individual?

A. 24 h vs 8 h
B. 24 h vs 12 h
C. 48 h vs 20 h
D. 72 h vs 24 h

Answer: D.

A study by Williams et al. (2012) compared gastric motility times for individuals with SCI with those without SCI. They showed delayed gastric emptying time in individuals with SCI compared to age and gender matched controls (10.6 vs 3.5 h) as well as delayed colonic transit time (52.3 vs 14.2 h) and delayed whole gut transit time (3.3 vs 1 days).

(Answers A, B, and C) Whole gut transit time was approximately 3 times as long (3 days vs. 1 day) in individuals with spinal cord injury compared with individuals without spinal cord injury.

Williams RE, Bauman WA, Spungen AM, Vinnakota RR, Farid RZ, Galea M, et al. SmartPill technology provides safe and effective assessment of gastrointestinal function in persons with spinal cord injury. Spinal Cord. 2012;50(1):81–4.

9. A 32-year-old female with T4 AIS A paraplegia is on your service. She has upper motor neuron neurogenic bowel and has been on a daily AM program with 17.2 mg of senna at night and a suppository in the morning. She reports daily medium Bristol type 1 stools. What adjustment should you make to her bowel program?

   A. Increase senna from 17.2 mg to 34.4 mg
   B. Add docusate and encourage her to drink more water
   C. Schedule senna in the morning instead of at night
   D. Add loperamide daily

   Answer: B.

   The goal consistency of stool for a patient with an upper motor neuron (UMN) bowel program is Bristol type 4 (like a sausage or snake, smooth and soft). If the stool is too hard (Bristol types 1–3), the patient will become constipated making it both challenging to move stool through the GI tract and also to evacuate stool. If the stool is too soft (Bristol types 5–6), the stool will become difficult to evacuate as it is not well formed. Docusate is a type of stool softener that acts to emulsify fat in the GI tract thereby decreasing reabsorption of water in the colon and causing increased water content in stool. Adequate fluid intake is important for stool softeners to be effective. Given that this patient has been having type 1 stools she would benefit from addition of a stool softener as well as increased fluid intake.

   (Answer A) Senna is a peristaltic stimulant that works directly on the enteric nervous system, specifically the myenteric plexus. Thus, increasing senna will increase peristalsis and increase the volume of stool produced. The goal volume for a patient with SCI is medium to large bowel movement daily or extra-large bowel movement every other day. Since this patient is having daily medium bowel movements she has achieved her goal in terms of frequency and volume of stools and does not require adjustments to her senna dosing.

   (Answer C) Bowel movements typically occur 6–12 h after ingesting senna, so the dosing schedule is usually based on the timing of the bowel program. This patient's nightly senna is timed appropriately for her AM bowel program.

   (Answer D) Bristol type 1 is a firm stool, therefore an anti-diarrheal medicine is not indicated.

Chen DA, Anschel A. Gastrointestinal disorders. In: Kirshblum S, Campagnolo DI, editors. Spinal cord medicine. 2nd ed. Philadelphia: Lipincott Williams & Wilkins; 2011. pp. 6–30

10. You are rounding on a 48-year-old male with T1 AIS B paraplegia and note that he is having small daily Bristol type 4 bowel movements and occasionally skips a day. He is on an AM bowel program with suppository and digital stimulation. He also takes 8.6 mg of senna at night and polyethylene glycol in the morning. What should your next step be to manage this patient?

A. Increase senna from 1 tab to 2 tabs
B. Change senna to the morning
C. Increase polyethylene glycol to BID
D. Have the patient drink more water

Answer: A.

Senna is a peristaltic stimulant that works directly on the enteric nervous system, specifically the myenteric plexus. Thus, increasing senna will increase peristalsis and increase the volume of stool produced. The goal volume for a patient with SCI is daily medium to large bowel movement daily or extra-large bowel movement every other day. Since this patient is having small daily stools and occasionally skipping a day, he would most benefit from increased dosing of his peristaltic stimulant agent to increase the propulsion of stool.

(Answer B) Bowel movements typically occur 6–12 h after ingesting senna, so the dosing schedule is usually based on the timing of the bowel program. This patient's nightly senna is timed appropriately for his AM bowel program.

(Answer C) The goal consistency of stool for a patient with an UMN bowel program is Bristol type 4 (like a sausage or snake, smooth and soft). If the stool is too hard (Bristol types 1–3), the patient will become constipated making it both challenging to move stool through the GI tract and also to evacuate stool. If the stool is too soft (Bristol types 5–6), the stool will become difficult to evacuate as it is not well formed. Polyethylene glycol is a type of laxative that acts by drawing fluid into the intestinal lumen and stimulating colonic motility thereby softening the consistency of the stool. This patient is currently having Bristol type 4 bowel movements, which is the goal consistency for UMN programs. Therefore, no changes are needed to the patient's laxative dosing.

(Answer D) As discussed above, the patient does not require changes made to the consistency of his stools, but rather to the amount and frequency of his stools. Therefore, he does not require changes to his fluid intake or laxative dosing.

Chen DA, Anschel A. Gastrointestinal disorders. In: Kirshblum S, Campagnolo DI, editors. Spinal cord medicine. 2nd ed. Philadelphia: Lipincott Williams & Wilkins; 2011. pp. 6–30

11. A 34-year-old female with T4 AIS B paraplegia presents with UMN neurogenic bowel. On rectal exam she has absent voluntary anal contraction, positive deep anal pressure, and present but impaired perianal sensation. She also has a positive bulbocavernosus reflex and significant discomfort with rectal exam. What is the best medication per rectum to trial for this patient?

A. Vegetable based bisacodyl suppository
B. Water based bisacodyl suppository
C. Docusate mini enema with benzocaine
D. Docusate mini enema

Answer: C.

Contact irritants stimulate the colonic mucosa directly and are available in a variety of forms including suppositories (semi-solid formulation) and enemas (liquid formulation). One of the benefits of docusate enemas is that the liquid formulation may be less uncomfortable than the semi-solid suppository formulation and also may take less time (up to 15 min vs 32 min for polyethylene glycol (PEG) suppository). Additionally, some docusate enemas are formulated with benzocaine, which can numb the rectal area to decrease pain with digital stimulation. In this patient with partially preserved rectal sensation, a docusate mini enema with benzocaine would be preferred due to these benefits.

(Answers A and B) Bisacodyl suppositories come in variety of forms, including vegetable oil based bisacodyl and polyethylene glycol (water based) bisacodyl. A study by Glen House et al. (1997) showed that water-based suppositories resulted in faster results due to improved bioavailability. Reported time to defecation is 58 min for the vegetable base versus 32 min for the PEG base. As discussed above, a docusate mini enema with benzocaine would be more beneficial in this patient with rectal sensation given its liquid form and anesthetic properties.

(Answer D) In this patient with partially preserved rectal sensation, a docusate mini enema with benzocaine would be preferred over a docusate mini enema without benzocaine given its added benefit of anesthetic properties.

House JG, Stiens SA. Pharmacologically initiated defecation for persons with spinal cord injury: effectiveness of three agents. Arch Phys Med Rehabil. 1997;78(10):1062–5. https://doi.org/10.1016/s0003-9993(97)90128-3.

Stiens SA. Reduction in bowel program duration with polyethylene glycol based bisacodyl suppositories. Arch Phys Med Rehabil. 1995;76(7):674–7. https://doi.org/10.1016/s0003-9993(95)80638-5.

12. You are consulted on a 32-year-old male status post gunshot wound to his left flank and spine. MRI showed fractures of T11, T12, and L1 vertebrae with complete transection of the cord from T11 to T12. On exam, the patient has 5/5 strength in bilateral UEs and 0/5 strength in hip flexion, knee extension, big toe extension, dorsiflexion, and plantarflexion. Light touch and pinprick are most caudally intact at the level of the inguinal ligament and then distally absent bilaterally. On rectal exam, the patient has absence of voluntary anal contraction, absence of deep anal pressure, positive rectal tone, and positive bulbocavernosal reflex. What kind of bowel regimen will you select for this patient?

A. Daily bowel program with suppository with digital stimulation
B. BID bowel program without digital stimulation
C. BID bowel program with suppository, but without digital stimulation
D. Daily bowel program without suppository or digital stimulation

Answer: A.

The two clinical presentations of bowel dysfunction following spinal cord injury include injury above the conus medullaris, which results in UMN bowel syndrome and injury at the conus medullaris or cauda equina, which results in LMN bowel syndrome. UMN bowel is diagnosed based on the presence of rectal tone as well as reflexes, such as bulbocavernosal reflex or anal wink. This patient with 5/5 strength in his bilateral upper extremities and 0/5 strength in his lower extremities and last intact sensation at the inguinal ligament (T12) presents with T12 AIS A paraplegia. His positive rectal tone and bulbocaverno-sal reflex suggest UMN neurogenic bowel. It is important to note that the UMN bowel pattern may not emerge until spinal shock has resolved, which may be up to 6 weeks after injury.

In an UMN bowel pattern, management focuses on using preserved reflexes to promote colonic activity and relax the contracted external anal sphincter (EAS). The bowel program is performed 20–30 min after a meal to take advantage of the gastrocolic reflex and rectal contact irritant, such as a suppository or mini enema, is used for rectal stimulation to take advantage or the recto-colic reflex. This reflex is then further enhanced with digital stimulation that involves inserting a lubricated gloved finger or adaptive device into the rectum and per-forming rotational movements to stretch the anus and stimulate the rectal wall (Answer A). This technique can be performed a variety of different ways. One example includes performing rotational movements for 15–60 s every 10–15 min until no additional stool is present in the rectal vault or there are no further results after two consecutive rounds of digital stimulation. UMN neuro-genic bowel management also typically consists of pharmacologic intervention, such as stimulants (i.e. senna) administered 6–12 h prior to scheduled supposi-tory with stool softeners (i.e. docusate) or laxatives (i.e. polyethylene glycol) scheduled up to three times daily. Goals of an UMN bowel program include having daily medium to large bowel movements or every other day extra large bowel movements. Goal consistency is Bristol type 4 stool.

(Answer B) Individuals with lumbar and sacral level injuries typically demonstrate LMN bowel programs. These injuries are typically T12 or below but may vary based on type of injury to the spinal cord. LMN bowel can be ascertained partially based on level of injury, but mostly based on flaccid rectal tone and lack of reflexes, such as bulbocavernosal reflex or anal wink. Treatment of LMN bowel consists of manual evacuation of stool from the flaccid rectum with bulking of stool consistency via fiber to facilitate easy removal of stool. Programs are often performed multiple times per day to ensure complete evacuation of stool between programs and prevent involun-tary bowel movements from the flaccid anal sphincter. This patient presents with UMN bowel program and thus would likely not benefit from twice a day (BID) bowel programs.

(Answer C) BID bowel programs are often part of LMN bowel programs, which would not be appropriate for this patient with UMN bowel. Furthermore, unlike in UMN bowel management suppositories are not effective since their mechanism of action is through the stimulation of the spinal reflex arc in the rectum which is no longer intact in a patient with LMN neurogenic bowel.

(Answer D) While daily bowel programs without suppositories or digital stimulation may be possible, especially in individuals with incomplete injuries, a patient with acute complete paraplegia should be started on a bowel program with digital stimulation and suppository.

Krassioukov A, Eng JJ, Claxton G, Sakakibara BM, Shum S. Neurogenic bowel management after spinal cord injury: a systematic review of the evidence. Spinal Cord. 2010;48(10):718–33. https://doi.org/10.1038/sc.2010.14. Epub 2010 Mar 9.
Chen DA, Anschel A. Gastrointestinal disorders. In: Kirshblum S, Campagnolo DI, editors. Spinal cord medicine. 2nd ed. Philadelphia: Lippincott Williams & Wilkins; 2011. pp. 6–30

13. A 42-year-old male with C6 AIS A tetraplegia is on an UMN bowel program at night. His senna is scheduled in the morning with docusate at night. You note that he has been having an extra-large bowel movement every other day. The bowel movements are consistently Bristol type 4. What should your next steps be to manage this?

A. Inquire about his bowel habits at home and consider every other day program
B. Increase senna
C. Add magnesium citrate
D. Increase docusate dosing

Answer: A.

The patient's bowel movements are at goal consistency with Bristol type 4 stools and goal volume with extra-large bowel movement every other day. It is always important to inquire about bowel habits as part of the neurogenic bowel history, since some individuals may not have had daily bowel movements prior to their injuries, which can inform bowel management. Since this patient is consistently having bowel movements every other day with a daily program, it is reasonable to consider switching him to an every other day program as long as he continues to have adequate results (Answer A).

(Answer B) The goal stool volume and frequency for a patient with SCI is medium to large bowel movement daily or extra-large bowel movement every other day. Since this patient is having extra-large bowel movements every other day, he is at goal for his senna dosing.

(Answer C) Magnesium citrate is a saline laxative thought to work by increasing fluid in the small intestine and typically takes between 30 min and 3 h to take effect. While this medication can be useful for clean outs for significant constipation, it is not typically used on a daily basis as its effect is stronger and less predictable than other laxatives, such as polyethylene glycol.

(Answer D) This patient is at goal stool consistency for UMN bowel management (Bristol type 4). Therefore, adjusting the consistency of his stools with docusate is not necessary.

Chen DA, Anschel A. Gastrointestinal disorders. In: Kirshblum S, Campagnolo DI, editors. Spinal cord medicine. 2nd ed. Philadelphia: Lippincott Williams & Wilkins; 2011. pp. 6–30
Vanner S, Hookey LC. Timing and frequency of bowel activity in patients ingesting sodium picosulphate/magnesium citrate and adjuvant bisacodyl for colon cleansing before colonoscopy. Can J Gastroenterol. 2011;25(12):663–6. https://doi.org/10.1155/2011/950263.

14. A 46-year-old male with C4 AIS D incomplete tetraplegia reports new neurogenic bowel complaints. He was initially on a bowel program directly following his injury but has progressed to being continent without requiring a daily program. He now reports multiple days of incontinent episodes with small liquid stools. He began refusing senna and polyethylene glycol a week ago as he was having regular stools at that time. Strength and sensory exam is consistent from the prior week. On rectal exam he has voluntary anal contraction, deep anal pressure, and normal perianal sensation. What should your next step be to work up the cause of his new incontinence?

A. Order a lumbar spine MRI
B. Order a kidney-ureter-bladder (KUB) x-ray
C. Start twice daily fiber
D. Restart senna

Answer: B.

This patient with C4 AIS D tetraplegia presents with voluntary anal contraction, deep anal pressure, and normal perianal sensation. Given his intact rectal exam, it is not surprising that he has become independent with bowel movements and progressed beyond needing a bowel program. You are clued into the possibility of constipation by the fact that the patient began refusing bowel medications a week ago. Furthermore, new incontinence with small liquid stools is concerning for overflow incontinence whereby watery stools leak around hard stool blocking the rectal vault. The best next step would be to order a KUB to evaluate for constipation and if constipation is present perform a bowel clean out followed by re-initiation of daily bowel regimen (stool softeners and possibly bowel stimulants). This can also be used as a tool to educate the patient regarding bowel function. After all, a picture is worth a thousand words.

(Answer A) In a patient with new incontinence it is important to consider spinal cord compression in the differential diagnosis. Red flags concerning for spinal cord compression include motor or sensory changes, saddle distribution sensory disturbance, and bowel or bladder dysfunction. This patient does not have any changes to strength, sensation, or urinary habits; therefore, spinal cord compression should be lower on your differential.

(Answer C) This patient presents with clinical picture concerning for overflow incontinence secondary to constipation. Fiber would serve to bulk his stool likely worsening his constipation.

(Answer D) While restarting senna will likely ultimately be part of the treatment plan, in this patient with new incontinence it is important to first confirm the diagnosis of constipation, and likely the need for a bowel cleanout, prior to initiating treatment.

Krassioukov A, Eng JJ, Claxton G, Sakakibara BM, Shum S. Neurogenic bowel management after spinal cord injury: a systematic review of the evidence. Spinal Cord. 2010;48(10):718–33. https://doi.org/10.1038/sc.2010.14. Epub 2010 Mar 9.

15. Which statement is INCORRECT regarding performing an effective bowel program?

A. Bowel programs are most effective after a meal.
B. Upright and seated bowel program on a padded commode is preferred when possible.
C. Left lateral decubitus position is preferred when a bowel program is performed in bed.
D. Digital stimulation cannot be used alone without a suppository.

Answer: D.

After a patient achieves regular results with his or her bowel program, aspects of the program can be adjusted. In chronic spinal cord injury, digital stimulation alone may be adequate for effective evacuation of stool. Kirshblum et al. (1998) studied 100 individuals with chronic SCI and found that 56% were using oral medications, 72% were using suppositories, and 80% using digital stimulation as components of the bowel program. Most patients who used a suppository also needed digital stimulation for effective evacuation, however they found that digital stimulation could be performed without other interventions.

(Answer A) Bowel programs are typically performed shortly after a meal to utilize the gastrocolic reflex.

(Answers B and C) Ideal bowel program positioning is upright and seated, such as on a padded commode, to allow for gravity to assist with bowel evacuation. However, often patients are unable to tolerate an upright position, especially in the acute phase of injury, and may need to perform the bowel program in bed. When a bowel program is performed in bed, the left lateral decubitus position is preferred to also allow gravity to assist with evacuating stool along the natural curvature of the bowel.

Kirshblum SC, Gulati M, O'Connor KC, Voorman SJ. Bowel care practices in chronic spinal cord injury patients. Arch Phys Med Rehabil. 1998;79(1):20–3. https://doi.org/10.1016/s0003-9993(98)90201-5.
Stiens SA, Luttrel W, Binard JE. Polyethylene glycol versus vegetable oil based bisacodyl suppositories to initiate side-lying bowel care: A clinical trial in persons with spinal cord injury. Spinal Cord. 1998;36(11):777–81.

16. A 52-year-old male with T6 AIS A paraplegia is on your service. His neurogenic bowel is managed with a daily AM bowel program with digital stimulation, daily senna every morning, and daily polyethylene glycol every morning. Nursing staff reports that he has been having daily involuntary bowel movements with variable timing throughout the day. Which of the following should NOT be part of your next steps in management?

A. Discuss the patient's fluid intake including caffeine consumption
B. Change the timing of senna

C. Discuss the patient's dietary habits
D. Eliminate digital stimulation

Answer: D.

In this patient who is having daily involuntary bowel movements with variable timing throughout the day, it would be beneficial to discuss his dietary habits (Answer A), discuss his caffeine consumption (Answer C), and change the timing of his senna (Answer B). The patient will likely need digital stimulation as part of his upper motor neuron bowel program.

(Answer A) The ingestion of caffeine has been suggested to facilitate stool evacuation through its laxative effects by drawing water into the colon and stimulating colonic motility. It would be prudent to discuss caffeine consumption with this patient as it could be contributing to involuntary bowel movements if the patient is drinking it throughout the day as well as dehydration due to caffeine being a diuretic. Thus, timing and quantity of caffeine are important. His caffeine intake may facilitate better results when taken prior to his program.

(Answer B) Bowel movements typically occur 6–12 h after ingesting senna, so the dosing schedule is usually based on the timing of the bowel program. This patient's senna is timed in the morning, which would not take effect until 6–12 h after his bowel program and may be contributing to his daily involuntary bowel movements. Therefore, senna dosing should be changed to nighttime so that its effect will be timed with the AM bowel program.

(Answer C) When a patient is having involuntary bowel movements, it is important to discuss their dietary habits. For example, foods with high fat and spice content have been known to cause diarrhea in individuals with neurogenic bowel sometimes leading to incontinence. Discussion of both the contents of this patient's diet and the timing of certain foods would be beneficial to determine if any particular foods are contributing to his incontinence.

Stiens SA. Reduction in bowel program duration with polyethylene glycol based bisacodyl suppositories. Arch Phys Med Rehabil. 1995;76(7):674–7. https://doi.org/10.1016/s0003-9993(95)80638-5.

Chen DA, Anschel A. Gastrointestinal disorders. In: Kirshblum S, Campagnolo DI, editors. Spinal cord medicine. 2nd ed. Philadelphia: Lipincott Williams & Wilkins; 2011. pp. 6–30

17. A 26-year-old male with L1 AIS B paraplegia presents with decreased rectal tone on exam. You start him on an evening bowel program with manual evacuation with good results. After five days you notice that he is having daily involuntary Bristol type 3 bowel movements with activities in the afternoon. What is the next step clinically?

A. Prescribe fiber
B. Prescribe senna
C. Prescribe polyethylene glycol
D. Schedule BID bowel program

Answer: D.

Individuals with lumbar and sacral level injuries typically demonstrate LMN bowel programs. These injuries are typically T12 or below but may vary based on type of injury to the spinal cord. LMN bowel can be ascertained partially based on level of injury, but mostly based on flaccid rectal tone and lack of reflexes, such as bulbocavernosal reflex or anal wink. Treatment of LMN bowel consists of manual evacuation of stool from the flaccid rectum and are often performed multiple times per day to ensure complete evacuation of stool between programs and prevent involuntary bowel movements from the flaccid anal sphincter. Since this patient has been having involuntary bowel movements later in the day with activity, he would likely benefit from a twice per day bowel program to ensure stool is not present in the rectal vault throughout the day.

(Answer A) The patient is having Bristol type 3 stools, which is the goal consistency for a LMN bowel program. Thus, he does not need a prescription of fiber to further bulk up his stools. Prescribing fiber to this patient would likely lead to constipation and more difficult evacuation of stools.

(Answer B) This patient is having good results with his nighttime bowel program, thus adding senna is not necessary since it acts to stimulate the colonic mucosa. Furthermore, additional stimulation of the colonic mucosa would likely worsen this patient's involuntary bowel movements.

(Answer C) The patient is having Bristol type 3 stools, which is the goal consistency for a LMN bowel program. Thus, prescribing polyethylene glycol which is a laxative drawing water in to the stool would serve to loosen the consistency of the stools making it less ideal for a LMN bowel program. Furthermore, polyethylene glycol stimulates colonic motility and may worsen this patient's involuntary bowel movements.

Chen DA, Anschel A. Gastrointestinal disorders. In: Kirshblum S, Campagnolo DI, editors. Spinal cord medicine. 2nd ed. Philadelphia: Lippincott Williams & Wilkins; 2011. pp. 6–30

Krassioukov A, Eng JJ, Claxton G, Sakakibara BM, Shum S. Neurogenic bowel management after spinal cord injury: a systematic review of the evidence. Spinal Cord. 2010;48(10):718–33. https://doi.org/10.1038/sc.2010.14. Epub 2010 Mar 9.

18. A 48-year-old male with chronic L5 complete paraplegia is seen in your office for chronic constipation. He reports only having a bowel movement every 4–5 days despite attempting twice daily programs with manual evacuation as prescribed. On interview, he reports that it has been 6 days since his last bowel movement. KUB x-ray shows rectal impaction. What might you consider for this patient?

A. Colostomy
B. Large volume retrograde enema
C. Malone anterograde continence enema (MACE)
D. Magnesium citrate

Answer: B.

A retrograde continence enema is comprised of a specially designed catheter that is inserted into the rectum and held in place by an inflated balloon. The enema is administered through the catheter into the rectum after which the balloon is deflated and the catheter removed with the goal of evacuation of stool from the rectum. In this patient who has not had a bowel movement in 6 days with KUB confirming rectal impaction large volume retrograde enema would be an appropriate next step.

(Answer A) A colostomy is considered if conservative measures are not successful to achieve a regulated bowel program. It is typically reserved for patients with ongoing incontinence in the setting of pressure injuries or severe constipation. However, a study by Coggrave et al. (2012) studied 92 individuals with chronic SCI who underwent ileostomy or colostomy and found that the main reasons for intervention were prolonged bowel care (61%), fecal incontinence (47%, and constipation (26%). Other studies have had similar findings, especially supporting the reduced time for bowel care as a major reason that individuals with SCI undergo colostomy. This patient has not yet tried less invasive procedures, such as retrograde enemas or transanal irrigation, thus colostomy is not the appropriate next step to manage his constipation.

(Answer C) The MACE procedure involves a surgical operation to pull the appendix through the skin forming an appendicostomy. An anterograde enema (ACE) can then be introduced through the abdominal wall stoma producing a wash-out effect and stimulating colonic peristalsis to evacuate the contents of the colon. The MACE procedure is an option for patients with neurogenic bowel with chronic, refractory constipation, however this patient should first try less invasive option, such as a large volume retrograde enema.

(Answer D) The KUB revealed rectal impaction making distal cleanout, such as an enema, the most effective treatment. An oral agent would worsen the impaction. However, if the KUB had instead shown large stool burden in the more proximal colon, the provider may consider an oral cleanout with a laxative.

Luther SL, Nelson AL, Harrow JJ, Chen F, Goetz LL. A comparison of patient outcomes and quality of life in persons with neurogenic bowel: standard bowel care program vs colostomy. J Spinal Cord Med. 2005;28(5):387–93. https://doi.org/10.1080/1079026 8.2005.11753838.

Kelly S, Shashidharan M, Borwell B, Tromans A, Finnis D, Grundy D. The role of intestinal stoma in patients with spinal cord injury. Spinal Cord. 1999;37(3):211–4.

Coggrave MJ, Ingram RM, Gardner BP, Norton CS. The impact of stoma for bowel management after spinal cord injury. Spinal Cord. 2012;50(11):848–52.

Christensen P, Kvitzau B, Krogh K, Buntzen S, Laurberg S. Neurogenic colorectal dysfunction—use of new antegrade and retrograde colonic wash-out methods. Spinal Cord. 2000;38(4):255–61.

Worsøe J, Christensen P, Krogh K, Buntzen S, Laurberg S. Long-term results of antegrade colonic enema in adult patients: assessment of functional results. Dis Colon Rectum. 2008;51(10):1523–8. https://doi.org/10.1007/s10350-008-9401-6. Epub 2008 Jul 12.

Christensen P, Bazzocchi G, Coggrave M, Abel R, Hulting C, Krogh K, Media S, Laurberg S. Outcome of transanal irrigation for bowel dysfunction in patients with spinal cord injury. J Spinal Cord Med. 2008;31(5):560–7. https://doi.org/10.1080/10790268.200 8.11754571.

Christensen P, Krogh K, Buntzen S, Payandeh F, Laurberg S. Long-term outcome and safety of transanal irrigation for constipation and fecal incontinence. Dis Colon Rectum. 2009;52(2):286–92. https://doi.org/10.1007/DCR.0b013e3181979341.

Christensen P, Bazzocchi G, Coggrave M, Abel R, Hultling C, Krogh K, Media S, Laurberg S. A randomized, controlled trial of transanal irrigation versus conservative bowel management in spinal cord-injured patients. Gastroenterology. 2006;131(3):738–47. https://doi.org/10.1053/j.gastro.2006.06.004.

19. A 52-year-old male with C4 AIS A tetraplegia presents for a follow up visit. He reports that his bowel program has been going well and bladder spasticity has been improved with oxybutynin. His spasticity has been well controlled with oral baclofen and he denies neuropathic pain. He initially had issues with dysphagia and was on a soft diet with honey thick liquids but has now progressed to regular diet and thin liquids. He is now enjoying his thin liquids with soda three times per day. On review of systems, he notes that five cavities were discovered during his last dentist appointment. He never had a cavity prior to his injury. Which of the following is LEAST likely to contribute to his poor dentition?

    A. Inability to maintain daily mechanical plaque removal
    B. Current medication regimen
    C. Dietary considerations
    D. Progression from soft to solid foods

Answer: D.

Animal studies have suggested that a soft consistency diet may lead to weaker gingiva, increased bacterial plaque, and decreased tooth strength leading to an increased risk of periodontal disease. Thus, progression from soft to solid foods may actually provide benefit for lowering the risk of periodontal disease.

   (Answer A) Depending on their level of injury, patients with tetraplegia are often dependent on caregivers or assistive devices for daily oral care. The inability to maintain daily mechanical plaque removal may be the most important factor in poor dentition following SCI. Individuals who are dependent on caregivers have been found to have more severe gingivitis, poorer oral hygiene, and greater periodontal disease compared to those capable of performing independent dental hygiene.

   (Answer B) Xerostomia is one of the causes of poor dentition often seen in individuals with SCI. This is often the result of medications administered to individuals with SCI. Antispasmodics and anticholingerics are two frequent culprits of xerostomia. Two of this patient's medications, baclofen and oxybutynin, respectively, fall under these categories.

   (Answer C) Dental carries have shown to be linked the consumption of foods high in extrinsic sugars, especially if consumed greater than four times per day or if sugar levels exceed 60g per day. Dental carries may also be linked to foods rich in starch. Additionally, lower levels of dietary vitamin C have been found to increase the risk of periodontal disease. Dental carries may also be worsened by foods and drinks high in acid.

Nishida M, Grossi SG, Dunford RG, Ho AW, Trevisan M, Genco RJ. Dietary vitamin C and the risk for periodontal disease. J Periodontol. 2000;71(8): 1215–23. https://doi.org/10.1902/jop.2000.71.8.1215.

Stiefel DJ, Truelove EL, Persson RS, Chin MM, Mandel LS. A comparison of oral health in spinal cord injury and other disability groups. Spec Care Dentist. 1993;13(6):229–35. https://doi.org/10.1111/j.1754-4505.1993.tb01473.x.

Sheiham A. Dietary effects on dental diseases. Public Health Nutr. 2001;4(2b):569–91.

20. You are caring for a 29-year-old female with T1 AIS A tetraplegia. She is noted to have a distended abdomen with nausea and vomiting. Her vital signs are stable. Which statement is INCORRECT regarding acute abdomen in this patient?

A. Acute abdomen has been reported in approximately 5% of patients in the acute phase following injury.
B. The majority of individuals with SCI who experience acute abdominal emergencies have neurological levels above T6.
C. Clinical signs and symptoms of acute abdomen include abdominal pain, referred shoulder pain, increased spasticity, fever, nausea, vomiting and autonomic dysreflexia.
D. Initial workup should include CT abdomen and pelvis.

Answer: D.

In an individual with spinal cord injury and concern for acute abdomen, a physical exam should be performed to assess for abdominal tenderness and distention, which can guide assessment. Initial workup should then include a KUB to rule out constipation or stones. If the KUB is normal, further workup can then include basic labs, such as a complete blood count (CBC) and comprehensive metabolic panel (CMP), as well as a CT abdomen and pelvis to aid in establishing the diagnosis. If the patient has other symptoms, such as fever and nausea, or the patient is unstable, the provider may choose to proceed with the CT abdomen and pelvis sooner.

(Answer A) In the acute phase following spinal cord injury acute abdomen has been reported in approximately 5% of patients with mortality rates reported as 9.5% in individuals with subacute to chronic SCI.

(Answer B) The majority of individuals with spinal cord injury who develop acute abdomen have neurological levels above T6. These patients are more likely to have impaired abdominal sensation leading to higher risk of further development of the abdominal process leading to acute abdomen on presentation.

(Answer C) Clinical signs and symptoms of acute abdomen include abdominal pain, referred shoulder tip pain, increased spasticity, fever, nausea, vomiting, abdominal distention and autonomic dysreflexia. A retrospective study of 237 individuals with SCI in the acute phase of rehabilitation found that the most frequent patient complaints were abdominal pain, fever, and abdominal discomfort. The most common signs were abdominal distention, leukocytosis, and abdominal tenderness to palpation. Juler and Eltorai (1985) performed a retrospective review to assess the signs and symptoms of acute abdomen in individuals with SCI who underwent emergent surgical intervention for acute abdomen and found that autonomic dysreflexia and shoulder pain were the most common symptoms in these individuals, however presentation was greatly affected with level of neurologic injury.

Sarıfakıoğlu B, Afşar SI, Yalbuzdağ ŞA, Ustaömer K, Ayaş Ş. Acute abdominal emergencies and spinal cord injury; our experiences: a retrospective clinical study. Spinal Cord. 2014;52(9):697–700.

Juler GL, Eltorai IM. The acute abdomen in spinal cord injury patients. Spinal Cord. 1985;23(2):118–23.

21. The most common causes of acute abdomen in the initial period following spinal cord injury include all of the following EXCEPT:

    A. Peptic ulcer perforation
    B. Acute cholecystitis
    C. Gastrointestinal (GI) bleed
    D. Appendicitis

Answer: D.

Based on studies of individuals with SCI in acute inpatient rehabilitation, the most common causes of acute abdomen in the initial period following injury are peptic ulcer perforation, acute cholecystitis, and GI bleed (Answers A, B, and C). Following injury, peptic ulcer perforation has the highest occurrence in the first 10–30 days. A retrospective study by Sarıfakıoğlu et al. (2014) of 237 individuals with SCI who were in acute inpatient rehabilitation found that 9 patients developed acute abdomen with acute cholecystitis being the most common cause. Other causes of acute abdomen in both the acute and chronic periods after spinal cord injury include intestinal obstruction, pancreatitis, appendicitis, and peritonitis.

Sarıfakıoğlu B, Afşar SI, Yalbuzdağ ŞA, Ustaömer K, Ayaş Ş. Acute abdominal emergencies and spinal cord injury; our experiences: a retrospective clinical study. Spinal Cord. 2014;52(9):697–700.

Juler GL, Eltorai IM. The acute abdomen in spinal cord injury patients. Spinal Cord. 1985;23(2):118–23.

Chen D, Apple DF Jr, Hudson LM, Bode R. Medical complications during acute rehabilitation following spinal cord injury–current experience of the Model Systems. Arch Phys Med Rehabil. 1999;80(11):1397–401. https://doi.org/10.1016/s0003-9993(99)90250-2.

22. A 48-year-old female with T3 AIS B sensory incomplete paraplegia secondary to a motor vehicle accident 3 weeks ago has recently transferred to your inpatient rehabilitation facility from acute care. On her second day in rehabilitation, she develops melena and has a drop in her hemoglobin. Which prophylaxis

regimen is recommended by the Consortium of Spinal Cord Injury Medicine to prevent her current situation?

A. 8 weeks of an H2 blocker
B. 12 weeks of an H2 blocker
C. 4 weeks of a proton pump inhibitor (PPI)
D. 2 weeks of a PPI

Answer: C.

The Consortium of Spinal Cord Injury Medicine recommends 4 weeks of stress ulcer prophylaxis since patients with acute SCI are at high risk of gastrointestinal bleeding in the first 4 weeks after injury. Patients should not be placed on prophylaxis longer than 4 weeks unless other risk factors are present, such as respiratory failure or coagulopathy. Patients with cervical complete injuries have consistently shown a higher risk of GI bleeding compared to individuals with thoracic or incomplete injuries, however the guidelines remain the same for all individuals with acute SCI. Thus, based on the guidelines, this patient would have benefited from 4 weeks of an H2 blocker or PPI for stress ulcer prophylaxis.

PPIs have been suggested to be more effective in preventing bleeding in high-risk patients. A meta-analysis comparing the therapeutic effectiveness of H2 blockers vs PPIs following endoscopy for upper GI bleed found that PPIs had statistically significant decreased rate of recurrent bleeding and surgery, however clostridium difficile infections occur at higher rates following PPI use. Ultimately guidelines recommend either H2 blocker or PPI for prophylaxis, which is left to the discretion of the provider.

In this patient with symptoms of GERD, treatment with lifestyle modifications, such as remaining upright during and after meals, smoking cessation if applicable, and reduced caffeine, chocolate, peppermint, and alcohol intake would be prudent first steps. It is also important to consider constipation as a possible contributing cause and treat this accordingly. If conservative measures fail, the patient should be started on a PPI.

(Answers A, B, C) The correct timeline for stress ulcer prophylaxis following an acute spinal cord injury is 4 weeks.

Consortium for Spinal Cord Medicine. Early acute management in adults with spinal cord injury: a clinical practice guideline for health-care professionals. J Spinal Cord Med. 2008;31(4):403–79. https://doi.org/10.1043/1079-0268-31.4.408.

Zhang Y-S. Proton pump inhibitors therapy vs H 2 receptor antagonists therapy for upper gastrointestinal bleeding after endoscopy: a meta-analysis. WJG. 2015;21(20):6341.

McDonald EG, Milligan J, Frenette C, Lee TC. Continuous proton pump inhibitor therapy and the associated risk of recurrent Clostridium difficile infection. JAMA Intern Med. 2015;175(5):784.

Dial S, Alrasadi K, Manoukian C, Huang A, Menzies D. Risk of Clostridium difficile diarrhea among hospital inpatients prescribed proton pump inhibitors: cohort and case-control studies. CMAJ. 2004;171(1):33–8. https://doi.org/10.1503/cmaj.1040876.

Chen DA, Anschel A. Gastrointestinal disorders. In: Kirshblum S, Campagnolo DI, editors. Spinal cord medicine. 2nd ed. Philadelphia: Lipincott Williams & Wilkins; 2011. pp. 6–30

23. A 56-year-old male with chronic tetraplegia comes to the emergency department with abdominal distention, nausea, and vomiting. He reports not having had a bowel movement for 6 days and a KUB x-ray reveals an ileus. You admit the patient, make him nothing by mouth and start intravenous fluids. The next day his nausea and vomiting persist and he becomes tachycardic with a fever to 102F. In addition to a CBC and CMP, what other workup should you consider next?

A. Blood cultures, Urinalysis, amylase, and lipase
B. CT abdomen and pelvis
C. MRI spine
D. Pharmacologic stress test

Answer: A.

Additional labs are the next best step in working up this patient with refractory ileus and new sepsis (criteria = fever and tachycardia). Workup should include CBC, CMP, blood cultures, urinalysis, amylase, and lipase. In patients with non-resolving ileus, co-existing intra-abdominal processes, such as pancreatitis, urinary tract infection, pyelonephritis, and cholecystitis should be considered in the differential.

It is important to remember that an intra-abdominal process, such as pancreatitis, may present differently in a patient with tetraplegia who has impaired abdominal sensation. Furthermore, acute pancreatitis is present in at least 3% of individuals with SCI, however the incidence may be higher due to underdiagnosis of the disease. A prospective observational study by Pirolla et al. (2014) found acute pancreatitis in over 11% of 78 individuals admitted for acute SCI and was associated with adynamic ileus. Increased frequency of pancreatitis in individuals with SCI compared to those without SCI may be due to disturbance of the autonomic nervous system, which alters pancreatic gland secretion resulting in overstimulation of the sphincter of Oddi via unregulated parasympathetic input. Other suggested causes include activation of pancreatic trypsinogen form hypercalcemia of immobility and increased viscosity of pancreatic secretions due to pharmacologic or endogenous steroids.

(Answer B) CT abdomen and pelvis is not required for initial diagnosis of pancreatitis as the diagnosis can be made based on clinical presentation and elevation of lipase or amylase over three times the upper limit of normal. However, CT abdomen and pelvis may be obtained if diagnosis of pancreatitis is unclear or to aid in determining the underlying cause for the pancreatitis, especially if malignancy is suspected.

(Answer C) While epidural abscess is on the differential for a patient with new sepsis, initial workup for this patient with refractory ileus and sepsis should include basic labs to investigate more common intrabdominal causes.

(Answer D) Patients with spinal cord injury may present with more vague clinical manifestations of acute coronary syndrome (ACS), thus in patients with nausea and vomiting ACS should remain in the differential. However, this would be lower on the differential thus lab work up for sepsis would be a more appropriate next step.

Pirolla EH, de Barros Filho TE, Godoy-Santos AL, Fregni F. Association of acute pancreatitis or high level of serum pancreatic enzymes in patients with acute spinal cord injury: a prospective study. Spinal Cord. 2014;52(11):817–20.

Carey ME, Nance FC, Kirgis HD, Young HF, Megison LC Jr, Kline DG. Pancreatitis following spinal cord injury. J Neurosurg. 1977;47(6):917–22. https://doi.org/10.3171/jns.1977.47.6.0917.

Nobel D, Baumberger M, Eser P, Michel D, Knecht H, Stocker R. Nontraumatic pancreatitis in spinal cord injury. Spine. 2002;27(9):E228–32.

da Silva S, Rocha M, Pinto-de-Sousa J. Acute Pancreatitis Etiology Investigation: A Workup Algorithm Proposal. GE Port J Gastroenterol. 2017;24(3):129–36.

24. A 16-year-old male who is on your service with C2 complete tetraplegia is noted to have an SBP of 160 mmHg and HR of 50. His typical SBP is in the 100s–110s. He reports having back pain but denies other symptoms and is afebrile. You sit him up in bed, remove constrictive clothing, perform straight catheterization, and check his rectal vault for stool (once SBP below 150 mmHg), but cannot find obvious underlying causes for dysreflexia. CBC shows WBC of 14,000 and CMP, Urinalysis, amylase, lipase, KUB are unremarkable. Which of the following is most likely elucidate the cause of his presentation?

A. CT abdomen and pelvis
B. Electrocardiogram (EKG) and troponin
C. MRI spine
D. Erythrocyte sedimentation rate (ESR) and C-reactive protein (CRP)

Answer: A.

Autonomic dysreflexia is a phenomenon that occurs in individuals with injuries at the thoracic level T6 or above and results from noxious stimuli, which trigger sympathetic hyperactivity. It is defined by systolic blood pressure 20mmHg higher than baseline and diastolic blood pressure 10mmHg higher than baseline. Given that acute abdominal processes can present with vague abdominal symptoms or back pain and autonomic dysreflexia, this patient with non-resolving autonomic dysreflexia and back pain should trigger further abdominal workup. Given that initial labwork was not consistent with urinalysis, pancreatitis, ileus, obstruction, or constipation, the next best step would be to obtain a CT abdomen and pelvis to look for other intra-abdominal processes, such as appendicitis.

(Answer B) Patients with spinal cord injury may present with more vague clinical manifestations of acute coronary syndrome (ACS), thus in patients with back pain and autonomic dysreflexia ACS should remain in the differential. However, this would be lower on the differential for this patient and thus initial workup with CT abdomen and pelvis for intra-abdominal process is most appropriate.

(Answer C) In this patient with non-resolving autonomic dysreflexia and back pain intraspinal process, such as epidural abscess, is lower on the differential given that the patient is afebrile. CT abdomen and pelvis to investigate possible intra-abdominal process would be the best next step compared to MRI spine.

(Answer D) ESR and CRP are non-specific and will be elevated in many disease processes. Therefore, more specific investigation, such as CT abdomen and pelvis, is the more appropriate next step.

Eldahan KC, Rabchevsky AG. Autonomic dysreflexia after spinal cord injury: Systemic pathophysiology and methods of management. Auton Neurosci. 2018;209:59–70. https://doi.org/10.1016/j.autneu.2017.05.002. Epub 2017 May 8.

25. A 23-year-old female who sustained C5 AIS A tetraplegia secondary to a motor vehicle accident is in inpatient rehabilitation. She is noted to have significant weight loss and vomiting after meals. Upper GI series show abrupt termination of the barium in the area of the duodenum. The clinical scenario is most likely related to:

A. Superior mesenteric artery syndrome
B. Cholecystitis
C. Chronic pancreatitis
D. Ileus

Answer: A.

Superior mesenteric artery syndrome (SMAS) occurs when there is intermittent functional obstruction of the distal duodenum between the aorta and superior mesenteric artery. Clinical presentation typically includes postprandial fullness, nausea, epigastric pain or discomfort, nausea, recurrent vomiting following oral intake, and weight loss. Symptoms are often worse in a supine position. SMAS is most common in tetraplegia as opposed to paraplegia and in individuals who have lost a significant amount of weight post-injury. An upper GI series can confirm the diagnosis with abrupt termination of barium in the third part of the duodenum.

SMAS is treated by sitting the patient upright during and after meals, restoring weight, and utilizing a lumbosacral corset to elevate the contents of the abdomen. Metoclopramide may also be used prior to meals. Surgery, such as a duodenojejunostomy, is only indicated in refractory cases.

(Answer B) Acute cholecystitis is characterized by right upper quadrant (RUQ) or epigastric pain, nausea, vomiting, and/or right shoulder pain, but may have a vague clinical presentation in individuals with tetraplegia. The diagnosis is confirmed by RUQ ultrasound showing gallbladder wall thickening, stones, and/or pericholecystic fluid with sonographic murphy's sign.

(Answer C) Pancreatitis is diagnosed by characteristic abdominal pain, lipase or amylase elevated beyond three times the upper limit of normal, or characteristic imaging findings.

(Answer D) The diagnosis of ileus is made based on physical examination and plain radiography, which reveals dilated loops of small and large intestines.

Wilkinson R, Huang CT. Superior mesenteric artery syndrome in traumatic paraplegia: a case report and literature review. Arch Phys Med Rehabil. 2000;81(7):991–4. https://doi.org/10.1053/apmr.2000.3867.

Roth EJ, Fenton LL, Gaebler-Spira DJ, Frost FS, Yarkony GM. Superior mesenteric artery syndrome in acute traumatic quadriplegia: case reports and literature review. Arch Phys Med Rehabil. 1991;72(6):417–20.

26. A 45-year-old female with a history of C7 complete tetraplegia presents with intermittent right shoulder pain and nausea. She describes the pain as non-radiating and has a hard time describing the location and quality of the pain. Shoulder and neck exam are unremarkable, lungs are clear to auscultation, and heart is regular rate and rhythm. Abdomen is mildly tender on exam, worse in the right upper quadrant (RUQ). KUB is unrevealing. After obtaining a CBC, CMP, lipase, and amylase what imaging study will you obtain?

A. CT abdomen and pelvis with contrast
B. CT abdomen and pelvis without contrast
C. RUQ ultrasound (US)
D. Hepatobiliary iminodiacetic acid (HIDA) scan

Answer: C.

Altered sensation can lead to atypical clinical presentation of cholecystitis in individuals with spinal cord injury. The only presenting symptom may be right shoulder pain or abdominal tenderness. However, Tola et al. (2000) studied individuals with SCI undergoing cholecystectomy for gallbladder disease and found that RUQ pain and biliary pain were present in 66% and 63% of patients. In a patient who is suspected of having cholelithiasis or cholecystitis, RUQ US should be obtained to confirm presence of disease (Answer C).

(Answer A) CT abdomen and pelvis with contrast is not the best imaging study to evaluate for cholecystitis. Furthermore, it exposes the patient to contrast and radiation while an ultrasound does not making ultrasound the best next step. If labs and ultrasound were unrevealing, then it may be reasonable to pursue CT abdomen and pelvis with contrast to evaluate for other intra-abdominal processes, such as pancreatitis or pyelonephritis.

(Answer B) CT abdomen and pelvis without contrast is not the best imaging study to evaluate for cholecystitis. It would be useful to evaluate for other intra-abdominal processes in the case of recurrent flank pain concerning for stones.

(Answer D) HIDA scan is the most sensitive test for acute cholecystitis and may be obtained if ultrasound is unclear. However, ultrasound is less invasive and should be obtained first.

Tola VB, Chamberlain S, Kostyk SK, Soybel DI. Symptomatic gallstones in patients with spinal cord injury. J Gastrointest Surg. 2000;4(6):642–7. https://doi.org/10.1016/s1091-255x(00)80115-8.

27. What is INCORRECT regarding ileus following acute SCI?

    A. It is most frequently seen in the first 24–48 h of injury and can be associated with pancreatitis.
    B. It typically resolves spontaneously, no interventions are necessary.
    C. It is thought to be due to the acute loss of both sympathetic and parasympathetic activity during spinal shock.
    D. Laboratory testing assessing for electrolyte disorders should be ordered.

Answer: B.

An ileus describes functional obstruction of intestinal transit without the presence of mechanical obstruction. It typically does not resolve spontaneously and may require varying levels of intervention (Answer B). Management of ileus typically involves bowel rest and nasogastric decompression without suction until bowel sounds return. If the ileus persists a prokinetic agent, such as metoclopramide or erythromycin, may be initiated.

(Answer A) Ileus most frequently occurs in the first 24–48 h of spinal cord injury and resolves within 2–3 days of onset.

(Answer C) Ileus is thought to be due to the acute loss of both sympathetic and parasympathetic activity during spinal shock.

(Answer D) Electrolyte imbalances may underly the presence of ileus in patients with spinal cord injury and electrolytes should be checked routinely in the setting of ileus.

Chen DA, Anschel A. Gastrointestinal disorders. In: Kirshblum S, Campagnolo DI, editors. Spinal cord medicine. 2nd ed. Philadelphia: Lipincott Williams & Wilkins; 2011. pp. 6–30

28. A 28-year-old male with C4 AIS A tetraplegia has had improved and stable lower extremity (LE) spasticity since starting baclofen 5mg three times per day (TID). When you see him this morning you note increased tone on LE exam and he describes acutely worsened spasms overnight preventing him from sleeping. He has been afebrile and denies chills, fevers, or other infectious symptoms. Basic labs including urinalysis are unremarkable. What should your next steps be?

    A. Obtain CT abdomen and pelvis
    B. Inquire about changes in bowel program and check a KUB
    C. Obtain RUQ US
    D. Obtain an EKG

Answer: B.

In a patient with acutely worsened spasticity it is important to consider under-lying causes related to bowel and bladder, such as urinary tract infection or constipation. Given that the patient's UA was unremarkable it would be reason-able to inquire about the patient's recent bowel habits and obtain a KUB if the history is concerning for constipation. The patient also had a recent medication change that may be contributing to constipation.

(Answer A) Intra-abdominal infection can be a cause of acutely worsening spasticity, however bowel and bladder are more common causes and should be investigated first before obtaining more invasive imaging.

(Answer C) Acutely worsening spasticity can be one of the presenting signs of cholecystitis or cholelithiasis in a patient with tetraplegia and impaired abdominal sensation, however bowel and bladder are more common causes and should be investigated first unless history is more specific for cholecystitis.

(Answer D) Acute coronary syndrome (ACS) could present with acutely worsened spasticity in a patient with tetraplegia whose thoracic sensation is impaired, however bowel and bladder are more common causes and should be investigated first unless history is more specific for ACS.

Chen DA, Anschel A. Gastrointestinal disorders. In: Kirshblum S, Campagnolo DI, editors. Spinal cord medicine. 2nd ed. Philadelphia: Lipincott Williams & Wilkins; 2011. pp. 6–30

29. A 32-year-old female with T4 AIS A paraplegia reports new onset rectal bleed-ing. Rectal exam confirms hemorrhoids as the source of bleeding. Which of the following is NOT appropriate in the management of this patient?

    A. Prescribe stool softeners to improve the consistency of her stools
    B. Prescribe hydrocortisone suppositories
    C. Recommend that she stop her bowel program for the next 2 weeks to allow the area to heal
    D. Review proper technique for digital stimulation

Answer: C.

Stopping this patient's bowel program would likely lead to worsening bowel dysfunction including constipation ultimately worsening her hemorrhoids. Bowel programs should never be discontinued for patients with spinal cord injuries and instead other steps should be taken to improve the consistency of stool and directly treat the patient's hemorrhoids. Conservative treatment involves improving the consistency of stool, decreasing straining, and improv-ing digital stimulation technique. Hydrocortisone suppositories and creams can also be used at the end of the bowel program.

Due to frequent constipation and chronic digital stimulation during bowel care, hemorrhoids are a common occurrence for individuals with SCI. Symptomatic hemorrhoids have been reported in 36–74% of individuals with chronic SCI. However, a study by Han et al. (2016) did not find a significant difference in prevalence of hemorrhoids on colonoscopy in individuals with chronic SCI compared to patients without SCI, while Menter et al. (1997) reported higher rates of hemorrhoids in patients who used chemical stimulation for bowel management compared to physical manipulation and found increasing incidence with increasing age.

(Answer A) It is important to address underlying causes of hemorrhoid formation, such as irregular, hard consistency stools that may be contributing. The provider should take a history that includes a discussion of stool consistency and prescribe stool softeners if appropriate to decrease straining and anal trauma.

(Answer B) Hydrocortisone suppositories and creams can be used at the end of the bowel program to treat hemorrhoids.

(Answer D) In this patient with hemorrhoids, poor technique for digital stimulation may be contributing, thus digital stimulation technique should be reviewed to ensure that the patient is not causing unnecessary trauma to her rectal vault.

Stone JM, Nino-Murcia M, Wolfe VA, Perkash I. Chronic gastrointestinal problems in spinal cord injury patients: a prospective analysis. Am J Gastroenterol. 1990;85(9):1114–9.

Adriaansen JJ, van Asbeck FW, van Kuppevelt D, Snoek GJ, Post MW. Outcomes of neurogenic bowel management in individuals living with a spinal cord injury for at least 10 years. Arch Phys Med Rehabil. 2015;96(5):905–12. https://doi.org/10.1016/j.apmr.2015.01.011. Epub 2015 Jan 22.

Menter R, Weitzenkamp D, Cooper D, Bingley J, Charlifue S, Whiteneck G. Bowel management outcomes in individuals with long-term spinal cord injuries. Spinal Cord. 1997;35(9):608–12.

Han SJ, Kim CM, Lee JE, Lee TH. Colonoscopic lesions in patients with spinal cord injury. J Spinal Cord Med. 2009;32(4):404–7. https://doi.org/10.1080/10790268.2009.11753183.

30. What is true regarding colorectal cancer after spinal cord injury?

   A. Rates of colorectal carcinoma after SCI vary in the literature.
   B. The rate of colorectal carcinoma is higher in patients with SCI.
   C. Individuals with SCI undergo higher rates of screening colonoscopies than individuals without SCI.
   D. Rectal examination is recommended annually for individuals with SCI over age of 50.

Answer: A.

Rates of colorectal carcinoma following spinal cord injury vary in the literature. A study by Frisbie et al. (1984) reported that the risk of colorectal carcinoma was two to six times greater than in individuals without spinal cord injury and that disease was more advanced at the time of diagnosis in men with spinal cord injury. A more recent study by Kao et al. (2016) compared non-genitourinary cancer rates between patients with SCI and patients without SCI and found a lower risk of colorectal cancer in the SCI population. A smaller study demonstrated an equal rate of colorectal carcinoma in individuals with SCI compared to age and gender matched individuals undergoing colonoscopy. In individuals with spinal cord injury who undergo colorectal carcinoma resection, the tumor distribution and stage are similar to individuals without spinal cord injury.

A study by Morris, Kucchal, and Burgess (2015) revealed lower rates of screening colonoscopy in individuals with SCIs and limitations of the procedure due to difficulty with adequate bowel preparation. Thus, it is important that routine screening for colorectal cancer be performed according to guidelines for the general population. Rectal examination is recommended annually for individuals with SCI over age 40.

(Answers B, C, D) Rates of colorectal carcinoma following SCI vary in the literature as above.

Frisbie JH, Chopra S, Foo D, Sarkarati M. Colorectal carcinoma and myelopathy. J Am Paraplegia Soc. 1984;7(2):33–6. https://doi.org/10.1080/01952307.1984.11719600.

Kao CH, Sun LM, Chen YS, Lin CL, Liang JA, Kao CH, Weng MW. Risk of nongenitourinary cancers in patients with spinal cord injury: a population-based cohort study. Medicine (Baltimore). 2016;95(2):e2462. https://doi.org/10.1097/MD.0000000000002462.

Morris BP, Kucchal T, Burgess AN. Colonoscopy after spinal cord injury: a case–control study. Spinal Cord. 2015;53(1):32–5.

Stratton MD, McKirgan LW, Wade TP, Vernava AM, Virgo KS, Johnson FE, Longo WE. Colorectal cancer in patients with previous spinal cord injury. Dis Colon Rectum. 1996;39(9):965–8. https://doi.org/10.1007/BF02054682.

Genitourinary Issues in Spinal Cord Injury

9

Karishma Gupta, Kyle A. Scarberry, Ryan P. Terlecki, and R. Caleb Kovell

Questions

1. The parameter that most accurately measures renal function in a patient with a spinal cord injury (SCI) is:

   A. Creatinine clearance
   B. Fractional excretion of sodium
   C. Proteinuria
   D. Serum cystatin C

   Answer: D.

   In patients with spinal cord injury, determination and monitoring of kidney function is of great importance and glomerular filtration rate (GFR) is considered to be the best marker of renal function. Creatinine correlates with muscle mass· but in patients with SCI, creatinine may not provide the most accurate measurement as they may have experienced muscle atrophy. Cystatin C is a non-glycosylated low molecular weight protein produced by all nucleated cells

K. Gupta (✉) · K. A. Scarberry
Urology Institute, University Hospitals Cleveland Medical Center, Case Western Reserve University School of Medicine, Cleveland, OH, USA
e-mail: Karishma.gupta2@uhhospitals.org

R. P. Terlecki
Wake Forest University Baptist Health System, Winston-Salem, NC, USA
e-mail: rterlecki@wakehealth.edu

R. C. Kovell
Perelman School of Medicine, University of Pennsylvania & The Children's Hospital of Philadelphia, Philadelphia, PA, USA
e-mail: robert.kovell@pennmedicine.upenn.edu

© The Author(s), under exclusive license to Springer Nature Switzerland AG 2022
B. A. Abramoff et al. (eds.), *The Essential Spinal Cord Injury Medicine Question Bank*, https://doi.org/10.1007/978-3-031-07796-8_9

at a constant rate, freely filtered in the glomeruli and reabsorbed and catabolized in the proximal tubular cells. The serum concentration of cystatin C is mainly determined by GFR, making it a better marker of the GFR than serum creatinine and creatinine clearance in patients with SCI.

Elmelund M, Oturai PS, Biering-Sørensen F. 50 years follow-up on plasma creatinine levels after spinal cord injury. Spinal Cord. 2014;52(5):368–72. https://doi.org/10.1038/sc.2014.24. Epub 2014 Mar 11.

Dharnidharka VR, Kwon C, Stevens G. Serum cystatin C is superior to serum creatinine as a marker of kidney function: a meta-analysis. Am J Kidney Dis. 2002;40(2):221–6. https://doi.org/10.1053/ajkd.2002.34487.

Jenkins MA, Brown DJ, Ierino FL, Ratnaike SI. Cystatin C for estimation of glomerular filtration rate in patients with spinal cord injury. Ann Clin Biochem. 2003;40(Pt 4):364–8. https://doi.org/10.1258/000456303766476995.

2. A 42-year-old male with a sacral spinal cord injury is likely to have:

   A. Normal erections
   B. No seminal vesicle emission
   C. Reflexogenic erections
   D. Psychogenic erections

Answer: D.

The neural pathways necessary for sexual function are sympathetic (T10–L2), parasympathetic (S2–S4), and motor function to perineal muscles from somatic motor neurons (S2–S4). Cerebral induced erections occur via the parasympathetic pathway, which can also be stimulated by direct penile stimulation and activation of the S2–S4 sensory fibers causing reflex-induced erections. Patients with sacral spinal cord injury are more likely to have the ability to achieve psychogenic erections, but the ability of reflexogenic erections is decreased. Psychogenic erections, however, generally do not occur in patients with complete spinal cord injuries above T9. Additionally, SCI causing disruption of the sympathetic nerve fibers can cause loss of seminal vesicle emission. Thus, in addition to loss of ability to achieve an erection, they may lose the ability to ejaculate.

Alexander M, Rosen RC. Spinal cord injuries and orgasm: a review. J Sex Marital Ther. 2008;34(4):308–24. https://doi.org/10.1080/00926230802096341.

Anderson KD, Borisoff JF, Johnson RD, Stiens SA, Elliott SL. The impact of spinal cord injury on sexual function: concerns of the general population. Spinal Cord. 2007;45(5):328–37. https://doi.org/10.1038/sj.sc.3101977. Epub 2006 Oct 10.

Andersson KE, Wagner G. Physiology of penile erection. Physiol Rev. 1995;75(1):191–236. https://doi.org/10.1152/physrev.1995.75.1.191.

3. A 44-year-old man has anejaculation after a spinal cord injury and wants to have a biological child with his 40-year-old wife. He has been able to achieve ejaculation through penile vibratory stimulation although intravaginal semen injection failed. His testes are normal volume and serum testosterone and FSH are in normal range. Semen analysis is also normal. The next step is:

A. Electroejaculation
B. Evaluation of his wife
C. Testicular sperm extraction
D. Serum testing for prolactin

Answer: B.

Female fecundity declines significantly after age 37 and his wife should be evaluated before other more invasive investigations. Of note, semen analysis is also important step to determine any concerns for impaired sperm quality or viability, factors that commonly occur after spinal cord injury and may lower the rate of success with intravaginal insemination. Further evaluation of both male and female factors will help guide the next intervention for this couple, balancing factors of invasiveness, cost, and expected success rate.

Steiner AZ, Jukic AM. Impact of female age and nulligravidity on fecundity in an older repro-
    ductive age cohort. Fertil Steril. 2016;105(6):1584–8.e1. https://doi.org/10.1016/j.fertn-
    stert.2016.02.028. Epub 2016 Mar 5.
Ibrahim E, Lynne CM, Brackett NL. Male fertility following spinal cord injury: an update.
    Andrology. 2016;4(1):13–26. https://doi.org/10.1111/andr.12119. Epub 2015 Nov 4.

4. The micturition reflex is under voluntary control and originates in the:

A. Pons
B. Medulla
C. Periaqueductal gray
D. Onuf's nucleus

Answer: A.

Bladder filling activates the stretch receptors within the bladder wall, which in turn increase activity in the myelinated fibers reaching the spinal cord. The central branch of these fibers contacts neurons in the dorsal horn of the sacral spinal cord, which project to the periaqueductal grey (PAG), a midbrain area known for nociception and emotional responses. When the bladder is filled enough to initiate voiding, the PAG activates the pontine micturition center (PMC). Bladder emptying requires a coordinated contraction of the bladder and relaxation of the urethral and striated sphincter. Onuf's nucleus is involved with the micturition process but does not initiate it. The medulla is activated during urinary storage.

Andersson KE, Arner A. Urinary bladder contraction and relaxation: physiology and pathophysiology. Physiol Rev. 2004;84(3):935–86. https://doi.org/10.1152/physrev.00038.2003.

Beckel JM, Holstege G. Neurophysiology of the lower urinary tract. Handb Exp Pharmacol. 2011;(202):149–69. https://doi.org/10.1007/978-3-642-16499-6_8.

Fowler CJ, Griffiths D, de Groat WC. The neural control of micturition. Nat Rev Neurosci. 2008;9(6):453–66. https://doi.org/10.1038/nrn2401.

Yoshimura N, de Groat WC. Neural control of the lower urinary tract. Int J Urol. 1997;4(2):111–25. https://doi.org/10.1111/j.1442-2042.1997.tb00156.x.

5. A 38-year-old male with tetraplegia undergoes creation of an ileal conduit for urinary diversion. What is the serum parameter that best reflects renal function?

   A. Blood urea nitrogen (BUN)
   B. Creatinine clearance
   C. Urine osmolality
   D. Fractional excretion of sodium

   Answer: D.

   Intestinal absorption and secretion patterns will result in inaccuracy in most traditional measures of renal function, such as creatinine clearance. Sodium handling (fractional excretion of sodium) remains stable following ileal diversion.

Jin XD, Roethlisberger S, Burkhard FC, Birkhaeuser F, Thoeny HC, Studer UE. Long-term renal function after urinary diversion by ileal conduit or orthotopic ileal bladder substitution. Eur Urol. 2012;61(3):491–7. https://doi.org/10.1016/j.eururo.2011.09.004. Epub 2011 Sep 15.

6. A 55-year-old man with paraplegia suffering from erectile dysfunction presents to the emergency department with a 5-h erection following intracavernous injection of alprostadil. Penile injection of phenylephrine to help with detumescence may result in which combinations?

   A. Hypertension and bradycardia
   B. Hypotension and tachycardia
   C. Hypertension and tachycardia
   D. Premature atrial contractions

   Answer: A.

   Phenylephrine is an alpha agonist and can cause hypertension and reflex bradycardia. Patients should be placed on the monitor when this medication is administered.

Muruve N, Hosking DH. Intracorporeal phenylephrine in the treatment of priapism. J Urol. 1996;155(1):141–3.

7. A 32-year-old female with a complete T4 spinal cord injury underwent injection of 300U of onabotulinumtoxinA for lower extremity spasticity 1 month ago. She notes that she is bothered by ongoing urinary incontinence despite maximal medical therapy including an antimuscarinic and beta-3-agonist. The best next step is:

A. Intravesical injection of 200U onabotulinumtoxinA immediately
B. Intravesical injection of 200U onabotulinumtoxinA in 2 months
C. Pelvic floor physical therapy, patient is not a candidate for intravesical onabotulinumtoxin A injection.
D. Sacral neuromodulation

Answer: B.

After failure of medical therapy, the next option to improve urinary incontinence would be onabotulinumtoxinA. OnabotulinumtoxinA should generally not be performed more frequently than every 3 months and attempts should be made to coordinate the intravesicular injections with skeletal muscle injections. Since this patient has undergone 300U of injection for spasticity last month, she will be eligible for 200U in 2 months and not immediately. Pelvic floor physical therapy would not be useful in addressing urinary incontinence in a patient with complete spinal cord injury and sacral neuromodulation is not Food and Drug Administration (FDA) approved for neurogenic bladder and would not be the next step in treatment.

Chen CY, Liao CH, Kuo HC. Therapeutic effects of detrusor botulinum toxin A injection on neurogenic detrusor overactivity in patients with different levels of spinal cord injury and types of detrusor sphincter dyssynergia. Spinal Cord. 2011;49(5):659–64. https://doi.org/10.1038/sc.2010.179. Epub 2011 Jan 18.
Ge XT, Li YF, Wang Q, Zhao JN. Effect of intravesical botulinum neurotoxin-A injection on detrusor hyperreflexia in spinal cord injured patients. Drug Res (Stuttg). 2015;65(6):327–31. https://doi.org/10.1055/s-0034-1383573. Epub 2014 Oct 28.

8. A 28-year-old male with a complete T4 spinal cord injury manages his bladder with clean intermittent catheterization (CIC) every 4 h. He reports urinary leakage between cathing. He is on maximal anticholinergic therapy, and underwent a urodynamic evaluation in the office which demonstrated ongoing, high pressure, phasic, detrusor overactivity. The best next step in management is:

A. Increase frequency of CIC
B. Intravesical injection of 200U of onabotulinumtoxinA
C. Sacral neuromodulation
D. Artificial urinary sphincter

Answer: B.

This patient has symptoms refractory to medical therapy and therefore the next option to improve his symptoms would involve onabotulinumtoxinA or bladder augmentation. Sacral nerve stimulation is not FDA approved for the treatment of neurogenic bladder (it is approved for the treatment of urinary retention and the symptoms of overactive bladder in patients who have failed lifestyle modifications, pelvic floor exercises and medical therapy).

Patients with complete spinal cord injury may not benefit from neuromodulation because it is implied that an intact reflex arc should be in place for neuromodulation to work. While this has been suggested in basic science data, it has not been proven clinically. An artificial urinary sphincter is appropriate for stress urinary incontinence which is not the cause of incontinence in this level of injury. 200U of onabotulinumtoxinA injection is an effective starting point, and this dose can be increased to 300U for refractory cases. Studies have demonstrated that 2/3 of the volume injected into the detrusor muscle and 1/3 of the volume injected into the trigonal area provided better relief of symptoms and improved compliance compared to detrusor-only injections.

Cruz F, Herschorn S, Aliotta P, Brin M, Thompson C, Lam W, Daniell G, Heesakkers J, Haag-Molkenteller C. Efficacy and safety of onabotulinumtoxinA in patients with urinary incontinence due to neurogenic detrusor overactivity: a randomised, double-blind, placebo-controlled trial. Eur Urol. 2011;60(4):742–50. https://doi.org/10.1016/j.eururo.2011.07.002. Epub 2011 Jul 13.

Leitner L, Guggenbühl-Roy S, Knüpfer SC, Walter M, Schneider MP, Tornic J, Sammer U, Mehnert U, Kessler TM. More than 15 years of experience with intradetrusor Onabotulinumtoxin A injections for treating refractory neurogenic detrusor overactivity: lessons to be learned. Eur Urol. 2016;70(3):522–8. https://doi.org/10.1016/j.eururo.2016.03.052. Epub 2016 Apr 19.

9. An 18-year-old male with T10 ASIA A spinal cord injury who voids with the Credé maneuver when he feels fullness in his lower abdomen develops new onset bilateral hydroureteronephrosis. The best next step is:

   A. Computed Tomography (CT) urogram
   B. Initiate CIC
   C. Intravesical onabotulinumtoxinA injections
   D. Alpha-adrenergic blockers

Answer: B.

The exact cause of upper tract deterioration is unclear but may be related detrusor overactivity (DO) or detrusor sphincter dyssynergia (DSD) in this patient population. The use of CIC to ensure the bladder remains adequately drained in combination with antimuscarinic medications is the best next step to prevent upper tract deterioration. Urodynamics assessment may be helpful in tailoring the regimen going forward. Intravesical onabotulinumtoxinA may be an appropriate next step depending on response to CIC and oral medications.

Alpha-adrenergic blockers are unlikely to be effective in a young male with complete spinal cord injury. Given his bilateral hydroureteronephrosis, a more aggressive management plan with incorporation of CIC is needed.

Hansen RB, Biering-Sørensen F, Kristensen JK. Bladder emptying over a period of 10–45 years after a traumatic spinal cord injury. Spinal Cord. 2004;42(11):631–7. https://doi.org/10.1038/sj.sc.3101637.

Lapides J, Diokno AC, Silber SJ, Lowe BS. Clean, intermittent self-catheterization in the treatment of urinary tract disease. J Urol. 1972;107(3):458–61. https://doi.org/10.1016/s0022-5347(17)61055-3.

Wyndaele JJ, Brauner A, Geerlings SE, Bela K, Peter T, Bjerklund-Johanson TE. Clean intermittent catheterization and urinary tract infection: review and guide for future research. BJU Int. 2012;110(11 Pt C):E910–7. https://doi.org/10.1111/j.1464-410X.2012.11549.x. Epub 2012 Oct 4.

Yalçın S, Ersöz M. Urodynamic findings, bladder emptying methods and therapeutic approaches in patients with upper lumbar and lower lumbar-sacral spinal cord injury. Neurol Sci. 2015;36(11):2061–5. https://doi.org/10.1007/s10072-015-2311-1. Epub 2015 Jul 3.

10. A 32-year-old male with a T6 spinal cord injury is noted to have new onset hydroureteronephrosis. The finding most indicative of development of upper tract deterioration on urodynamics is:

A. Low bladder compliance
B. Low detrusor LPP
C. Functional bladder capacity of 200 mL
D. Involuntary bladder contractions

Answer: A.

Compliance is defined as the change in volume divided by the change in pressure. Most studies support that a bladder compliance <10–20 mL/cm H_2O would be abnormal. Patients with decreased bladder compliance are at great risk for upper tract deterioration, especially when patients maintain urinary volumes that are consistently in high pressure ranges. Detrusor LPP > 40 cm H_2O is a risk factor for upper tract deterioration; however, it is not as significant as poor bladder compliance. Low detrusor leak point pressures often indicates that the patient will experience incontinence, but it does provide a "pop off" mechanism for pressure rather than transmitting pressure to the upper tracts. A smaller bladder capacity is not an independent risk factor for hydronephrosis unless associated with elevated storage pressures.

McGuire EJ. Urodynamics of the neurogenic bladder. Urol Clin North Am. 2010;37(4):507–16. https://doi.org/10.1016/j.ucl.2010.06.002.

Weld KJ, Graney MJ, Dmochowski RR. Differences in bladder compliance with time and associations of bladder management with compliance in spinal cord injured patients. J Urol. 2000;163(4):1228–33.

11. A 34-year-old male with a C6 spinal cord injury managed with CIC every 4 h presents with headache, profuse sweating, and generalized back and abdominal pain. UA shows 25 red blood cells/high powered field (HPF), 25 white blood cells/HPF, and no bacteria. Bladder scan demonstrates 5cc. CT abdomen and pelvis without contrast demonstrates an obstructive 1.5 cm stone in the right renal pelvis. The next step is:

    A. Urgent stent placement
    B. Placement of an indwelling foley catheter
    C. Urine culture
    D. Urinary alkalinization

    Answer: A.

    Clinicians should have a high index of suspicion for stone disease in patients with SCI. Patients with SCI are at a higher risk of stone formation due to immobility, which can lead to hypercalciuria secondary to demineralization of bone. Additional causes of stone formation include urinary stasis despite attempts at complete bladder emptying. In this patient, stent placement will address the obstruction. While urinary alkalinization is useful for stone treatment, it may be more appropriate after addressing the patient's acute presentation.

    Chen Y, DeVivo MJ, Roseman JM. Current trend and risk factors for kidney stones in persons with spinal cord injury: a longitudinal study. Spinal Cord. 2000;38(6):346–53. https://doi. org/10.1038/sj.sc.3101008.
    Nabbout P, Slobodov G, Culkin DJ. Surgical management of urolithiasis in spinal cord injury patients. Curr Urol Rep. 2014;15(6):408. https://doi.org/10.1007/s11934-014-0408-3.
    Ramsey S, McIlhenny C. Evidence-based management of upper tract urolithiasis in the spinal cord-injured patient. Spinal Cord. 2011;49(9):948–54. https://doi.org/10.1038/ sc.2011.50. Epub 2011 May 31.
    Welk B, Fuller A, Razvi H, Denstedt J. Renal stone disease in spinal-cord-injured patients. J Endourol. 2012;26(8):954–9. https://doi.org/10.1089/end.2012.0063. Epub 2012 Apr 17.

12. A 42-year-old female with a T6 spinal cord injury with a history of recurrent urinary tract infections (UTI)s who just completed an antibiotic course for a UTI one week ago, presents to the Emergency Department with fevers, chills, nausea, and vomiting. She also has a history of a bladder augmentation. She reports successfully catheterizing 2 h ago. The best next step in management is antibiotics and:

    A. Placement of an indwelling Foley catheter
    B. CT Abdomen and Pelvis
    C. Immediate urologic consultation
    D. Suprapubic catheter placement

    Answer: B.

Both SCI and CIC are associated with an increased incidence of urinary tract lithiasis, particularly in the bladder. Patients with augmentations, especially those with catheterizable channels and those with bladder neck closures, are at increased risk of stone formation due to mucus production, difficulty with complete emptying, and changes to urine electrolyte composition. In patients with refractory, persistent, or recurrent UTIs, a nidus of infection should be suspected and stone disease would be high on the differential. Therefore, imaging should be performed to rule out urinary obstruction.

Chen Y, DeVivo MJ, Roseman JM. Current trend and risk factors for kidney stones in persons with spinal cord injury: a longitudinal study. Spinal Cord. 2000;38(6):346–53. https://doi. org/10.1038/sj.sc.3101008.
DeVivo MJ, Fine PR, Cutter GR, Maetz HM. The risk of renal calculi in spinal cord injury patients. J Urol. 1984;131(5):857–60. https://doi.org/10.1016/s0022-5347(17)50680-1.

13. A 26-year-old patient with a history of L1 spinal cord injury and neurogenic bladder with a history of augmentation cystoplasty, bladder neck closure and catheterizable channel formation has been struggling with persistent bladder stone formation. Which of the following has been shown to decrease the rate of bladder stone formation in this patient population:

    A. Daily potassium citrate supplementation
    B. Daily antibiotic therapy
    C. Daily irrigation of the bladder with at least 240cc
    D. Daily antimuscarinic therapy

    Answer: C.

    Daily irrigation has been shown to decrease the rate of bladder stone formation in patients with augmented bladders. This has also been correlated with volume of irrigation, with increasing irrigation volumes inversely correlated with stone formation rates over time. None of the other options has been shown to decrease stone formation, although mitigating infections or upper tract calculi may decrease lower tract stone rates in certain populations.

Husmann DA. Long-term complications following bladder augmentations in patients with spina bifida: bladder calculi, perforation of the augmented bladder and upper tract deterioration. Transl Androl Urol. 2016;5(1):3–11. https://doi.org/10.3978/j.issn.2223-4683.2015.12.06.

14. A 32-year-old male with a history of a T10 spinal cord injury has a urine culture sent at a routine office visit which returns as >100k Klebsiella pneumoniae. Isolates are sensitive to ceftriaxone, ciprofloxacin, and Fosfomycin. He has a history of a bladder augmentation. He catheterizes through a catheterizable channel every 4 h without difficulty. His creatinine is 0.5 mg/dL. Recent bladder ultrasound shows no stones. He is asymptomatic. What is the appropriate treatment:

A. No antibiotic management
B. Oral antibiotic management for 5 days with fosfomycin
C. Oral antibiotic management for 14 days with ciprofloxacin
D. Intravenous (IV) antibiotic management for 14 days with ceftriaxone

Answer: A.

Diagnosis of a urinary tract infection in patients with spinal cord injuries can be challenging. The classic symptoms of dysuria, suprapubic pain, and frequency may be absent and clinical symptoms can be vague. Asymptomatic bacteriuria is very common in patients who self-catheterize, have indwelling tubes, or urinary diversions. In the absence of symptoms or clinical signs of infection, a positive urine culture generally does not require antibiotic treatment. Judicious use of antibiotics in this patient population can help prevent development of resistant organisms which make treatment of future infections more challenging.

Lewis RI, Carrion HM, Lockhart JL, Politano VA. Significance of asymptomatic bacteriuria in neurogenic bladder disease. Urology. 1984;23(4):343–7. https://doi.org/10.1016/0090-4295(84)90136-5.
Nicolle LE, Bradley S, Colgan R, Rice JC, Schaeffer A, Hooton TM; Infectious Diseases Society of America; American Society of Nephrology; American Geriatric Society. Infectious Diseases Society of America guidelines for the diagnosis and treatment of asymptomatic bacteriuria in adults. Clin Infect Dis. 2005;40(5):643–54. https://doi.org/10.1086/427507. Epub 2005 Feb 4. Erratum in: Clin Infect Dis. 2005;40(10):1556.

15. The strongest indication for antimicrobial therapy in a patient with a spinal cord injury is:

A. Bacteriuria on UA
B. >100,000 colony-forming units/mL on urine culture
C. Foul-smelling urine
D. Flank and abdominal discomfort

Answer: D.

Asymptomatic bacteriuria is commonly present in patients with spinal cord injury and generally does not need to be treated. Symptomatic infectious, however, should be treated and usually manifest as increased leakage between catheterizations if managed by CIC, increased spasticity, increased flank or abdominal discomfort, fevers, presence of autonomic dysreflexia, and malaise or lethargy. Malodorous urine alone is not indicative for infection meriting treatment.

Biering-Sørensen F, Bagi P, Høiby N. Urinary tract infections in patients with spinal cord lesions: treatment and prevention. Drugs. 2001;61(9):1275–87. https://doi.org/10.2165/00003495-200161090-00004.
Siroky MB. Pathogenesis of bacteriuria and infection in the spinal cord injured patient. Am J Med. 2002;113(Suppl. 1A):67S–79S. https://doi.org/10.1016/s0002-9343(02)01061-6.

16. A 46-year-old male with a T6 spinal cord injury and a history of recurrent UTIs reports intermittent episodes of gross hematuria and increased bladder spasms. His bladder has been managed with a chronic indwelling foley catheter since diagnosis 17 years ago. The best next step is:

    A. Evaluation with imaging and cystoscopy
    B. Have the patient change to CIC
    C. Initiate broad-spectrum antibiotic therapy
    D. Urodynamic study

    Answer: A.

    Bladder cancer is a rare but serious occurrence in SCI patients and is more common than in the general population. Physicians need to have a high index of suspicion for bladder cancer, particularly among those patients managed with long-term indwelling catheters. Bladder cancer is the third leading cause of cancer death in the SCI population. Historical studies have reported a 2.5–10% incidence of squamous cell carcinoma in the spinal cord-injured population. In this case, a hematuria workup would be warranted with imaging to rule out calculi and flexible cystoscopy to evaluate for bladder lesions.

Kaufman JM, Fam B, Jacobs SC, Gabilondo F, Yalla S, Kane JP, Rossier AB. Bladder cancer and squamous metaplasia in spinal cord injury patients. J Urol. 1977;118(6):967–71. https://doi.org/10.1016/s0022-5347(17)58266-x.

West DA, Cummings JM, Longo WE, Virgo KS, Johnson FE, Parra RO. Role of chronic catheterization in the development of bladder cancer in patients with spinal cord injury. Urology. 1999;53(2):292–7. https://doi.org/10.1016/s0090-4295(98)00517-2.

Welk B, McIntyre A, Teasell R, Potter P, Loh E. Bladder cancer in individuals with spinal cord injuries. Spinal Cord. 2013;51(7):516–21. https://doi.org/10.1038/sc.2013.33. Epub 2013 Apr 23.

17. A 24-year-old male with a complete T4 spinal cord injury underwent intra-vesical injection of 200U of onabotulinumtoxinA for urinary incontinence 5 days ago. He presents to the emergency department with a chief complaint of increased bladder spasms and urinary leakage. Post-void residual is 5cc. The best next step is:

    A. Check a urine culture
    B. Place an indwelling foley catheter
    C. Repeat injection of 200 units onabotulinumtoxinA in 1 month
    D. Counsel patient on need for augmentation cystoplasty

    Answer: A.

    There are several risks associated with intravesical onabotulinumtoxinA therapy, including urinary tract infection, hematuria, and urinary retention. The rate of UTI after intradetrusor injections ranges from 2% to 32%, with Escherichia coli being the most common pathogen. This presence of bladder spasms and urinary leakage indicate that the patient should undergo evaluation for a possible UTI, and are not necessarily indicators of failure of therapy.

Leitner L, Sammer U, Walter M, Knüpfer SC, Schneider MP, Seifert B, Tornic J, Mehnert U, Kessler TM. Antibiotic prophylaxis may not be necessary in patients with asymptomatic bacteriuria undergoing intradetrusor onabotulinumtoxinA injections for neurogenic detrusor overactivity. Sci Rep. 2016;6:33197. https://doi.org/10.1038/srep33197.

Mouttalib S, Khan S, Castel-Lacanal E, Guillotreau J, De Boissezon X, Malavaud B, Marque P, Rischmann P, Gamé X. Risk of urinary tract infection after detrusor botulinum toxin A injections for refractory neurogenic detrusor overactivity in patients with no antibiotic treatment. BJU Int. 2010;106(11):1677–80. https://doi.org/10.1111/j.1464-410X.2010.09435.x.

18. A 28-year-old male with tetraplegia and a history of recurrent UTIs and bladder stones requiring surgical treatment every 6 months was noted to have a positive urine culture for *Proteus mirabilis*. He is currently managed with a 14Fr indwelling urethral catheter. The best next step is treatment of current urine culture and:

A. Prophylactic antibiotics
B. Upsize urethral catheter
C. Suprapubic tube
D. Sphincterotomy and condom catheter

Answer: D.

UTIs and chronic bacteriuria is a risk factor for stone formation in the SCI population. Daily suppressive antibiotics are not enough; management involves eliminating potential sources of infection. Proteus mirabilis is a urease producing bacteria, associated with bacterial biofilm. The patient cannot perform CIC on his own and any indwelling catheter will be associated with colonization and bacteriuria. Of the options available, sphincterotomy with condom catheter drainage is his best chance of minimizing chronic bacteriuria. Patients must accept that they will be incontinent from below after the procedure. Patients also should be monitored to assure emptying after the procedure. Although urinary diversion would be the best long-term solution, most patients initially prefer sphincterotomy as it the least-invasive option.

Noll F, Sauerwein D, Stöhrer M. Transurethral sphincterotomy in quadriplegic patients: long-term-follow-up. Neurourol Urodyn. 1995;14(4):351–8. https://doi.org/10.1002/nau.1930140409.

Perkash I. Transurethral sphincterotomy provides significant relief in autonomic dysreflexia in spinal cord injured male patients: long-term follow-up results. J Urol. 2007;177(3):1026–9. https://doi.org/10.1016/j.juro.2006.10.066.

19. A 32-year-old female with a T10 spinal cord injury has chronic, asymptomatic
    Escherichia coli bacteriuria unresponsive to antimicrobial therapy. She is man-
    aged by CIC with volumes of 400 mL. The best next step in management is:

    A. Reassurance
    B. Urine culture
    C. Urinary acidification
    D. Prophylactic antibiotics

Answer: A.

Asymptomatic bacteriuria is a frequent finding in spinal cord injured patients
managed by CIC. There is no indication to perform routine urine culture in
these patients. The patient needs reassurance that chronic bacteriuria is not concerning, provided that his urine storage pressures are low, the patient is symptom free and the bacteria is not a urease producing bacteria. Asymptomatic
bacteriuria should not be treated, except in cases when the patient must undergo
surgical or endoscopic manipulations. Urine acidification has not been proven
to decrease the risk of bacteriuria in spinal cord injured patients. Routine antibiotic prophylaxis is not required because there is no evidence that it reduces
symptomatic UTIs.

Biering-Sørensen F, Bagi P, Høiby N. Urinary tract infections in patients with spinal cord
    lesions: treatment and prevention. Drugs. 2001;61(9):1275–87. https://doi.org/10.216
    5/00003495-200161090-00004.
Siroky MB. Pathogenesis of bacteriuria and infection in the spinal cord injured patient. Am
    J Med. 2002;113(Suppl. 1A):67S–79S. https://doi.org/10.1016/s0002-9343(02)01061-6.
Wyndaele JJ, Brauner A, Geerlings SE, Bela K, Peter T, Bjerklund-Johanson TE. Clean inter-
    mittent catheterization and urinary tract infection: review and guide for future research.
    BJU Int. 2012;110(11 Pt C):E910–7. https://doi.org/10.1111/j.1464-410X.2012.11549.x.
    Epub 2012 Oct 4.

20. In addition to good hygiene, the best method to reduce the incidence of catheter-
    associated UTIs in individuals with indwelling catheters is:

    A. Daily prophylactic antibiotics
    B. Catheter irrigation
    C. Maintenance of a closed drainage system
    D. Weekly catheter changes

Answer: C.

Among UTIs acquired in the hospital, approximately 75% are associated with
a urinary catheter. An indwelling catheter is also an option utilized for bladder
management in patients with SCI. Indwelling urethral catheters are generally
reserved for patients unable or unwilling to perform CIC. Catheter-associated

UTIs (CAUTI) result in increased morbidity and mortality among these patients. There are several methods to minimize the risk of CAUTI. In addition to good hygiene and care of equipment, a closed drainage system and an aseptic insertion technique is recommended to reduce risk of CAUTI. Catheter irrigation and daily prophylactic antibiotics are not recommended for routine use in patients with indwelling urethral catheters, and have not been shown to reduce risk of CAUTI. Catheters are changed approximately every 4–6 weeks, and weekly catheter changes are not feasible from a practical perspective.

Averch TD, Stoffel J, Goldman HB, et al. AUA White Paper on catheter-associated urinary tract infections: Definitions and significance in the urologic patient. Urol Pract. 2015;2:321–328.

Hooton TM, Bradley SF, Cardenas DD, Colgan R, Geerlings SE, Rice JC, Saint S, Schaeffer AJ, Tambayh PA, Tenke P, Nicolle LE; Infectious Diseases Society of America. Diagnosis, prevention, and treatment of catheter-associated urinary tract infection in adults: 2009 International Clinical Practice Guidelines from the Infectious Diseases Society of America. Clin Infect Dis. 2010;50(5):625–63. https://doi.org/10.1086/650482.

Centers for Disease Control and Prevention. Catheter-associated urinary tract infection. Available from: https://www.cdc.gov/hai/ca_uti/uti.html [Accessed December 8, 2020].

21. A 40-year-old woman with tetraplegia and frequent plugging of her 20 French suprapubic catheter from sediment is now requiring catheter changes nearly every two weeks. Which of the following represents the next best course of action?

    A. Magnetic Resonance Imaging (MRI) of the pelvis
    B. Video urodynamics
    C. Increase size of suprapubic tube to 24 French
    D. Urine culture for urease producing bacteria

    Answer: D.

    Organisms producing urease (e.g., Proteus) are associated with frequent catheter encrustation. Eradication through antibiotic therapy may prove effective as a long-term strategy.

Jacobsen SM, Stickler DJ, Mobley HL, Shirtliff ME. Complicated catheter-associated urinary tract infections due to Escherichia coli and Proteus mirabilis. Clin Microbiol Rev. 2008;21(1):26–59. https://doi.org/10.1128/CMR.00019-07.

22. A 42-year-old female with a history of a T12 spinal cord injury is brought to the emergency room with abdominal distension and diffuse abdominal pain. She has a history of a bladder augmentation in the past. She admits to binge drinking last night and has not catheterized in over 16 h. Her serum creatinine is 3.2 mg/dL from a baseline of 0.9 mg/dL. Her blood pressure is 90/50 mmHg and heart rate is 140 beats per minute (bpm). A CT scan shows free fluid in the abdomen. A catheter is placed and returns 200cc of blood-tinged urine. In addition to fluid resuscitation and antibiotics coverage, the next step in management is:

A. Admission for observation
B. Abdominal drain placement
C. Immediate urologic consultation for operative management
D. Initiation of emergent dialysis

Answer: C.

Bladder perforation is a risk for any patient with an augmented bladder or neo-bladder. Catheterization must be done consistently to keep the bladder drained as these patients may not have a "pop-off" mechanism to leak urine otherwise. As the bladder becomes distended and pressure builds, the suture line where the bowel and bladder are sewn together or the bowel segment itself can become relatively ischemic. If this area weakens, perforation can occur leading to urine entering the peritoneum leading to peritonitis and possible sepsis. Immediate decompression of the pouch with a catheter may be helpful, but ultimately, these patients generally require operative exploration, abdominal drainage, and repair of the perforated area. Creatinine elevation can be multifactorial from absorption of urine across the peritoneum, dehydration, sepsis, etc. This situation is more common in patients who abuse alcohol or use IV drugs and individuals with mental health issues. Catheterization regimens should be monitored especially closely in these populations.

Chartier-Kastler EJ, Mongiat-Artus P, Bitker MO, Chancellor MB, Richard F, Denys P. Long-term results of augmentation cystoplasty in spinal cord injury patients. Spinal Cord. 2000;38(8):490–4. https://doi.org/10.1038/sj.sc.3101033.
Husmann DA. Long-term complications following bladder augmentations in patients with spina bifida: bladder calculi, perforation of the augmented bladder and upper tract deterioration. Transl Androl Urol. 2016;5(1):3–11. https://doi.org/10.3978/j.issn.2223-4683.2015.12.06.

23. A 40-year-old female with a history of a complete C8 spinal cord injury has a neurogenic bladder. On urodynamics testing, she has a 500cc capacity with good compliance throughout filling. She has no hydronephrosis on ultrasound. She has had minimal urinary tract infections over the last 5 years. She is catheterized via urethra every 4 h by the staff at her nursing facility. Catheterization requires multiple caregivers to position her for access to the urethra. This is creating a tremendous burden on both her and the staff at the facility. Which would be the best option going forward?

A. Creation of an ileal chimney (ileovesicostomy)
B. Creation of an ileal loop urinary diversion
C. Creation of a catheterizable channel
D. Indwelling foley catheter

Answer: C.

This patient is doing quite well with intermittent catheterization but the process of performing catheterization via urethra is challenging. She has good bladder capacity, no upper tract changes and minimal infections. Creation of a catheterizable channel using appendix or bowel to the level of the umbilicus or to an area on the abdomen tailored to her positioning may allow for ongoing catheterization in a much simpler fashion if she is a reasonable candidate for surgery.

An ileal chimney involves placing a piece of ileum onto the native bladder with drainage to the skin as a stoma. For patients with a compliant native bladder of reasonable capacity who are not ambulatory, these systems often do not drain well and may be a set up for infection, stone formation and urinary stasis. An ileal loop may be a reasonable option if CIC were not working for her, but the complication rate is higher than catheterizable channel creation, the diversion is incontinent by nature, and may leave her with a potentially higher rate of UTIs. Indwelling foley catheter placement is likely to increase her rate of UTIs, increase her chances of development of squamous changes/carcinoma and result in urethral erosion over time. Suprapubic tube placement can be considered in some patients although CIC is preferred whenever possible.

Leslie B, Lorenzo AJ, Moore K, Farhat WA, Bägli DJ, Pippi Salle JL. Long-term follow-up and time to event outcome analysis of continent catheterizable channels. J Urol. 2011;185(6):2298–302. https://doi.org/10.1016/j.juro.2011.02.601. Epub 2011 Apr 21.

24. A 48-year-old female with a history of T6 spinal cord injury has been managed with a chronic indwelling foley catheter for the last 15 years. She frequently has substantial urinary leakage around her indwelling 16Fr foley catheter and inquires about options to manage her incontinence. Physical examination reveals a widely dilated urethra around the foley catheter. Urodynamic study shows no detrusor overactivity. The best next step is:

A. Upsizing the foley catheter to 2-Fr with 30cc in foley balloon
B. Suprapubic (SP) catheter
C. Bladder neck closure and suprapubic catheter
D. Antimuscarinic medications

Answer: C.

The patient is exhibiting signs of an eroded urethra secondary to long-term indwelling catheter placement. Placement of a larger indwelling catheter with a greater volume in the foley balloon will likely worsen the erosion without improvement in urinary incontinence. A suprapubic catheter alone is unlikely to address the leakage per urethra. The best management option is bladder neck closure with suprapubic tube placement, as a suprapubic tube alone will not prevent dependent leakage if the bladder neck and sphincter mechanism have been compromised. Additional options that can be considered include urinary diversion, with the type of diversion (continent vs. non-continent) depending on the patient's dexterity, level of independence, and willingness to perform CIC.

Ginger VA, Miller JL, Yang CC. Bladder neck closure and suprapubic tube placement in a debilitated patient population. Neurourol Urodyn. 2010;29(3):382–6. https://doi. org/10.1002/nau.20751.

Levy JB, Jacobs JA, Wein AJ. Combined abdominal and vaginal approach for bladder neck closure and permanent suprapubic tube: urinary diversion in the neurologically impaired woman. J Urol. 1994;152(6 Pt 1):2081–2. https://doi.org/10.1016/s0022-5347(17)32313-3.

Rovner ES, Goudelocke CM, Gilchrist A, Lebed B. Transvaginal bladder neck closure with posterior urethral flap for devastated urethra. Urology. 2011;78(1):208–12. https://doi. org/10.1016/j.urology.2010.11.054.

25. A 17-year-old male with T4 spinal cord injury develops hypotension and tachycardia during a left ureteroscopy for treatment of an obstructive 1.2 cm stone in the renal pelvis. He had a history of struvite stones in the past. His preoperative urine culture was negative and he received IV prophylactic antibiotics prior to the start of the procedure. The next step is:

A. Empty the bladder
B. Place ureteral stent and abort
C. Decrease the fluid pressure
D. Pressor support

Answer: B.

The symptoms of hypotension and tachycardia are more likely to be related to sepsis caused by treatment of an infectious or struvite stone. Continuation of the procedure may cause more release of bacteria and endotoxins and lead to further bacteremia. Therefore, the upper tract should be drained and the procedure should be aborted. Definitive stone management can be undertaken at a later date when he has stabilized. Autonomic dysreflexia can occur in patients with spinal cord injury levels above T6 but generally presents with hypertension and reflex bradycardia.

Donnellan SM, Bolton DM. The impact of contemporary bladder management techniques on struvite calculi associated with spinal cord injury. BJU Int. 1999;84(3):280–5.

Karlsson AK. Autonomic dysreflexia. Spinal Cord. 1999;37(6):383–91. https://doi. org/10.1038/sj.sc.3100867.

Liu N, Zhou M, Biering-Sørensen F, Krassioukov AV. Iatrogenic urological triggers of autonomic dysreflexia: a systematic review. Spinal Cord. 2015;53(7):500–9. https://doi. org/10.1038/sc.2015.39. Epub 2015 Mar 24.

Shergill IS, Arya M, Hamid R, Khastgir J, Patel HR, Shah PJ. The importance of autonomic dysreflexia to the urologist. BJU Int. 2004;93(7):923–6. https://doi.org/10.1111/j.1464-41 0X.2003.04756.x.

26. A 28-year-old female with T6 spinal cord injury underwent a left ureteral stent placement for an obstructive 9 mm left ureteropelvic junction stone 8 months ago. She manages her bladder with CIC every 6 h. She missed a few clinic appointments due to lack of available transportation. However, she reports feeling well, denies flank pain, and has minimal leakage between catheterizations. The next step is:

   A. Urinary alkalization
   B. 24-h urine collection
   C. Referral to urology for retained stent
   D. Renal bladder US

Answer: C.

A retained ureteral stent is defined as a stent in place for more than 6 months. While this patient underwent management to decompress the kidney and upper tract that was being blocked by the stone, she did not undergo definitive stone treatment. Retained stents pose a significant problem and can lead to severe encrustation, stone formation, and recurrent urinary tract infections. If left unaddressed, retained stents can lead to irreversible nephron damage and cause significant morbidity and mortality.

Lam JS, Gupta M. Tips and tricks for the management of retained ureteral stents. J Endourol. 2002;16(10):733–41. https://doi.org/10.1089/08927790260472881.
Vajpeyi V, Chipde S, Khan FA, Parashar S. Forgotten double-J stent: Experience of a tertiary care center. Urol Ann. 2020;12(2):138–143. https://doi.org/10.4103/UA.UA_73_19. Epub 2020 Apr 14.

27. A 24-year old male with quadriplegia has urinary incontinence on high-dose medical therapy and an onabotulinumtoxinA regimen. Video urodynamics demonstrate a detrusor leak point pressure (DLPP) of 70 cm H_2O at 75 mL capacity without vesicouretral reflux (VUR). The best next step is:

   A. Continue current management
   B. Ileovesicostomy
   C. Augmentation cystoplasty
   D. Clean intermittent catheterization

Answer: B.

Ileovesicostomy is an incontinent diversion, consisting of the interposition of a segment of ileum between the bladder and the skin. This patient has dangerously elevated intravesical pressures and a continuously draining ileovesicostomy will permit low pressure bladder emptying. The incompetent outlet of the ileovesicostomy acts as a "pop off" valve as the bladder fills, which would allow the intravesical pressures to remain low. Ileovesicostomy should always be undertaken with care given its high complication rate. If chosen, the ideal patient for an ileovesicostomy has a low capacity, high pressure bladder to prevent stasis in the system, but this option should always be chosen with care due to the risk of complications (mucus production, stone formation, infections, poor drainage, ongoing need for catheterization, etc.). Urinary diversion with ileal conduit would also be a reasonable option (although this comes with a higher risk of ureteroenteric anastomotic strictures).

Continuing current management may lead to injury to the upper urinary tract. The patient is also a quadriplegic and would not be able to physically handle catheterization without substantial assistance; thus, augmentation with its requirement to CIC may not be an ideal option for this patient. An indwelling catheter would another potential option although would be associated with a risk of UTI, stones, cancer, and urethral erosion.

Gauthier AR Jr, Winters JC. Incontinent ileovesicostomy in the management of neurogenic bladder dysfunction. Neurourol Urodyn. 2003;22(2):142–6. https://doi.org/10.1002/nau.10093.
Tan HJ, Stoffel J, Daignault S, McGuire EJ, Latini JM. Ileovesicostomy for adults with neurogenic bladders: complications and potential risk factors for adverse outcomes. Neurourol Urodyn. 2008;27(3):238–43. https://doi.org/10.1002/nau.20467.
Schwartz SL, Kennelly MJ, McGuire EJ, Faerber GJ. Incontinent ileo-vesicostomy urinary diversion in the treatment of lower urinary tract dysfunction. J Urol. 1994;152(1):99–102. https://doi.org/10.1016/s0022-5347(17)32826-4.

28. The most likely cause of spontaneous bladder perforation following enterocystoplasty is:

    A. Mucous plug
    B. Presence of malignancy
    C. Inconsistent catheterization
    D. Chronic inflammation

Answer: C.

Bladder perforation is a serious complication of enterocystoplasty, as they are likely to be intraperitoneal and may lead to sepsis, peritonitis, and death. Ischemic necrosis of the augmented bladder wall may result from inefficient bladder emptying and chronic overdistension. Therefore, perforation is the result of poor compliance with the catheterization regimen. This may be an especially high risk in patients with substance abuse or mental health issues.

While mucous plugs and chronic inflammation may be contributing factors, they are not the primary cause of bladder rupture following augmentation cystoplasty. Bladder malignancy following enterocystoplasty is rare and not associated with spontaneous bladder perforation.

Chartier-Kastler EJ, Mongiat-Artus P, Bitker MO, Chancellor MB, Richard F, Denys P. Long-term results of augmentation cystoplasty in spinal cord injury patients. Spinal Cord. 2000;38(8):490–4. https://doi.org/10.1038/sj.sc.3101033.

Chen JL, Kuo HC. Long-term outcomes of augmentation enterocystoplasty with an ileal segment in patients with spinal cord injury. J Formos Med Assoc. 2009;108(6):475–80. https://doi.org/10.1016/S0929-6646(09)60095-4.

Gurung PM, Attar KH, Abdul-Rahman A, Morris T, Hamid R, Shah PJ. Long-term outcomes of augmentation ileocystoplasty in patients with spinal cord injury: a minimum of 10 years of follow-up. BJU Int. 2012;109(8):1236–42. https://doi.org/10.1111/j.1464-410X.2011.10509.x. Epub 2011 Aug 18.

29. An obese 27-year-old male with tetraplegia and a chronic suprapubic catheter elects to undergo creation of an ileal conduit. Antibiotic prophylaxis for surgery should involve which of the following:

A. Ampicillin and gentamicin 24 h before incision and continued after 72 h
B. Third generation cephalosporin + metronidazole 30 min before incision and discontinued within 24 h
C. Triple antibiotic therapy 30 min before incision and discontinued after 1 week
D. First generation cephalosporin 30 min before incision and discontinued within 24 h.

Answer: B.

For abdominal surgery with entrance into the urinary tract, the American Urological Association antibiotics best practice statement recommends a 2nd or 3rd generation cephalosporin (or aminoglycoside) and metronidazole as standard therapy to be discontinued within 24 h.

Alternative regimens for allergic patients include ampicillin/sulbactam, ticarcillin/clavulanate, piperacillin/tazobactam or a fluoroquinolone.

Consideration should be given to the patient's preoperative urine culture and antibiotics may need to be adjusted based on the patient's specific condition or local sensitivity patterns. For complicated patients with resistance patterns, an infectious disease team consultation can be helpful.

Lightner DJ, Wymer K, Sanchez J, Kavoussi L. Best Practice Statement on Urologic Procedures and Antimicrobial Prophylaxis. J Urol. 2020;203(2):351–6. https://doi.org/10.1097/JU.0000000000000509. Epub 2019 Aug 23.

30. A 61-year-old woman with paraplegia presents to the urology clinic 6 months after creation of an Indiana pouch (continent cutaneous diversion with a neo-bladder) with complaints of some abdominal fullness and low-grade fevers. Imaging shows mild bilateral hydronephrosis. Her creatinine is normal and urine culture is positive for Klebsiella. After antibiotic therapy, which of the following measures should be taken?

A. Placement of a suprapubic catheter
B. Conversion to incontinent diversion
C. Regimen of mechanical pouch irrigation
D. Potassium Citrate with meals

Answer: C.

Pouchitis can occur from mucus accumulation and infection. This can be improved with an irrigation regimen of the neobladder.

Patients may have a difficult time describing their symptoms after bowel interposition given the nerve supply to the neobladder will be that of the bowel. They will no longer describe a classic sensation of needing to void, but may complain of a sense of fullness or bloating.

Defoor W, Ferguson D, Mashni S, Creelman L, Reeves D, Minevich E, Reddy P, Shel-
   don C. Safety of gentamicin bladder irrigations in complex urological cases. J Urol.
   2006;175(5):1861–4. https://doi.org/10.1016/S0022-5347(05)00928-6.
Shen B, Lashner BA. Diagnosis and treatment of pouchitis. Gastroenterol Hepatol (N Y).
   2008;4(5):355–61.

31. A 29-year old woman is taken to the operating room for revision of the catheterizable limb of her Indiana pouch created 5 years earlier for neurogenic bladder secondary to SCI. Hemostasis is quite challenging as increased bleeding is encountered. The bleeding is likely related to:

A. Thrombocytopenia
B. Decreased prothrombin time
C. Decreased factors VII and X
D. Decreased Factor VIII

Answer: C.

Loss of terminal ileum results in less absorption of Vitamin K over time, which is necessary for production of factors VII and X, which are part of the extrinsic pathway and measured by prothrombin time (which would be elevated).

Patients in whom terminal ileum has been used should also be checked periodically for vitamin B12 levels as this is the site of B12 absorption in the bowel.

Perrouin-Verbe MA, Chartier-Kastler E, Even A, Denys P, Rouprêt M, Phé V. Long-term
   complications of continent cutaneous urinary diversion in adult spinal cord injured
   patients. Neurourol Urodyn. 2016;35(8):1046–1050. https://doi.org/10.1002/nau.22879.
   Epub 2015 Sep 23.
Plancke HR, Delaere KP, Pons C. Indiana pouch in female patients with spinal cord injury.
   Spinal Cord. 1999;37(3):208–10. https://doi.org/10.1038/sj.sc.3100731.

32. A 48-year-old man with chronic kidney disease (CKD) (GFR 25 mL/s) and neurogenic bladder resulting from a T11 SCI 30 years prior is referred for surgical management of his incontinence which is resulting in skin breakdown. He had successful urethral sphincterotomy 5 years ago but his condom catheter can no longer stay on due to obesity. His manual dexterity is intact and he feels confident he can catheterize without issue. His best option would be:

A. Incontinent diversion with ileal conduit
B. Ileal augmentation cystoplasty and bladder neck closure
C. Continent colon pouch with catheterizable channel (Indiana pouch)
D. Suprapubic catheter placement

Answer: A.

Continent urinary diversion with bowel is contraindicated in patients with advanced CKD due to the risk of significant metabolic abnormalities. This occurs as a longer segment of bowel is used for augmentations & continent diversions and the urine dwells within the system longer. This leads to much more contact time between the urine and bowel mucosa than in an incontinent urinary diversion.

An ileal conduit allows rapid transport of urine into a stoma bag, limiting the bowel's reabsorption of urine metabolites. A suprapubic catheter would not adequately relieve this patient's incontinence as urine would continue to leak via the urethra given the lack of outlet resistance from his prior sphincterotomy.

Skinner DG, Studer UE, Okada K, Aso Y, Hautmann H, Koontz W, Okada Y, Rowland RG, Van Velthoven RF. Which patients are suitable for continent diversion or bladder substitution following cystectomy or other definitive local treatment? Int J Urol. 1995;2(Suppl. 2):105–12. https://doi.org/10.1111/j.1442-2042.1995.tb00483.x.

33. An 18-year-old with a C6 spinal cord injury 6 months prior comes to the office for urodynamic testing to establish baseline bladder function. He has been managed with a suprapubic tube since his injury. As the bladder is filled to 200cc, the patient becomes diaphoretic and flushed. His blood pressure is found to be 200/120 mgHg and his heart rate is 48 bpm. The next step in management is:

A. Administer a bolus of NS
B. Administer intravenous nifedipine and continue the test
C. Administer intramuscular atropine and clamp the infusion catheter
D. Open the suprapubic tube and drain the bladder

Answer: D.

Patients with high spinal cord lesions (usually above the T6 level) are susceptible to autonomic dysreflexia. Urologic causes such as a distended bladder, clogged catheter or urologic testing are the most common triggers for the condition. Similar pathology can occur with a distended rectum. In autonomic dysreflexia, stimulation below the level of the injury leads to reflex sympathetic activity which initiates vasoconstriction leading to a rapid rise in blood pressure which triggers a parasympathetic response above the level of the injury, leading to bradycardia and vasodilation (above the level of injury). Decompression of the offending hollow viscus (the bladder or rectum) can rapidly reverse the autonomic dysreflexia. The hypertension and bradycardia should be monitored and potentially treated with agents if persistent and the patient should be put in an upright position with clothes and braces loosened.

Consortium for Spinal Cord Medicine. Acute management of autonomic dysreflexia: individuals with spinal cord injury presenting to health-care facilities. J Spinal Cord Med. 2002;25(Suppl. 1):S67–88.

34. A 20-year-old male with a history of an T12 spinal cord injury from a gunshot wound 4 years ago complains of bothersome urinary incontinence. He currently catheterizes every 2–3 h but leaks in between catheterization. He has tried antimuscarinics, beta 3 agonists, and botox injections with minimal improvement. His US shows moderate bilateral hydronephrosis. His urodynamics testing is shown below (Fig. 9.1).

   He begins leaking on the study when he reaches 130cc of filling. What is the best next step in management?

   A. Augmentation cystoplasty
   B. Placement of artificial urinary sphincter
   C. Bladder neck closure without augmentation
   D. Increase catheterization to every 1 h

   Answer: A.

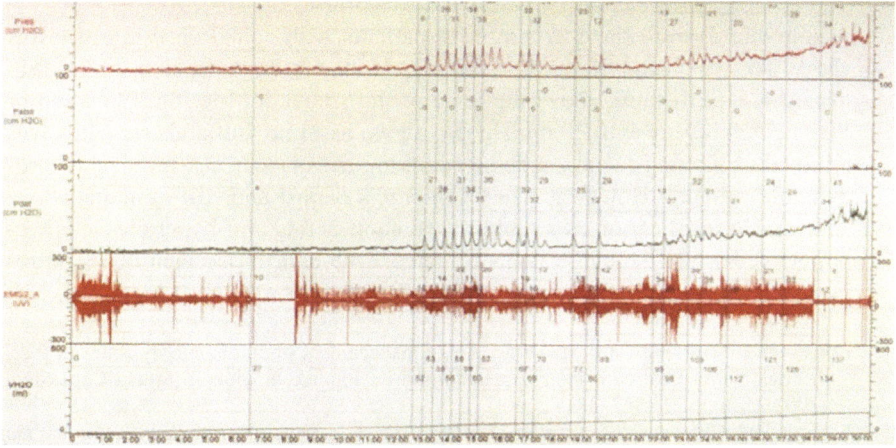

Fig. 9.1 Urodynamic testing results in a 20-year old patient with a T12 spinal cord injury

This patient has a poorly compliant bladder on urodynamics with a rise in pressure starting around 50cc with pressures rapidly increasing into a dangerous range. He has upper tract changes and leakage that occurs at high pressure. He has not had improvement with medications or botox injection, which are reasonable first options. This is a hostile bladder and is a set up for renal deterioration. Options that increase resistance (B and C) may decrease his leakage, but come at the cost of higher pressures and further renal damage. Catheterizing more than every 2–3 h is extremely difficult for most patients and most patients will not be able to stick to a regimen of every hour catheterization consistently. This patient would benefit from a procedure that increases his bladder capacity and compliance. Augmentation cystoplasty would be the best choice for him. Given his leakage occurs at high pressures, his outlet may be providing enough resistance to keep him continent without bladder neck closure or reconstruction if he would like to avoid these procedures.

Flood HD, Malhotra SJ, O'Connell HE, Ritchey MJ, Bloom DA, McGuire EJ. Long-term results and complications using augmentation cystoplasty in reconstructive urology. Neurourol Urodyn. 1995;14(4):297–309. https://doi.org/10.1002/nau.1930140402.

35. A 28-year-old male with T5 spinal cord injury is undergoing a urodynamic evaluation in the clinic. During the procedure, the patient develops a headache, profuse sweating, hypertension, and bradycardia. The bladder was emptied and the catheter was removed, but his symptoms persist. Vital signs are repeated and systolic blood pressure (SBP) remains elevated at 180mm Hg. The next step is:

A. Oral hydralazine
B. Sublingual nifedipine
C. Topical 2% nitropaste
D. IV atropine

Answer: C.

Autonomic dysreflexia is common in patients with spinal cord injury levels above T6, which manifests as sweating, headache, hypertension, reflex bradycardia, and flushing above the level of the spinal cord lesion. Elevation of SBP occurs begins with 20 mmHg rise above baseline. Initial therapy involves removal of inciting factors such as emptying the bladder and removal of urodynamic catheter. However, when symptoms persist and SBP remains above 150 mmHg, application of a rapid-onset, short-acting anti-hypertensive is recommended while the cause is investigated. One-half to one inch of 2% nitropaste should be applied above the level of the lesion.

Consortium for Spinal Cord Medicine. Acute management of autonomic dysreflexia: individuals with spinal cord injury presenting to health-care facilities. J Spinal Cord Med. 2002;25(Suppl. 1):S67–88.

Faaborg PM, Christensen P, Krassioukov A, Laurberg S, Frandsen E, Krogh K. Autonomic dysreflexia during bowel evacuation procedures and bladder filling in subjects with spinal cord injury. Spinal Cord. 2014;52(6):494–8. https://doi.org/10.1038/sc.2014.45. Epub 2014 Apr 29.

Solinsky R, Bunnell AE, Linsenmeyer TA, Svircev JN, Engle A, Burns SP. Pharmacodynamics and effectiveness of topical nitroglycerin at lowering blood pressure during autonomic dysreflexia. Spinal Cord. 2017;55(10):911–914. https://doi.org/10.1038/sc.2017.58. Epub 2017 Jun 6.

36. A 32-year-old man is brought to the hospital after a fall from a roof with imaging concerning for a significant T6 injury. He has been leaking urine from the penis intermittently. Urinalysis shows no hematuria. On imaging his bladder appears to be distended to 500cc. Which of the following would be expected to be normal at this point?

   A. Detrusor muscle contractility
   B. Guarding reflex
   C. Internal sphincter function
   D. Maximum urethral closure pressure

Answer: C.

The patient is experiencing spinal shock after the injury. This condition involves autonomic and somatic nerve activity suppression. The bladder becomes areflexic and acontractile during this period with patients experiencing urinary retention that results in overflow incontinence. The detrusor muscle contraction is impaired and volitional voiding is interrupted. The guarding reflex (function of the striated, external urethral sphincter during filling/increases in intravesical pressure) is also absent, leading to overflow urinary incontinence. The maximum urethral closure pressure is decreased during this time. The smooth muscle, internal sphincter (bladder neck) remains intact and functional during the period of spinal shock.

Ditunno JF, Little JW, Tessler A, Burns AS. Spinal shock revisited: a four-phase model. Spinal Cord. 2004;42(7):383–95. https://doi.org/10.1038/sj.sc.3101603.

37. A 21-year-old male is admitted to the hospital following a motor vehicle collision and was found to have a complete T6 spinal cord injury. Urology is consulted because the patient has not been able to void on his own. He currently has an indwelling foley catheter in place. The best next step for evaluation is:

   A. MRI head
   B. Voiding cystourethrogram
   C. Urodynamic evaluation while inpatient
   D. Urodynamic evaluation in 3 months

Answer: D.

The initial phase following acute SCI is that of spinal shock. In addition to the effects on skeletal muscle, spinal shock may result in an acontractile/hypocontractile detrusor. The duration of spinal shock varies widely, from several days to several months. Urodynamics should be performed after spinal shock has ended. The average period of spinal shock in patients is approximately 90 days or, more exactly, when the bulbocavernosus reflex returns.

As a young male individual with paraplegia, he likely will be able to learn independent self CIC. While awaiting further testing, the patient should likely be taught CIC rather than continuing with a indwelling catheter. Potential benefits of CIC over an indwelling catheter include decreased rate of UTIs, improved bladder compliance, decreased interference with sexual function and improved body image/quality of life.

Ditunno JF, Little JW, Tessler A, Burns AS. Spinal shock revisited: a four-phase model. Spinal Cord. 2004;42(7):383–95. https://doi.org/10.1038/sj.sc.3101603.

Pavese C, Schneider MP, Schubert M, Curt A, Scivoletto G, Finazzi-Agrò E, Mehnert U, Maier D, Abel R, Röhrich F, Weidner N, Rupp R, Kessels AG, Bachmann LM, Kessler TM. Prediction of bladder outcomes after traumatic spinal cord injury: a longitudinal cohort study. PLoS Med. 2016;13(6):e1002041. https://doi.org/10.1371/journal.pmed.1002041.

Welk B, Liu K, Shariff SZ. The use of urologic investigations among patients with traumatic spinal cord injuries. Res Rep Urol. 2016;8:27–34. https://doi.org/10.2147/RRU.S99840.

38. A 45-year-old man has an incomplete cervical spinal cord injury and a weak urinary stream. On videourodynamics he generates a detrusor contraction during voiding of 70 cm H_2O and has an elevated postvoid residual of 250cc. There is no reflux, a normal electromyography (EMG), and the bladder neck is closed during voiding. He is not having infections and has normal creatinine. Which medication should be considered?

    A. Tamsulosin
    B. Bethanechol
    C. Baclofen
    D. Oxybutynin

Answer: A.

SCI above lower thoracic levels can cause internal sphincter dyssynergia. Tamsulosin, an alpha blocker, relaxes the internal sphincter and may be helpful to some degree.

Kakizaki H, Ameda K, Kobayashi S, Tanaka H, Shibata T, Koyanagi T. Urodynamic effects of alpha1-blocker tamsulosin on voiding dysfunction in patients with neurogenic bladder. Int J Urol. 2003;10(11):576–81. https://doi.org/10.1046/j.1442-2042.2003.00710.x.

Lee KK, Lee MY, Han DY, Jung HJ, Joo MC. Effects of bladder function by early tamsulosin treatment in a spinal cord injury rat model. Ann Rehabil Med. 2014;38(4):433–42. https://doi.org/10.5535/arm.2014.38.4.433. Epub 2014 Aug 28.

39. A 40-year-old male with a history of a spinal cord injury (level unknown) is admitted to the hospital with mental status changes. He is found to have a severe hyperchloremic, hypokalemic metabolic acidosis. His family is not able to provide much history other than "he had a procedure in the past where they used bowel because of his bladder problems." Based on his

metabolic issues, which procedure is he most likely to have undergone in the past?

A. Bladder augmentation with ileum
B. Bladder augmentation with stomach
C. Incontinent loop diversion with jejunum
D. Appendicovesicostomy into native bladder

Answer: A.

Procedures where there is a longer dwell time of urine (augmentation cystoplasty, neobladder creation, ileovesicostomy, etc.) are more likely to result in metabolic complications than those with shorter dwell times (incontinent loop diversions), as the urine is in contact with the bowel mucosa for longer periods of time and potentially at higher pressure.

Use of terminal ileum can result in long term issues with B12 handling, and B12 levels should be checked periodically starting about 5 years after surgery. Diversions or augmentations involving the ileum or colon most commonly lead to hyperchloremic, hypokalemic metabolic acidosis. Those involving jejunum lead to a hypochloremic hyperkalemic metabolic acidosis. Those involving stomach cause hypochloremic, hypokalemia, metabolic alkalosis. Hematuria/dysuria syndrome occurred in patients for whom stomach was used, limiting the use of this tissue in most modern urinary reconstructions.

Gerharz EW, Turner WH, Kälble T, Woodhouse CR. Metabolic and functional consequences of urinary reconstruction with bowel. BJU Int. 2003;91(2):143–9. https://doi.org/10.1046/j.1464-410x.2003.04000.x.

40. A 44-year-old woman with paraplegia previously underwent creation of an Indiana (ileocolonic) pouch in her 20s. She is complaining of numbness in the hands and feet. Her blood work will likely demonstrate elevation of which of the following?

A. Homocysteine
B. Creatinine
C. Potassium
D. Lead

Answer: A.

Use of terminal ileum results in B12 deficiency and pernicious anemia. Elevated homocysteine is a sensitive marker for significant B12 deficiency.

Vashi P, Edwin P, Popiel B, Lammersfeld C, Gupta D. Methylmalonic acid and homocysteine as indicators of vitamin B-12 deficiency in cancer. PLoS One. 2016;11(1):e0147843. https://doi.org/10.1371/journal.pone.0147843.

Sexuality and Reproductive Health After Spinal Cord Injury

10

Christine Krull, Aaron J. Lin, and Jennifer E. Mast

Questions

1. Patients with spinal cord injury and which of the following levels of injury are the least likely to experience a reflexogenic erection?

   A. C4 American Spinal Injury Association Impairment Scale (AIS) A
   B. T6 AIS B
   C. L1 AIS B
   D. S1 AIS A

   Answer: D.

   For men with spinal cord injury, the majority of individuals are able to experience a reflexogenic erection if they have an upper motor neuron lesion (complete or incomplete) or an incomplete lower motor neuron lesion. This is due to the parasympathetic sacral reflex arc (S2–S4) remaining intact. For those with complete lower motor neuron lesions, reflexogenic erections are often not possible due to damage of the sacral reflex arc.

C. Krull (✉)
Spinal Cord Injury/Dysfunction Service, VA St. Louis Health Care System, St. Louis, MO, USA

Department of Physical Medicine and Rehabilitation, Baylor College of Medicine, TIRR Memorial Hermann, Houston, TX, USA
e-mail: Christine.krull@va.gov

A. J. Lin
Department of Physical Medicine and Rehabilitation, University of Texas Medical School at Houston, Houston, TX, USA

J. E. Mast
Department of Physical Medicine and Rehabilitation, OhioHealth Neurological Physicians, Columbus, OH, USA
e-mail: jennifer.mast2@ohiohealth.com

© The Author(s), under exclusive license to Springer Nature Switzerland AG 2022
B. A. Abramoff et al. (eds.), *The Essential Spinal Cord Injury Medicine Question Bank*, https://doi.org/10.1007/978-3-031-07796-8_10

Bors E. Neurological disturbances of sexual function with special reference to 529 patients with spinal cord injury. Urol Surv. 1960;10:191–221.

2. A 45-year-old male with history of spinal cord injury (C7 AIS A) and sexual dysfunction requiring sildenafil has sudden onset of a headache during sexual activity that is concerning for autonomic dysreflexia (AD). Regarding AD in this patient, which next step below is NOT recommended?

   A. Loosen any constrictive clothing.
   B. Stop the activity and sit upright.
   C. Apply nitroglycerin paste topically if blood pressure remains elevated.
   D. Attempt straight catheterization with lidocaine jelly to reduce bladder volume.

   Answer: C.

   Explanation: Nitrates, such as nitroglycerin paste or sublingual nitroglycerine, are contraindicated in patients who take phosphodiesterase-5 inhibitors (PDE5i) such as sildenafil, vardenafil, and tadalafil, due to the high risk of hypotension as a result of vasodilation from both medications.

Lue TF, Giuliano F, Montorsi F, Rosen RC, Andersson KE, Althof S, Christ G, Hatzichristou D, Hirsch M, Kimoto Y, Lewis R, McKenna K, MacMahon C, Morales A, Mulcahy J, Padma-Nathan H, Pryor J, de Tejada IS, Shabsigh R, Wagner G. Summary of the recommendations on sexual dysfunctions in men. J Sex Med. 2004;1(1):6–23. https://doi.org/10.1111/j.1743-6109.2004.10104.x.

3. Which of the following reflexes is the LEAST helpful in estimating a spinal cord injury patient's sexual function?

   A. Abdominal reflex
   B. Bulbocavernosus reflex
   C. Hip flexion reflex
   D. Anal wink

   Answer: A.

   The abdominal reflex tests segments T7–T12 and can be helpful in determining the level of a central nervous system lesion but is not used to help predict sexual functioning after spinal cord injury. The bulbocavernosus reflex and anal wink reflex both demonstrate the intactness of the sacral cord reflex (pudendal nerve and sacral segments, S2–S4), along with genital sensation, which are promising signs for the potential of reflexogenic genital arousal in women and strong predictors for ejaculation with penile vibratory stimulation (PVS) and orgasm in men. The hip flexion reflex measures the integrity of L2–L4 reflex arc and presumes the integrity of the spinal cord segments immediately above S2–S4, so it is a positive sign for successful PVS.

Bird VG, Brackett NL, Lynne CM, Aballa TC, Ferrell SM. Reflexes and somatic responses as predictors of ejaculation by penile vibratory stimulation in men with spinal cord injury. Spinal Cord. 2001;39(10):514–9. https://doi.org/10.1038/sj.sc.3101200.

4. A 28-year-old female with a history of complete cauda equina syndrome has questions during an outpatient clinic visit regarding sexual functioning. Which of the following is most likely to be intact for this patient?

A. Reflexogenic arousal
B. Psychogenic arousal
C. Orgasm
D. Genital sensation

Answer: B.

The psychogenic pathway for arousal is supplied by T11–L2, which is above this patient's level of injury. Reflexogenic arousal, orgasm, and genital sensation are more dependent on the sacral nerve roots, S2–S4, being intact. These sacral nerve roots would be damaged for a patient who has complete cauda equina syndrome.

Sipski ML, Alexander CJ, Rosen R. Sexual arousal and orgasm in women: effects of spinal cord injury. Ann Neurol. 2001;49(1):35–44. https://doi.org/10.1002/1531-8249(200101)4 9:1<35::aid-ana8>3.0.co;2-j.

5. Which of the following is NOT a validated model for assessing sexual dysfunction?

A. Bring up, Explain, Tell, Time, Educate, and Record (BETTER)
B. Permission, Limited Information, Specific Suggestions, and Intensive Therapy (PLISSIT)
C. Ask, Legitimize, Limitations, Open up, and Work together (ALLOW)
D. Study, Ask, Formulate a Plan, Empathy (SAFE)

Answer: D.

The BETTER, PLISSIT, and ALLOW models have been validated for assessing sexual dysfunction. There is no SAFE model to assess for sexual dysfunction.

Frank JE, Mistretta P, Will J. Diagnosis and treatment of female sexual dysfunction. Am Fam Physician. 2008;77(5):635–42. Erratum in: Am Fam Physician. 2009;79(3):180.
Hatzichristou D, Rosen RC, Broderick G, Clayton A, Cuzin B, Derogatis L, Litwin M, Meuleman E, O'Leary M, Quirk F, Sadovsky R, Seftel A. Clinical evaluation and management strategy for sexual dysfunction in men and women. J Sex Med. 2004;1(1):49–57. https://doi.org/10.1111/j.1743-6109.2004.10108.x.
Hordern A. Intimacy and sexuality after cancer: a critical review of the literature. Cancer Nurs. 2008;31(2):E9–17.
Hordern A. Intimacy and sexuality after cancer: a critical review of the literature. Cancer Nurs. 2008;31(2):E9–17. https://doi.org/10.1097/01.NCC.0000305695.12873.d5.

6. In which of the following situations would it be safest to use a penile constriction band with vacuum device to promote the development of erections during sexual activity?

   A. A patient using a penile constriction band in place for 60 min
   B. A patient on anticoagulation
   C. A patient with absent penile sensation
   D. A patient with a penile hematoma

Answer: C.

Absent penile sensation is not a contraindication to using a penile constriction band with vacuum device, but the penis should be monitored carefully for ischemia, bruising, and skin breakdown. The penile constriction bands can be used for up to 30 min safely. Patients who use anticoagulation or have a penile hematoma should not use a penile constriction band.

Ganem JP, Lucey DT, Janosko EO, Carson CC. Unusual complications of the vacuum erection device. Urology. 1998;51(4):627–31.

7. A 30-year-old male with spinal cord injury (T12 AIS A) presents with his spouse to an outpatient clinic to discuss options for conception. Sperm retrieval using penile vibratory stimulation with one vibrator has been unsuccessful in producing antegrade ejaculation. There has been an absence of any response, such as abdominal contractions, to indicate the presence of any ejaculation. What is the next best step in attempting sperm retrieval?

   A. Penile vibratory stimulation using the "sandwich" technique
   B. Electroejaculation
   C. Surgical aspiration
   D. Prostate massage

Answer: B.

Electroejaculation should be the next step. The decision to attempt further penile vibratory stimulation (PVS) is dependent upon the neurologic level of injury and somatosensory function. For injuries at T10 or rostral and when there is evidence of somatic responses to PVS (increased spasticity, abdominal contractions, or possible erection), there has been a report of an 86% success rate for anterograde ejactulation using PVS. However, for injuries caudal to T10, there was only a 17% success rate. This may be due to adjacent interrupted reflex arcs involving the dorsal nerve of the penis, which arises from the pudendal nerve and is innervated by S2–S4. An algorithm has been suggested for treatment of ejaculation dysfunction, which may be referenced below.

Brackett NL, Ibrahim E, Iremashvili V, Aballa TC, Lynne CM. Treatment for ejaculatory dysfunction in men with spinal cord injury: an 18-year single center experience. J Urol. 2010;183(6):2304–8. https://doi.org/10.1016/j.juro.2010.02.018. Epub 2010 Apr 18.

8. A 26-year-old male with spinal cord injury (T4 AIS B) presents with his spouse to an outpatient clinic to request treatment for infertility. They have been unsuccessful in conceiving at home using the method of ejaculation via masturbation and attempting intravaginal insemination with an eye dropper. What is the next best next step for this couple to attempt conception?

   A. Intracytoplasmic sperm injection
   B. Intrauterine insemination
   C. In vitro fertilization
   D. Semen analysis

   Answer: D.

   Semen analysis should be offered as the next step for this couple. When surveyed, many institutions do not offer penile vibratory stimulation or electroejaculation, often due to lack of training or equipment. While sperm evaluation is not routinely done, it could guide couples on whether to attempt intravaginal insemination at home or intrauterine insemination. Sperm evaluation is typically a more cost-effective next step than advanced fertilization techniques, such as in vitro fertilization or intracytoplasmic sperm injection.

   Kafetsoulis A, Brackett NL, Ibrahim E, Attia GR, Lynne CM. Current trends in the treatment of infertility in men with spinal cord injury. Fertil Steril. 2006; 86(4):781–9. https://doi.org/10.1016/j.fertnstert.2006.01.060. Epub 2006 Sep 11.

9. When comparing men who use different bladder management strategies after spinal cord injury, which strategy is associated with the highest level of sperm motility?

   A. Intermittent catheterization
   B. Foley catheter
   C. Suprapubic catheter
   D. Volitional voiding

   Answer: A.

   Intermittent catheterization is the bladder management strategy that is associated with the highest level of sperm motility (27%), followed by volitional voiding (15%), and then indwelling catheter (5%). Although men with spinal cord injury who perform intermittent catheterization are the most likely to have motile sperm, it is important to note that bladder management is not the sole reason for low sperm motility.

   Ibrahim E, Lynne CM, Brackett NL. Male fertility following spinal cord injury: an update. Andrology. 2016;4(1):13–26. https://doi.org/10.1111/andr.12119. Epub 2015 Nov 4.
Ohl DA, Denil J, Fitzgerald-Shelton K, McCabe M, McGuire EJ, Menge AC, Randolph JF. Fertility of spinal cord injured males: effect of genitourinary infection and bladder management on results of electroejaculation. J Am Paraplegia Soc. 1992;15(2):53–9. https://doi.org/10.1080/01952307.1992.11735862.

10. A man who has a spinal cord injury (SCI) submitted his semen for analysis due to infertility issues, and the semen appears brown. When compared to the general population, what is the most characteristic semen profile after SCI?

A. Normal sperm concentration, low sperm motility
B. Normal sperm concentration, normal sperm motility
C. Low sperm concentration, low sperm motility
D. Low sperm concentration, normal sperm motility

Answer: A.

Normal sperm concentration and low sperm motility is the most characteristic semen profile after with SCI. Additionally, sperm viability is typically below normal as well. This is a unique profile, because low sperm motility usually occurs at the same time as low sperm concentration. The low sperm motility after SCI is thought to be due to inflammatory cytokines and inflammasome components. Semen analysis also yields leukocytospermia, which when typed, are activated T-cells. These cytokines are likely deleterious to sperm motility.

Patki P, Woodhouse J, Hamid R, Craggs M, Shah J. Effects of spinal cord injury on semen parameters. J Spinal Cord Med. 2008;31(1):27–32. https://doi.org/10.1080/10790268.2008.11753977.

11. For men with spinal cord injury who cannot produce antegrade ejaculation and require medical assistance to retrieve sperm, which of the following is the best initial method?

A. Penile vibratory stimulation
B. Electroejaculation
C. Prostate massage
D. Surgery

Answer: A.

There are several methods for obtaining sperm from men with spinal cord injury (SCI) who do not have obvious antegrade ejaculation. It is initially helpful to determine if there is any ejaculation with penile vibratory stimulation (PVS) or electroejaculation (EEJ) and if there is retrograde ejaculation. PVS is commonly used first and is successful in 86% of men with SCI at T10 or rostral and 17% of men with SCI caudal to T10. EEJ is a reasonable next choice in sperm retrieval, but it is associated with a higher rate of retrograde ejaculation and may require sedation/anesthesia. Prostate massage is not well-studied, and the few reports that have been published show inconsistent results. It may be reasonable to try due to drastically lower cost when compared to procedures that require anesthesia. Surgical sperm retrieval is the last option when all other methods have failed, which may be done through fine needle aspiration or microsurgery, but there are no clear guidelines regarding the surgical technique for optimal retrieval. Sperm yields from surgical retrieval are reported to be low, and this is an invasive and expensive option.

Ibrahim E, Lynne CM, Brackett NL. Male fertility following spinal cord injury: an update. Andrology. 2016;4(1):13–26. https://doi.org/10.1111/andr.12119. Epub 2015 Nov 4.

12. A 33-year-old man with history of spinal cord injury (T10 AIS B) presents to an outpatient clinic for erectile dysfunction. He has tried sildenafil, and it has not produced a satisfactory response. He agrees to trial intracavernosal injection. What is the mechanism of action for alprostadil?

    A. Phosphodiesterase-5 inhibitor
    B. Prostaglandin E1 analog
    C. Nonselective alpha-adrenergic antagonist
    D. Selective serotonin reuptake inhibitor

Answer: B.

Both intracavernosal injections and urethral suppositories commonly use alprostadil, a prostaglandin E1 analog (PGE1). Papaverine, hypothesized to be a phosphodiesterase-5 inhibitor (PDE5i), and phentolamine, a non-selective alpha-adrenergic antagonist, may be used in combination with alprostadil for intracavernosal injections. In concert, these drugs create an environment with high concentrations of cyclic AMP, which is a potent vasodilator of the corpora cavernosa. Men with spinal cord injury may be limited in the ability to perform injections due to limited functional hand movement. Urethral delivery methods are not optimal due to variable urethral mucosal absorption and lower efficacy. Sildenafil, vardenafil, and tadalafil are phosphodiesterase-5 inhibitors, which result in an increase in cyclic GMP. In turn, cyclic GMP is thought to be important in activating protein kinase G to allow for a cascade of signals to relax smooth muscle and promote blood flow into the penis, which result in tumescence. Note that some medications, such as selective serotonin reuptake inhibitors (SSRIs) may have a side effect of erectile dysfunction.

Ibrahim E, Lynne CM, Brackett NL. Male fertility following spinal cord injury: an update. Andrology. 2016;4(1):13–26. https://doi.org/10.1111/andr.12119. Epub 2015 Nov 4.

13. Which of the following is true about pregnancy/fertility for women after spinal cord injury?

    A. Fertility for women is largely unaffected by chronic spinal cord injury.
    B. Amenorrhea often occurs after spinal cord injury, and menses usually never return.
    C. Most women who have had a spinal cord injury will need medical procedures/assistance for conception.
    D. Contraception is not typically necessary after spinal cord injury.

Answer: A.

Fertility is not significantly affected by chronic spinal cord injury for women (unlike men, where it can be significantly affected). Women will typically have a period of amenorrhea for 2–8 months after SCI, then menses and fertility resume. Most women do not require medical procedures to conceive. Contraception is an important consideration due to preserved female fertility after spinal cord injury, as well as other benefits of certain contraceptive methods, such as lowering the risk of sexually transmitted infections.

Sipski ML. The impact of spinal cord injury on female sexuality, menstruation and pregnancy: a review of the literature. J Am Paraplegia Soc. 1991;14(3):122–6. https://doi.org/1 0.1080/01952307.1991.11735841.

14. Which symptoms may some women with a spinal cord injury experience during menstruation?

    A. None, since menstruation never returns after spinal cord injury
    B. None, due to lack of sensation
    C. Decreased muscle spasticity
    D. Autonomic symptoms, such as sweating and headaches

Answer: D.

Premenstrual and menstrual symptoms, such as cramping, might be exacerbated after spinal cord injury. Although the usual sensation of menstrual symptoms may be limited, the body may still react to the symptoms. For instance, menstrual symptoms may cause autonomic symptoms (sweating, headaches, flushing, etc.), increase of muscle spasticity, and increase in the frequency of bladder spasms. Feminine hygiene products may be more difficult to use/manage after SCI, so education may be included in the rehab process, such as using mirrors for insertion, using splinting to improve self-management, and instructing attendants about how to use these products. After an initial phase of amenorrhea following spinal cord injury, menstruation usually returns around 6 months post injury on average. However, women nearing menopause already may develop permanently amenorrhea after SCI.

Consortium for Spinal Cord Medicine. Sexuality and reproductive health in adults with spinal cord injury: a clinical practice guideline for health-care professionals. J Spinal Cord Med. 2010;33(3):281–336. https://doi.org/10.1080/10790268.2010.11689709.
Sipski ML. The impact of spinal cord injury on female sexuality, menstruation and pregnancy: a review of the literature. J Am Paraplegia Soc. 1991;14(3):122–6. https://doi.org/1 0.1080/01952307.1991.11735841.

15. Which method of contraception generally has the lowest risk and is generally the first recommendation for women with spinal cord injury?

A. Intrauterine devices
B. Basal body temperature
C. Contraceptive pills
D. Condoms

Answer: D.

Each form of contraception has pros and cons, and there are some additional considerations after spinal cord injury (SCI) relative to the general population. Condoms are generally the recommended birth control method after SCI, as they are considered the safest method, and they provide some protection against many sexually transmitted infections.

Hormonal methods, such as contraceptive pills, have an association with increased DVT incidence and are, therefore, less recommended after SCI. Patients should generally avoid hormonal birth control for the first year after injury and altogether in women who smoke or have history of cardiovascular/circulatory problems. Of the hormonal options, progesterone-only options may be preferred. Combined oral contraception containing estrogen is thought to carry a higher risk of VTE compared to progesterone alone.

Intrauterine devices (IUDs) are generally less recommended due to the potential difficulty in detecting complications, such as pelvic inflammatory disease or device migration, due to impaired sensation.

There is risk of vaginal wall breakdown with devices such as diaphragms, cervical caps, and vaginal sponges due to the pressure applied to the vaginal tissue and impaired sensation. These may also be more difficult to place if manual dexterity is impaired.

Basal body temperature methods are not recommended due to higher rates of unintended pregnancy with this method.

Permanent sterilization methods may be considered if there is no desire for children in the future. When weighing the risks and benefits of various forms of contraception after SCI, another consideration is how much difficulty a patient has with menstrual cramps and menstrual hygiene. If these challenges limit quality of life or cause frequent autonomic dysreflexia, then it may make hormonal methods more desirable (while weighing benefits and risks).

Consortium for Spinal Cord Medicine. Sexuality and reproductive health in adults with spinal cord injury: a clinical practice guideline for health-care professionals. J Spinal Cord Med. 2010;33(3):281–336. https://doi.org/10.1080/10790268.2010.11689709.

Jackson AB, Wadley V. A multicenter study of women's self-reported reproductive health after spinal cord injury. Arch Phys Med Rehabil. 1999;80(11):1420–8. https://doi.org/10.1016/s0003-9993(99)90253-8.

Sipski ML. The impact of spinal cord injury on female sexuality, menstruation and pregnancy: a review of the literature. J Am Paraplegia Soc. 1991;14(3):122–6. https://doi.org/10.1080/01952307.1991.11735841.

16. For an expectant woman who is a wheelchair user, which of the following adjustments is anticipated as her pregnancy progresses?

    A. Increased seat-to-back angle
    B. Firmer cushion
    C. Decreased camber
    D. Reduced seat height

Answer: A.

A woman who uses a wheelchair will likely need adjustments as her pregnancy progresses. Changes in the body that are relevant to seating needs include: increased weight, change in body shape (necessitating an increase in the seat-to-back angle), and increased risks to skin integrity (due to rapid weight gain, fatigue, stretching of skin, and hyperdynamic circulation). The cushion interface should be monitored to ensure that the changes in body habitus and increased weight do not lead to problems with pressure distribution. Seating adjustments are needed to adapt to the increased abdominal size and are also important to maximize respiratory function, because posture/positioning may affect lung expansion with the increased abdominal pressure on the diaphragm from the growing gravid uterus. It is recommended to maintain a near vertical backrest, but progressively increase the downward slope of the seat plane (front lower) throughout pregnancy. In the future, these seating configuration changes will need to be reverted back to the previously appropriate settings postpartum.

Other changes in equipment needs and mobility techniques may also need to be addressed by PT and OT, such as increasing difficulty with transfers as pregnancy progresses. Upcoming needs for holding the baby and breastfeeding may also factor into equipment modifications. It is recommended to have PT and OT services involved during and after pregnancy to meet these evolving needs.

Consortium for Spinal Cord Medicine. Sexuality and reproductive health in adults with spinal cord injury: a clinical practice guideline for health-care professionals. J Spinal Cord Med. 2010;33(3):281–336. https://doi.org/10.1080/10790268.2010.11689709.

17. Which of the following statements is NOT true regarding routine health maintenance for women after spinal cord injury?

    A. The guidelines for screening for cervical cancer after spinal cord injury are different from the guidelines for the general population.
    B. The guidelines for screening for breast cancer after spinal cord injury are the same as the guidelines for the general population.
    C. Women should continue to follow with their primary care provider or gynecologist on a routine basis after spinal cord injury.

D. There are a number of limitations for women accessing routine women's health services after spinal cord injury, such as inaccessible clinics, exam tables, and radiology centers for mammograms.

Answer: A.

The guidelines for screening for both cervical and breast cancer after spinal cord injury are the same as the guidelines for the general population. All of the other answers are true and should not be overlooked when caring for women with spinal cord injury despite the barriers to accessing care.

Consortium for Spinal Cord Medicine. Sexuality and reproductive health in adults with spinal cord injury: a clinical practice guideline for health-care professionals. J Spinal Cord Med. 2010;33(3):281–336. https://doi.org/10.1080/10790268.2010.11689709.

Welner SL, Foley CC, Nosek MA, Holmes A. Practical considerations in the performance of physical examinations on women with disabilities. Obstet Gynecol Surv. 1999;54(7):457–62. https://doi.org/10.1097/00006254-199907000-00025.

Welner SL. Screening issues in gynecologic malignancies for women with disabilities: critical considerations. J Womens Health. 1998;7(3):281–5. https://doi.org/10.1089/jwh.1998.7.281.

18. Which of the following challenges after spinal cord injury is generally NOT worsened during pregnancy?

    A. Risk of urinary tract infections and urinary incontinence
    B. Spasticity
    C. Cognitive dysfunction
    D. Constipation

Answer: C.

There are a number of changes that occur due to pregnancy that overlap with complications of SCI, which include increased risk of constipation, venous thromboembolism, pedal edema, pressure sores, anemia, increased spasticity, and possible inferior vena cava compression. Respiratory difficulty may arise from diaphragmatic restriction. Bladder management challenges may occur, particularly as there is increasing pressure from the gravid uterus, and there may be a need to do more frequent intermittent catheterization. There is an increased risk of urinary tract infections and leakage as well. There is also risk of autonomic dysreflexia, which may have an overlapping presentation with preeclampsia and must be differentiated carefully. Autonomic dysreflexia is episodic, while preeclampsia tends to cause persistent blood pressure elevation. There is no evidence of increased cognitive dysfunction in pregnant women with spinal cord injury.

Dawood R, Altanis E, Ribes-Pastor P, Ashworth F. Pregnancy and spinal cord injury. Obstet Gynaecol. 2014;16(2):99–107.

Wenzel LR, Vrooman A, Hammill HA. Acute spinal cord injury. Crit Care Obstetr. 2018:369–89.

19. A 28-year-old female with a history of spinal cord injury (T2 AIS A) is pregnant and preparing for labor and delivery. Which of the following is the appropriate counseling to offer this patient?

    A. She should proceed with routine obstetric care and no modifications compared to the general population.
    B. She will likely not need epidural anesthesia.
    C. She should plan for a cesarean section due to her spinal cord injury.
    D. She may not feel contractions in the same way as a woman without a spinal cord injury.

Answer: D.

There are special considerations for pregnancy, labor, and delivery in a woman who has a spinal cord injury. It is recommended that women with spinal cord injury have more frequent checkups, particularly towards the end of pregnancy. During labor and delivery, there are additional considerations, such as the need to prevent autonomic dysreflexia, perform frequent turns/repositioning to protect from skin breakdown, and use of a Foley catheter to avoid the need for intermittent catheterization during labor.

Autonomic dysreflexia, an issue for those with injuries at T6 and above, is a high-risk complication during labor and delivery. The recommended management is epidural anesthesia initiated early in labor. In some cases, combined spinal epidural or continuous spinal anesthesia may be needed. There have been cases of severe morbidity and mortality reported related to autonomic dysreflexia in pregnancy/delivery. For women with lesions below T6, there is a broader choice for analgesia during labor. Of note, epidurals may be difficult to insert in the setting of prior lumbar or lower thoracic spine surgery. Lesions above T10 (but below T6) may not require analgesia, because the sensory nerves for the uterus involve segments T11–L1.

Cesarean sections should be performed for obstetric indications only, as women with spinal cord injury can often still deliver vaginally. However, the observed rate of cesarean section remains higher in the spinal cord injured population compared to the general population. An institution's familiarity with managing labor after SCI may influence the likelihood of cesarean section.

Due to impaired sensation after spinal cord injury, it may be difficult to recognize the signs when labor has begun, and those signs may be different than observed in a woman without a spinal cord injury. Uterine sensory afferent signals synapse at T11–L2. Women with lesions above the level of T10 have been reported to have an absence of nociceptive uterine contractions and may be unaware at the beginning of labor. However, other signs of labor include: sympathetically-induced symptoms, strong abdominal spasms, leg spasms, difficulty breathing, and back or abdominal pain.

Sipski ML. The impact of spinal cord injury on female sexuality, menstruation and pregnancy: a review of the literature. J Am Paraplegia Soc. 1991;14(3):122–6. https://doi.org/1
0.1080/01952307.1991.11735841.
Dawood R, Altanis E, Ribes-Pastor P, Ashworth F. Pregnancy and spinal cord injury. Obstet
Gynaecol. 2014;16(2):99–107.

20. Spinal cord injury above which level may cause a woman to have the most relative difficulty with breastfeeding?

A. T4
B. T8
C. T12
D. L2

Answer: A.

Breastfeeding may be more difficult after spinal cord injury, especially for
women with injuries at or above T6, since they may experience decreased milk
production, possibly due to a lack of nipple sensation with resultant decrease in
neurologic communication to the pituitary gland, which is necessary for milk
production. The afferent pathway of the milk ejection reflex is triggered by
infant suckling, carried via the tactile receptors to the dorsal roots of T4–T6.
The initiation of breastfeeding may be delayed and require additional stimulation for a woman with a complete injury above T4. Visual stimulation or oxy-
tocin nasal spray may help with initiation of lactation. An association has been
identified between a higher level of injury and shorter breastfeeding duration.
Difficulty with positioning and holding the baby during breastfeeding has been
identified as a key challenge for mothers after spinal cord injury. Autonomic
dysreflexia is a possible occurrence during breastfeeding, especially with
higher level spinal cord injuries. Early breastfeeding support is essential, as
well as pre-counseling about potential challenges for prospective mothers.

Sipski ML. The impact of spinal cord injury on female sexuality, menstruation and pregnancy: a review of the literature. J Am Paraplegia Soc. 1991;14(3):122–6. https://doi.org/1
0.1080/01952307.1991.11735841.
Dawood R, Altanis E, Ribes-Pastor P, Ashworth F. Pregnancy and spinal cord injury. The
Obstet Gynaecol. 2014;16(2):99–107.
Holmgren T, Lee AHX, Hocaloski S, Hamilton LJ, Hellsing I, Elliott S, Hultling C, Krassioukov AV. The influence of spinal cord injury on breastfeeding ability and behavior.
J Hum Lact. 2018;34(3):556–65. https://doi.org/10.1177/0890334418774014. Epub
2018 May 22.

Musculoskeletal Issues in Spinal Cord Injury

11

Allison Kessler, Vivian Roy, and Sushil Singla

Questions

1. For a person with a C8 American Spinal Injury Association Impairment Scale (AIS) A spinal cord injury, which area will likely have the most bone loss in the first 3 months after injury and be at higher risk for subsequent fracture?

   A. Proximal humerus
   B. Proximal femur
   C. Distal humerus
   D. Distal femur

   Answer: D.

   After spinal cord injury there is significant bone loss more pronounced distal to the neurological level of injury. The areas of highest bone density loss occur in the distal femur and proximal tibia. Areas with higher bone loss are at higher risk of fracture.

   Bauman WA, Cardozo CP. Osteoporosis in individuals with spinal cord injury. PM R. 2015;7(2):188–201; quiz 201. https://doi.org/10.1016/j.pmrj.2014.08.948. Epub 2014 Aug 27.

A. Kessler (✉) · V. Roy
Division of Spinal Cord Injury Medicine, Shirley Ryan Abilitylab, Chicago, IL, USA

Department of Physical Medicine and Rehabilitation, Northwestern University, Chicago, IL, USA
e-mail: akessler@sralab.org

S. Singla
Division of Spinal Cord Injury Medicine, Shirley Ryan Abilitylab, Chicago, IL, USA

© The Author(s), under exclusive license to Springer Nature Switzerland AG 2022
B. A. Abramoff et al. (eds.), *The Essential Spinal Cord Injury Medicine Question Bank*, https://doi.org/10.1007/978-3-031-07796-8_11

Jiang SD, Dai LY, Jiang LS. Osteoporosis after spinal cord injury. Osteoporos Int. 2006;17(2):180–92. https://doi.org/10.1007/s00198-005-2028-8. Epub 2005 Oct 11. Erratum in: Osteoporos Int. 2006;17(8):1278–81.

Jiang SD, Jiang LS, Dai LY. Mechanisms of osteoporosis in spinal cord injury. Clin Endocrinol (Oxf). 2006;65(5):555–65. https://doi.org/10.1111/j.1365-2265.2006.02683.x.

2. In the first 2 months after spinal cord injury, the weekly rate of bone loss below the neurological level of injury is approximately:

   A. 0.1%
   B. 1.0%
   C. 5.0%
   D. 10.0%

Answer: B.

Beginning a few weeks following a spinal cord injury, the weekly rate of bone loss (absorption) can approach 1% at some sites distal to the neurological level of injury. This absorption reaches a steady state between absorption and formation approximately 2 years after a spinal cord injury.

Battaglino RA, Lazzari AA, Garshick E, Morse LR. Spinal cord injury-induced osteoporosis: pathogenesis and emerging therapies. Curr Osteoporos Rep. 2012;10(4):278–85. https://doi.org/10.1007/s11914-012-0117-0.

Bauman WA, Cardozo CP. Osteoporosis in individuals with spinal cord injury. PM R. 2015;7(2):188–201; quiz 201. https://doi.org/10.1016/j.pmrj.2014.08.948. Epub 2014 Aug 27.

Jiang SD, Dai LY, Jiang LS. Osteoporosis after spinal cord injury. Osteoporos Int. 2006;17(2):180–92. https://doi.org/10.1007/s00198-005-2028-8. Epub 2005 Oct 11. Erratum in: Osteoporos Int. 2006;17(8):1278–81.

Jiang SD, Jiang LS, Dai LY. Mechanisms of osteoporosis in spinal cord injury. Clin Endocrinol (Oxf). 2006;65(5):555–65. https://doi.org/10.1111/j.1365-2265.2006.02683.x.

3. Which of the following areas will show the least amount of bone density loss after spinal cord injury?

   A. Distal humerus in a person with a C4 AIS A spinal cord injury
   B. Distal femur in a person with a T12 AIS A spinal cord injury
   C. Distal humerus in a person with a T12 AIS A spinal cord injury
   D. Thoracic vertebra in a person with a C4 AIS A spinal cord injury

Answer: C.

Bone mineral density loss is most prominent distal to the neurological level of injury. Upper extremities in persons with paraplegia do not show significant bone mineral density loss after spinal cord injury. Relative to long bones and distal sites, the vertebral column shows less loss of bone mineral density.

Jiang SD, Dai LY, Jiang LS. Osteoporosis after spinal cord injury. Osteoporos Int. 2006;17(2):180–92. https://doi.org/10.1007/s00198-005-2028-8. Epub 2005 Oct 11. Erratum in: Osteoporos Int. 2006;17(8):1278–81.

Jiang SD, Jiang LS, Dai LY. Mechanisms of osteoporosis in spinal cord injury. Clin Endocrinol (Oxf). 2006;65(5):555–65. https://doi.org/10.1111/j.1365-2265.2006.02683.x.

Garder DR, Ajit BP. Metabolic disorders. In: Kirshblum S, Campagnolo DI, editors. Spinal cord medicine. 2nd ed. Philadelphia: Lipincott Williams & Wilkins; 2011. p. 185–210.

4. Which of the following is associated with higher rates of observed osteoporosis following spinal cord injury?

A. Younger age at time of injury
B. Absence of spasticity
C. Lower spinal level of injury
D. Acute injury

Answer: B.

Although studies are small, older age, higher spinal level of injury, and longer time since injury have been shown to be associated with higher amount of bone mineral density loss and osteoporosis after spinal cord injury. Higher degrees of spasticity have been associated with lower amounts of bone mineral density loss.

Jiang SD, Dai LY, Jiang LS. Osteoporosis after spinal cord injury. Osteoporos Int. 2006;17(2):180–92. https://doi.org/10.1007/s00198-005-2028-8. Epub 2005 Oct 11. Erratum in: Osteoporos Int. 2006;17(8):1278–81.

Jiang SD, Jiang LS, Dai LY. Mechanisms of osteoporosis in spinal cord injury. Clin Endocrinol (Oxf). 2006;65(5):555–65. https://doi.org/10.1111/j.1365-2265.2006.02683.x.

Bauman WA, Cardozo CP. Osteoporosis in individuals with spinal cord injury. PM R. 2015;7(2):188–201; quiz 201. https://doi.org/10.1016/j.pmrj.2014.08.948. Epub 2014 Aug 27.

5. Which of the following patients with a new traumatic spinal cord injury is most likely to develop clinically relevant scoliosis which might require surgical intervention?

A. 8-year-old boy with a T3 AIS C spinal cord injury
B. 17-year-old girl with a C3 AIS A spinal cord injury
C. 38-year-old man with a T3 AIS C spinal cord injury
D. 76-year-old woman with a C3 AIS A spinal cord injury

Answer: A.

Neuromuscular scoliosis is most often progressive and clinically relevant potentially requiring surgery in people who sustain a spinal cord injury in childhood prior to puberty and skeletal maturity. Neurological level, motor level, and severity of injury are not strong predictors of scoliosis.

Mulcahey MJ, Gaughan JP, Betz RR, Samdani AF, Barakat N, Hunter LN. Neuromuscular sco-liosis in children with spinal cord injury. Top Spinal Cord Inj Rehabil. 2013;19(2):96–103. https://doi.org/10.1310/sci1902-96.

6. Which of the following is the best predictor of progression of neuromuscular scoliosis in people with pediatric spinal cord injuries?

   A. Age <12
   B. Neurological level of injury
   C. Severity or complete injury
   D. Motor level of injury

Answer: A.

Neuromuscular scoliosis is most often progressive and clinically relevant poten-tially requiring surgery in people who sustain a spinal cord injury in childhood prior to puberty and skeletal maturity (with highest odds in individuals under age 12). Neurological level, motor level, and severity of injury are not strong predictors of scoliosis. Virtually all children with a traumatic spinal cord injury before the age of 10 will develop scoliosis.

Mulcahey MJ, Gaughan JP, Betz RR, Samdani AF, Barakat N, Hunter LN. Neuromuscular sco-liosis in children with spinal cord injury. Top Spinal Cord Inj Rehabil. 2013;19(2):96–103. https://doi.org/10.1310/sci1902-96.

7. A 10-year-old boy sustained a T4 AIS B spinal cord injury 3 years ago and pres-ents to your outpatient clinic for his yearly exam. He describes mild back pain with prolonged sitting in his wheelchair. Neurological exam today is consistent with the exam documented at the patient's annual visit last year. You obtain plain film x-rays of his spine and note a cobb angle of 40°. All of the following are appropriate treatment options EXCEPT:

   A. Physical Therapy
   B. Evaluation of a custom molded backrest for his wheelchair
   C. Refer for surgical intervention
   D. Refer for bracing intervention

Answer: C.

Almost 100% of adolescents with a traumatic spinal cord injury before skeletal maturity will develop scoliosis. Scoliosis is likely to continue to worsen until skeletal maturity is reached. Scoliosis may or may not cause clinically significant complications depending on the severity of the scoliosis. Although bracing can help with symptomatic management in the pediatric population, unlike idiopathic scoliosis it generally does not halt progression of neuromuscular scoliosis. Surgical management is generally not indicated unless a cobb angle is >50°, there is cardiopulmonary compromise, neurological compromise, or significant decrease in functional activities such as ability to sit in a wheelchair. As this patient has advanced scoliosis at a young age, he should be established with a surgeon for monitoring and consideration of intervention.

Mulcahey MJ, Gaughan JP, Betz RR, Samdani AF, Barakat N, Hunter LN. Neuromuscular scoliosis in children with spinal cord injury. Top Spinal Cord Inj Rehabil. 2013;19(2):96–103. https://doi.org/10.1310/sci1902-96.
Murphy RF, Mooney JF 3rd. Current concepts in neuromuscular scoliosis. Curr Rev Musculoskelet Med. 2019;12(2):220–227. https://doi.org/10.1007/s12178-019-09552-8.
Zidek K, Srinivasan R. Rehabilitation of a child with a spinal cord injury. Semin Pediatr Neurol. 2003;10(2):140–50. https://doi.org/10.1016/s1071-9091(03)00022-6.

8. A 78-year-old woman with a history of osteoporosis comes to your office for evaluation of acute onset back pain after a low velocity fall at home. She has point tenderness over the 6th thoracic vertebra with no changes in lower extremity strength or sensation. Plain radiographs show an anterior wedge deformity of the 6th thoracic vertebra. In addition to prescribing physical therapy, which of the following braces would you prescribe to help with short term pain management?

A. Milwaukee brace
B. Charleston bending brace
C. Jewett brace
D. Minerva brace

Answer: C.

Osteoporotic compression fractures do not necessarily need bracing although bracing can be used acutely to help with symptomatic management. Appropriate bracing for a thoracic fracture would provide thoracic extension and stabilization. Examples of thoracolumbar orthosis include cruciform anterior spinal hyperextension (CASH) braces, Jewett braces, and Taylor braces. The Milwaukee brace and Charleston bending braces are used for scoliosis treatment. The Minerva brace is a type of cervicothoracic brace and does not provide adequate thoracic extension.

Wong CC, McGirt MJ. Vertebral compression fractures: a review of current management and multimodal therapy. J Multidiscip Healthc. 2013;6:205–14. https://doi.org/10.2147/JMDH.S31659.
Ensrud KE, Schousboe JT. Clinical practice. Vertebral fractures. N Engl J Med. 2011;364(17):1634–42. https://doi.org/10.1056/NEJMcp1009697.

9. A 65-year-old man with osteoporosis suffers a fall with a fracture of T1. Which of the following is the most appropriate orthosis to provide post-operatively which would provide spinal stabilization with the least restriction for physical therapy?

A. Philadelphia collar
B. Sterno-Occipital Mandibular Immobilizer
C. Cervicothoracic orthosis
D. Cruciform anterior spinal hyperextension (CASH) brace

Answer: C.

Adequate bracing after a spinal injury should span the level of injury and provide at least 3 contact points with the body. A soft cervical collar and Philadelphia collar are both cervical orthosis, which would not adequately stabilize a thoracic vertebral fracture. A sterno-occipital mandibular immobilizer (SOMI) would stabilize the fracture but is more restrictive of the cervical spine than is necessary. In this case a cervicothoracic orthosis (CTO) would be most appropriate. A CASH brace is a thoracolumbar orthosis and would not adequately stabilize T1.

Uustal H, Baerga E, Joki J. Prosthetics and Orthotics. In: Cuccurullo, S. Physical medicine and rehabilitation board review. New York: Demos Medical; 2010. p. 471–549.
Sandler AJ, Dvorak J, Humke T, Grob D, Daniels W. The effectiveness of various cervical orthoses. An in vivo comparison of the mechanical stability provided by several widely used models. Spine (Phila Pa 1976). 1996;21(14):1624–9. https://doi.org/10.1097/00007632-199607150-00002.

10. An 85-year-old woman with long-standing rheumatoid arthritis presents to the emergency room with progressive gait instability and falls. Imaging in the emergency room revealed anterior subluxation of C1 on C2 measuring 10mm. Which of the following removable orthoses would provide the most stabilization of his fracture?

A. Halo device
B. Minerva Brace
C. Soft collar
D. Philadelphia Collar

Answer: B.

Although the Halo brace provides the most restriction of movement for the cervical spine, it is not removable. Cervical braces in order of least to most restrictive: soft collar, Philadelphia collar, SOMI brace, four poster brace, Minerva brace.

Uustal H, Baerga E, Joki J. Prosthetics and Orthotics. In: Cuccurullo, S. Physical medicine and rehabilitation board review. New York: Demos Medical; 2010. p. 471–549.

Richter D, Latta LL, Milne EL, Varkarakis GM, Biedermann L, Ekkernkamp A, Ostermann PA. The stabilizing effects of different orthoses in the intact and unstable upper cervical spine: a cadaver study. J Trauma. 2001;50(5):848–54. https://doi.org/10.1097/00005373-200105000-00012.

11. Which of the following orthoses provides the most stability in terms of reduction of rotational range of motion?

A. Soft Collar
B. Yale Cervicothoracic Brace
C. SOMI Brace
D. Philadelphia Collar

Answer: B.

Cervical braces in order of least to most restrictive: soft collar, Philadelphia collar, SOMI brace, four poster brace, Yale cervicothoracic brace, Minerva brace, halo device.

Uustal H, Baerga E, Joki J. Prosthetics and Orthotics. In: Cuccurullo, S. Physical medicine and rehabilitation board review. New York: Demos Medical; 2010. p. 471–549.

12. Which of the following is NOT a risk for developing heterotopic ossification?

A. Male sex
B. Older age
C. Complete injury
D. Absence of spasticity

Answer: D.

Risk factors for development of heterotopic ossification include male sex, older age, complete neurologic injuries, presence of DVT, presence of spasticity, and presence of pressure ulcer.

Banovac K, Gonzalez F. Evaluation and management of heterotopic ossification in patients with spinal cord injury. Spinal Cord. 1997;35(3):158–62. https://doi.org/10.1038/sj.sc.3100380.

13. A 50-year-old morbidly obese male with T5 AIS A paraplegia after a motor vehicle accident 2 months ago develops fever and right hip swelling. Which imaging modality is most likely to be positive for heterotopic ossification in this patient?

A. Plain radiograph
B. Three-phase nuclear bone scan
C. Ultrasound
D. CT

Answer: B.

Three-phase nuclear bone scan is the gold standard in early diagnosis of heterotopic ossification. Plain radiographs may take weeks to months to show
changes. Ultrasound can be used for early detection; however, it is not ideal
given this patient's body habitus. CT scan is useful for surgical planning purposes but is not reliable in making early diagnosis. MRI can detect increased
tissue vascularization in the acute phase, but may also be challenging due to the
body habitus.

Meyers C, Lisiecki J, Miller S, Levin A, Fayad L, Ding C, Sono T, McCarthy E, Levi B, James
    AW. Heterotopic ossification: a comprehensive review. JBMR Plus. 2019;3(4):e10172.
    https://doi.org/10.1002/jbm4.10172.
Mujtaba B, Taher A, Fiala MJ, Nassar S, Madewell JE, Hanafy AK, Aslam R. Heterotopic
    ossification: radiological and pathological review. Radiol Oncol. 2019;53(3):275–84.
    https://doi.org/10.2478/raon-2019-0039.

14. An 18-year-old woman with C5 AIS A tetraplegia and spasticity after a gun-
    shot wound 6 months ago develops left hip pain, left leg swelling, and fever.
    Infectious workup is negative. Ultrasound dopplers of the left lower extremity
    are negative for DVT. Three-phase bone scan shows uptake on the third phase.
    What is the best treatment to prevent further progression of this condition?

    A. Bisphosphonates
    B. Radiation therapy
    C. Warfarin
    D. Surgical excision

Answer: A.

Bisphosphonates have been shown to halt the progression of new bone formation in those with heterotopic ossification (HO). The traditional choice of
bisphosphonates, Etidronate, is no longer available in some countries including
the United States, but it is thought that other bisphosphonates may have similar
benefit for HO treatment. Radiation therapy has been shown to be effective for
early HO, however, the long-term effects are not well established—therefore,
it should be avoided in an 18-year-old. A study by Buschbacher et al. (1992)
supported the use of warfarin for treatment of HO, but this has yet to be rep-
licated. Surgical excision is typically reserved for those who fail conservative
management.

Teasell RW, Mehta S, Aubut JL, Ashe MC, Sequeira K, Macaluso S, Tu L; SCIRE Research Team. A systematic review of the therapeutic interventions for heterotopic ossification after spinal cord injury. Spinal Cord. 2010;48(7):512–21. https://doi.org/10.1038/sc.2009.175. Epub 2010 Jan 5.

Buschbacher R, McKinley W, Buschbacher L, Devaney CW, Coplin B. Warfarin in prevention of heterotopic ossification. Am J Phys Med Rehabil. 1992;71(2):86–91. https://doi.org/10.1097/00002060-199204000-00005.

15. Which answer choice reflects the incidence in order of the most commonly affected joint to least commonly affected joint for heterotopic ossification after spinal cord injury (from highest to lowest)?

    A. Knee > shoulder > hip
    B. Knee > hip > shoulder
    C. Hip > shoulder > knee
    D. Hip > knee > shoulder

    Answer: D.

    After SCI, heterotopic ossification most commonly affects the hip (90%), followed in order by the knee, shoulder, and elbow.

    Kirshblum S, Nieves J, Clark D, Gonzalez P, Cuccurullo SJ, Luciano L. Spinal Cord Injuries. In: Cuccurullo, S. Physical medicine and rehabilitation board review. New York: Demos Medical; 2010. p. 551–62.

    van Kuijk AA, Geurts AC, van Kuppevelt HJ. Neurogenic heterotopic ossification in spinal cord injury. Spinal Cord. 2002;40(7):313–26. https://doi.org/10.1038/sj.sc.3101309.

16. Part 1. A 43-year-old morbidly obese woman with chronic C7 AIS C paraplegia sustained 20 years ago has insidious onset of pain in her anterior right shoulder with radiation toward the elbow. She is a manual wheelchair user. On physical examination, there is tenderness to palpation of the anterior glenohumeral joint and empty can test is positive for pain. There is stable weakness of the right finger flexors and finger abductors. Which diagnostic test should be ordered next?

    A. MRI of the shoulder
    B. MRI of the cervical spine
    C. X-ray of the shoulder
    D. EMG of the right arm

    Answer: C.

    Shoulder overuse syndrome is a common etiology of shoulder pain in persons with chronic spinal cord injuries. An X-ray can be obtained and may show glenohumeral joint narrowing or acromioclavicular joint arthritis. Studies have shown that 72% of individuals with chronic SCI and shoulder pain have degenerative changes on radiographs. There is no new weakness or numbness in the distal upper extremities to suggest a new issue with the spinal cord or nerve impingement—therefore, neither MRI of the cervical spine and EMG of the arm are warranted. MRI of the shoulder could be considered if pain persists despite treatment but should not be an initial step.

Sie IH, Waters RL, Adkins RH, Gellman H. Upper extremity pain in the post rehabilitation spinal cord injured patient. Arch Phys Med Rehabil. 1992;73(1):44–8.
Lal S. Premature degenerative shoulder changes in spinal cord injury patients. Spinal Cord. 1998;36(3):186–9. https://doi.org/10.1038/sj.sc.3100608.

Part 2: Which of the following is the greatest risk factor for developing this condition in this particular patient?

A. Age
B. Length of time from spinal cord injury
C. Body mass index
D. Gender

Answer: B.

Age, length of time from spinal cord injury, and body mass index have all been linked to development of shoulder overuse and pain syndrome. However, length of time from onset of spinal cord injury has been shown in multiple studies to be most predictive of upper extremity complications. Gender has not been linked to development of shoulder pain.

Nyland J, Quigley P, Huang C, Lloyd J, Harrow J, Nelson A. Preserving transfer independence among individuals with spinal cord injury. Spinal Cord. 2000;38(11):649–57. https://doi.org/10.1038/sj.sc.3101070.

17. All of the following are mechanisms of action of botulinum toxin EXCEPT:

A. Inhibits release of glutamate
B. Cleaves SNAP-25
C. Agonist of GABA-B
D. Suppresses secretion of calcitonin gene-related peptide

Answer: C.

Botulinum toxin's mechanism of action in regards to spasticity is cleavage of a portion of the SNARE complex, a group of proteins involved in vesicle fusion of acetylcholine at the presynaptic terminal; SNAP-25 is targeted by botulinum toxin A specifically. Botulinum toxins have also been shown to inhibit release of glutamate and suppress secretion of calcitonin gene-related peptide (CGRP) which are both involved in pain modulation pathways. Baclofen is a GABA-B agonist.

Ashkenazi A. Botulinum toxin type a for chronic migraine. Curr Neurol Neurosci Rep. 2010;10(2):140–6. https://doi.org/10.1007/s11910-010-0087-5.
Walker HW, Lee MY, Bahroo LB, Hedera P, Charles D. Botulinum toxin injection techniques for the management of adult spasticity. PM R. 2015;7(4):417–27. https://doi.org/10.1016/j.pmrj.2014.09.021. Epub 2014 Oct 8.

18. A 30-year-old man with T3 AIS A paraplegia develops erythema over the lateral aspect of both feet. He is a manual wheelchair user. On examination, he has a stage 1 pressure injury over the plantar aspect of the fifth metatarsal head. On Modified Ashworth Scale testing, his ankle plantarflexion and ankle inversion are noted to be 2 with clonus. Which is the best next step in management of his spasticity?

    A. Serial casting
    B. Botulinum toxin injection to posterior tibialis, gastrocnemius, and soleus
    C. Physical therapy for consideration of bracing
    D. Initiate oral baclofen

Answer: C.

Spasticity is a common sequelae of spinal cord injury. It has been shown to preserve muscle mass; however, this patient's spasticity of the ankle is likely impacting his positioning in the wheelchair causing pressure injuries over the lateral feet. Conservative management should be preferentially initiated with range of motion and evaluation for bracing. Botulinum toxin is a focal treatment which can improve spasticity, and could be considered if no improvement was seen with bracing/ROM. Serial casting would not be ideal in this patient due to his pressure injury. Oral baclofen would also not be ideal in this patient due to the focal nature of the spasticity.

Lin J, Chay W. Special considerations in assessing and treating spasticity in spinal cord injury. Phys Med Rehabil Clin N Am. 2018;29(3):445–453. https://doi.org/10.1016/j.pmr.2018.03.001. Epub 2018 May 28.
Adams MM, Hicks AL. Spasticity after spinal cord injury. Spinal Cord. 2005;43(10):577–86. https://doi.org/10.1038/sj.sc.3101757.

19. In the first 5 years after spinal cord injury, the incidence of shoulder pain in individuals with tetraplegia is approximately:

    A. 10–15%
    B. 25–40%
    C. 50–65%
    D. 75–90%

Answer: C.

In the first 5 years after spinal cord injury approximately 53% of individuals with tetraplegia experience shoulder pain. This is higher than the incidence of shoulder pain in individuals with paraplegia, which is potentially attributed to increased neuropathic pain in the shoulder region after cervical spinal cord injury.

Scelza WM, Dyson-Hudson TA. Neuromusculoskeletal complications of spinal cord injury. In: Kirshblum S, Campagnolo DI, editors. Spinal cord medicine. 2nd ed. Philadelphia: Lipincott Williams & Wilkins; 2011. p. 282–308.

20. In the first 5 years after spinal cord injury, the incidence of shoulder pain in individuals with paraplegia is approximately :

    A. 15–25%
    B. 25–40%
    C. 50–65%
    D. 75–90%

Answer: A.

In the first 5 years after spinal cord injury approximately 16% of individuals with paraplegia reported shoulder pain. In individuals less than 5 years post-spinal cord injury those with tetraplegia report a higher incidence of shoulder pain than those with paraplegia. This is higher than the incidence of shoulder pain in individuals with paraplegia which is potentially attributed to increased neuropathic pain in the shoulder region after cervical spinal cord injury.

Scelza WM, Dyson-Hudson TA. Neuromusculoskeletal complications of spinal cord injury. In: Kirshblum S, Campagnolo DI, editors. Spinal cord medicine. 2nd ed. Philadelphia: Lippincott Williams & Wilkins; 2011. p. 6–30.

21. Which individual is most likely to complain of shoulder pain with activities of daily living?

    A. An individual with tetraplegia who is 1 year post spinal cord injury
    B. An individual with paraplegia who is 1 year post spinal cord injury
    C. An individual with tetraplegia who is 20 years post spinal cord injury
    D. An individual with paraplegia who is 20 years post spinal cord injury

Answer: D.

In individuals less than 5 years post spinal cord injury, those with tetraplegia report a higher incidence of shoulder pain than those with paraplegia. This is higher than the incidence of shoulder pain in individuals with paraplegia which is potentially attributed to increased neuropathic pain in the shoulder region after cervical spinal cord injury. However, by 20 years post injury more than

70% of individuals with paraplegia reported shoulder pain which was higher than individuals with tetraplegia. This increase in shoulder pain in the paraplegic population is potentially attributed to repetitive stress on the shoulders in this population related to transfers and wheelchair propulsion.

Sie IH, Waters RL, Adkins RH, Gellman H. Upper extremity pain in the postrehabilitation spinal cord injured patient. Arch Phys Med Rehabil. 1992;73(1):44–8.
Gellman H, Sie I, Waters RL. Late complications of the weight-bearing upper extremity in the paraplegic patient. Clin Orthop Relat Res. 1988;(233):132–5.

22. The Painful Arc Test refers to what range of motion in the shoulder and is indicative of strain to which muscle

    A. Between 60° and 120° of abduction, Supraspinatus
    B. Between 120° and 180° of abduction, Infraspinatus
    C. Between 60° and 120° of external rotation, Teres Minor
    D. Between 120° and 180° of abduction, Supraspinatus

Answer: A.

Pain between 60° and 120° of active shoulder abduction (i.e., "Painful Arc Test"), or after resistance is applied with the patient's arm abducted to 90° and fully pronated within the scapular plane (i.e., "Empty Can Test"), may indicate supraspinatus tendinopathy. Rotator cuff pathology is a common overuse injury in persons with paraplegia due to over-use from transfers and wheelchair propulsion.

Flynn, T.W., Cleland, J.A., & Whitman, J.M. User's guide to the musculoskeletal examination: fundamentals for the evidence-based clinician. Buckner, Kentucky: Evidence in Motion; 2008.

23. Which of the following conditions should be included in the differential diagnosis of shoulder abnormalities in individuals with paraplegia as its prevalence is much higher than ambulatory individuals with shoulder pain?

    A. Distal clavicle osteolysis
    B. Clavicle fracture
    C. Acromioclavicular dislocation
    D. Proximal humeral fracture

Answer: A.

The prevalence of osteolysis of the distal clavicle is approximately 13% in individuals with paraplegia though not all individuals have shoulder pain associated with this finding. This is higher than in the non-spinal cord injury population. The increased prevalence is attributed to repetitive trauma to the shoulder due to transfers and wheelchair propulsion in the paraplegic population. Distal clavicular osteolysis should be on the differential for people with paraplegia who present with shoulder complaints.

Boninger ML, Towers JD, Cooper RA, Dicianno BE, Munin MC. Shoulder imaging abnormalities in individuals with paraplegia. J Rehabil Res Dev. 2001;38(4):401–8.
Roach NA, Schweitzer ME. Does osteolysis of the distal clavicle occur following spinal cord injury? Skeletal Radiol. 1997;26(1):16–9. https://doi.org/10.1007/s002560050184.

24. Which of the following is a risk factor for developing carpal tunnel syndrome after spinal cord injury?

    A. Longer time since injury
    B. Having tetraplegia
    C. Being male
    D. Younger age

Answer: A.

The prevalence of carpal tunnel syndrome after spinal cord injury is estimated to be between 49% and 73% depending on the study, compared to only 15% in the general population. Risk factors for carpal tunnel syndrome include higher body mass index, older age, longer duration of paralysis, and activities which cause overuse of the wrist and hand (such as wheelchair sports). Being female is a risk factor for carpal tunnel syndrome in the general population but has not been established in those with spinal cord injury.

Yang J, Boninger ML, Leath JD, Fitzgerald SG, Dyson-Hudson TA, Chang MW. Carpal tunnel syndrome in manual wheelchair users with spinal cord injury: a cross-sectional multicenter study. Am J Phys Med Rehabil. 2009;88(12):1007–16. https://doi.org/10.1097/PHM.0b013e3181bbddc9.

25. Which of the following propulsion patterns is preferred for injury prevention when using a manual wheelchair?

    A. Single looping over
    B. Double looping over
    C. Arched
    D. Elliptical or semi-circular

Answer: D.

The most appropriate pattern of wheelchair propulsion which provides the best ergonomic posture for propulsion with shoulder protection is the elliptical or semi-circular pattern.

Boninger ML, Koontz AM, Sisto SA, Dyson-Hudson TA, Chang M, Price R, Cooper RA. Pushrim biomechanics and injury prevention in spinal cord injury: recommendations based on CULP-SCI investigations. J Rehabil Res Dev. 2005;42(3 Suppl. 1):9–19. https://doi.org/10.1682/jrrd.2004.08.0103.

Boninger ML, Souza AL, Cooper RA, Fitzgerald SG, Koontz AM, Fay BT. Propulsion patterns and pushrim biomechanics in manual wheelchair propulsion. Arch Phys Med Rehabil. 2002;83(5):718–23. https://doi.org/10.1053/apmr.2002.32455.

Paralyzed Veterans of America Consortium for Spinal Cord Medicine. Preservation of upper limb function following spinal cord injury: a clinical practice guideline for health-care professionals. J Spinal Cord Med. 2005;28(5):434–70. https://doi.org/10.1080/1079026 8.2005.11753844.

26. Which of the following statements regarding wheelchairs is correct:

    A. Increasing camber creates a larger turning radius
    B. Decreasing the camber creates a larger base of support
    C. Shifting the rear axle forward improves curb navigation
    D. Shifting the rear axle backwards improves propulsion efficiency

Answer: C.

Camber is the angle created by the rear wheelchair wheel and a line perpendicular to the ground. Standard everyday use wheelchairs use a camber of 0–4°. Increasing the camber results in a wider base of support and smaller turning radius. Shifting the rear axle of a manual wheelchair forward decreases propulsion frequency, rate of rise of force and push angle making propulsion more efficient, but also decreases the base of support making it less stable (more likely to tip over backwards). As the wheelchair user's center of gravity is closer to the rear axle, achieving a wheelie position for curb navigation becomes easier.

Boninger ML, Souza AL, Cooper RA, Fitzgerald SG, Koontz AM, Fay BT. Propulsion patterns and pushrim biomechanics in manual wheelchair propulsion. Arch Phys Med Rehabil. 2002;83(5):718–23. https://doi.org/10.1053/apmr.2002.32455.

Paralyzed Veterans of America Consortium for Spinal Cord Medicine. Preservation of upper limb function following spinal cord injury: a clinical practice guideline for health-care professionals. J Spinal Cord Med. 2005;28(5):434–70. https://doi.org/10.1080/1079026 8.2005.11753844.

27. Which of the following is the best propulsive stroke adaptation to prevent overuse injuries while using a manual wheelchair?

    A. Increased stroke frequency
    B. Decreased stroke frequency
    C. Increased rate of loading
    D. Increased peak force

Answer: B.

Longer strokes, reduced stroke frequency, reduced peak forces, and reduced rate of loading are all strategies which can help prevent over-use injuries to the shoulder due to wheelchair propulsion. Elliptical push pattern with a slower recovery compared to push time results in lower stroke frequency.

Scelza WM, Dyson-Hudson TA. Neuromusculoskeletal complications of spinal cord injury. In: Kirshblum S, Campagnolo DI, editors. Spinal cord medicine. 2nd ed. Philadelphia: Lipincott Williams & Wilkins; 2011. p. 6–30.

Boninger ML, Koontz AM, Sisto SA, Dyson-Hudson TA, Chang M, Price R, Cooper RA. Pushrim biomechanics and injury prevention in spinal cord injury: recommendations based on CULP-SCI investigations. J Rehabil Res Dev. 2005;42(3 Suppl. 1):9–19. https://doi.org/10.1682/jrrd.2004.08.0103.

Boninger ML, Souza AL, Cooper RA, Fitzgerald SG, Koontz AM, Fay BT. Propulsion patterns and pushrim biomechanics in manual wheelchair propulsion. Arch Phys Med Rehabil. 2002;83(5):718–23. https://doi.org/10.1053/apmr.2002.32455.

28. According to the Subaxial Injury Classification System (SLICS), greater or equal to what score would indicate surgical intervention?

A. 3
B. 4
C. 5
D. 6

Answer: B.

The subaxial cervical spine injury classification system is a severity score for cervical spine trauma that can help determine treatment. No abnormality is 0 points. Simple compression fracture gives 1 point. Burst fracture gives 2 points. Distraction (e.g. perched facet joint, hyperextension cervical injuries) gives 3 points. Rotation/translation (e.g. facet discolation, unstable teardrop or advanced flexion compression injury) gives 4 points. A cumulative score of 4 points or above generally indicates the need for surgical intervention.

Samuel S, Lin JL, Smith MM, Hartin NL, Vasili C, Ruff SJ, Cree AK, Ball JR, Sergides IG, Gray R. Subaxial injury classification scoring system treatment recommendations: external agreement study based on retrospective review of 185 patients. Spine (Phila Pa 1976). 2015;40(3):137–42. https://doi.org/10.1097/BRS.0000000000000666.

Joaquim AF, Patel AA, Vaccaro AR. Cervical injuries scored according to the subaxial injury classification system: an analysis of the literature. J Craniovertebr Junction Spine. 2014;5(2):65–70. https://doi.org/10.4103/0974-8237.139200.

Dvorak MF, Fisher CG, Fehlings MG, Rampersaud YR, Oner FC, Aarabi B, Vaccaro AR. The surgical approach to subaxial cervical spine injuries: an evidence-based algorithm based on the SLIC classification system. Spine (Phila Pa 1976). 2007;32(23):2620–9. https://doi.org/10.1097/BRS.0b013e318158ce16.

29. According to the Denis Classification the spine is divided into columns. What structures are included in the posterior column?

   A. Pedicles, facet joints and articular processes, ligamentum flavum, neural arch and interconnecting ligaments
   B. Posterior one-third of the vertebral body, posterior one-third of the intervertebral disc, and posterior longitudinal ligament
   C. Pedicles, facet joints and articular processes, ligamentum flavum, neural arch, interconnecting ligaments, and posterior longitudinal ligament
   D. Posterior one-third of the vertebral body and posterior one-third of the intervertebral disc

Answer: A.

The pedicles, facet joints and articular processes, ligamentum flavum, neural arch and interconnecting ligaments are all included in the posterior column. The middle column consists of the posterior one-third of the vertebral body, posterior one-third of the intervertebral disc (annulus fibrosis) and the posterior longitudinal ligament. The anterior column consists of the anterior longitudinal ligament, anterior two-thirds of the vertebral body, and anterior two-thirds of the intervertebral disks. Disruption to two or more or the middle column of the spine generally leads to spinal instability.

Denis F. The three column spine and its significance in the classification of acute thoracolumbar spinal injuries. Spine (Phila Pa 1976). 1983;8(8):817–31. https://doi.org/10.1097/00007632-198311000-00003.

30. Following a traumatic spine fracture resulting in incomplete tetraplegia, surgical intervention for decompression of the spinal cord within what time period will likely provide the best chance of neurological recovery:

   A. Within 24 h (1 day)
   B. Within 72 h (3 days)
   C. Within 96 h (4 days)
   D. Within 168 h (7 days)

Answer: A.

Decompression of the spinal cord after traumatic fracture resulting in incomplete spinal cord injury within 24 h has shown to have improved neurological outcomes compared to delayed decompression.

Fehlings MG, Vaccaro A, Wilson JR, Singh A, W Cadotte D, Harrop JS, Aarabi B, Shaffrey C, Dvorak M, Fisher C, Arnold P, Massicotte EM, Lewis S, Rampersaud R. Early versus delayed decompression for traumatic cervical spinal cord injury: results of the Surgical Timing in Acute Spinal Cord Injury Study (STASCIS). PLoS One. 2012;7(2):e32037. https://doi.org/10.1371/journal.pone.0032037. Epub 2012 Feb 23.

Gupta DK, Vaghani G, Siddiqui S, Sawhney C, Singh PK, Kumar A, Kale SS, Sharma BS. Early versus delayed decompression in acute subaxial cervical spinal cord injury: a prospective outcome study at a Level I trauma center from India. Asian J Neurosurg. 2015;10(3):158–65. https://doi.org/10.4103/1793-5482.161193.

31. Which of the following would be considered an unstable fracture and require surgical stabilization?

    A. Disruption of the posterior longitudinal ligament
    B. Anterior wedge compression fracture
    C. Spinous process fracture
    D. Disruption of the anterior longitudinal ligament

Answer: A.

The pedicles, facet joints and articular processes, ligamentum flavum, neural arch and interconnecting ligaments are all included in the posterior column. The middle column consists of the posterior one-third of the vertebral body, posterior one-third of the intervertebral disc (annulus fibrosis) and the posterior longitudinal ligament. The anterior column consists of the anterior longitudinal ligament, anterior two-thirds of the vertebral body, and anterior two-thirds of the intervertebral disks. Disruption to two or more or the middle column of the spine generally leads to spinal instability.

Denis F. The three column spine and its significance in the classification of acute thoraco-lumbar spinal injuries. Spine (Phila Pa 1976). 1983;8(8):817–31. https://doi.org/10.109 7/00007632-198311000-00003.

32. A 65-year-old man falls down a flight of stairs. He is able to stand immediately afterwards but complains of significant neck pain. Upon evaluation in the emergency department, he is immediately placed in a hard cervical collar and taken for cervical spine imaging. Radiographs reveal an odontoid fracture. Which type of odontoid fracture is most likely to require surgical intervention?

    A. Type I fracture
    B. Type II fracture
    C. Type III fracture
    D. Type IV fracture

Answer: B.

Type I odontoid fractures are avulsions of the tip of the odontoid and are generally considered stable fractures. Type II fractures are through the base of the odontoid and are unstable. Type III fractures are through the junction of the odontoid and body of C2. Type II fractures have a higher rate of nonunion when treated non-operatively than type III fractures. Type IV is not a type of odontoid fracture.

Gornet ME, Kelly MP. Fractures of the axis: a review of pediatric, adult, and geriatric injuries. Curr Rev Musculoskelet Med. 2016;9(4):505–12. https://doi.org/10.1007/s12178-016-9368-1.

33. A woman with a C4 AIS A SCI returns to your clinic for routine follow up 1 year after her spinal cord injury. A general exam includes range of motion measurements of each joint. Which of the following joints is most likely to exhibit a decrease in range of motion from the year prior?

    A. Shoulder
    B. Elbow
    C. Hip
    D. Knee

Answer: A.

Contractures are a common sequelae of spinal cord injury resulting in a loss of range of motion of the joint. The prevalence of contracture is cited as between 11–50%. The shoulder, ankles and wrists are the most common joints affected, though any joint below the neurological level of injury may be affected.

Diong J, Harvey LA, Kwah LK, Eyles J, Ling MJ, Ben M, Herbert RD. Incidence and predictors of contracture after spinal cord injury—a prospective cohort study. Spinal Cord. 2012;50(8):579–84. https://doi.org/10.1038/sc.2012.25. Epub 2012 Mar 27.
Fergusson D, Hutton B, Drodge A. The epidemiology of major joint contractures: a systematic review of the literature. Clin Orthop Relat Res. 2007;456:22–9. https://doi.org/10.1097/BLO.0b013e3180308456.

34. Which of the following individuals is at highest risk for long bone fracture after spinal cord injury?

    A. A person with T12 AIS A SCI
    B. A person with T12 AIS C SCI
    C. A person with C4 AIS B SCI
    D. A person with C4 AIS D SCI

Answer: A.

Individuals with motor complete SCI are at higher risk than motor incomplete injuries for fractures after spinal cord injury. Individuals with paraplegia are at higher risk than those with tetraplegia for fractures after spinal cord injury, possibly due to increased activity level.

Edwards WB, Schnitzer TJ. Bone imaging and fracture risk after spinal cord injury. Curr Osteoporos Rep. 2015;13(5):310–7. https://doi.org/10.1007/s11914-015-0288-6.

35. Which of the following fracture types is the most stable fracture?

    A. Jefferson fracture
    B. Chance Fracture
    C. Hangman's fracture
    D. Clay-shoveler's fracture

Answer: D.

A clay-shoveler's fracture is an avulsion fracture of the spinous process only, which is the posterior column only therefore it is a stable fracture. A Jefferson fracture is a burst fracture resulting in fractures of the anterior and posterior arches of the Atlas (C1) vertebra and occurs most often due to falls or diving into shallow water. A Chance fracture (also known as a seatbelt fracture) is a flexion-distraction injury of the spine which occurs in the thoracic or lumbar vertebra and usually involves disruption of all three columns. A Hangman's fracture refers to a bilateral fracture of the posterior arch of the Axis (C2 vertebra) and disruption of C2–3 junction (pars interarticularis) and occurs most often due to falls.

Thomas Pope, Hans L. Bloem, Javier Beltran, William B. Morrison, David John Wilson. Musculoskeletal imaging. Philadelphia PA: Elsevier Saunders; 2014.
Posthuma de Boer J, van Wulfften Palthe AF, Stadhouder A, Bloemers FW. The clay Shoveler's fracture: a case report and review of the literature. J Emerg Med. 2016;51(3):292–7. https://doi.org/10.1016/j.jemermed.2016.03.020. Epub 2016 Jun 1.

Neurological Complications of Spinal Cord Injury

12

Peter Park and Katharine Tam

Questions

1. A 27-year-old male involved in a motor vehicle accident with resultant C7 AIS A spinal cord injury (SCI) is admitted to the intensive care unit. On hospital day 6, his vital signs are notable for a temperature of 97.8 °F, blood pressure of 197/110 mmHg and heart rate of 68 bpm. He appears uncomfortable lying on a pressure redistribution mattress and is diaphoretic. His abdomen is nontender but firm and distended. There is no visible stool in his diaper. Foley catheter is in place with clear urine draining into the bag with a urine output of 2100 mL over the past 24 h. What is the postulated mechanism for the phenomenon that this patient is experiencing?

   A. Compensatory increase in cardiac output due to peripheral vasodilation
   B. Physiologic response to hypovolemic status
   C. Disruption of the inhibitory descending vasomotor pathways
   D. Systemic manifestation of recurrent hydronephrosis

   Answer: C.

   Given the patient's elevated blood pressure and flushing in the setting of a complete SCI above T6, this presentation is consistent with autonomic dysreflexia

P. Park
Division of Rehabilitation, Department of Neurology, Washington University School of Medicine, Saint Louis, MO, USA

K. Tam (✉)
Division of Rehabilitation, Department of Neurology, Washington University School of Medicine, Saint Louis, MO, USA

Spinal Cord Injury and Disorders, Saint Louis VA Healthcare System, Saint Louis, MO, USA
e-mail: Katharine.Tam@va.gov

© The Author(s), under exclusive license to Springer Nature Switzerland AG 2022
B. A. Abramoff et al. (eds.), *The Essential Spinal Cord Injury Medicine Question Bank*, https://doi.org/10.1007/978-3-031-07796-8_12

(AD). Noxious stimuli such as tight clothing, over-distension of bowel and/or bladder, and pressure injuries can cause widespread sympathetic vasoconstriction (Option A) that should normally be compensated by descending vasomotor pathways to sympathetic preganglionic neurons. In a complete SCI, however, this compensatory mechanism is disrupted (Option C). In this patient, the firm distended abdomen is suggestive of constipation secondary to neurogenic bowel. While a kinked foley or other urinary tract obstruction (e.g. nephrolithiasis) can cause bladder distention or hydronephrosis and thereby precipitate AD; it is a specific reason that doesn't explain the underlying neurological mechanism of AD. Specifically, this patient's urine output has been adequate without evidence of hypovolemic status (Options B and D).

Eldahan KC, Rabchevsky AG. Autonomic dysreflexia after spinal cord injury: systemic pathophysiology and methods of management. Auton Neurosci. 2018;209:59–70. https://doi.org/10.1016/j.autneu.2017.05.002. Epub 2017 May 8.

2. A 67-year-old male with a C3 AIS C SCI secondary to a fall is admitted to the SCI unit. He has been complaining of increasing muscle spasms that are occurring every 20 min throughout the day. He has been participating in therapy with range-of-motion exercises daily, although these exercises have been limited by significant pain. Bedside passive range of motion of his bilateral elbows reveals catching of the joint at various speeds of elbow flexion and extension, and it is difficult, although possible, to complete the full range of motion. He is currently taking acetaminophen 500 mg QID, gabapentin 300 mg TID, and baclofen 5 mg daily. What is the most appropriate next step in this patient's management?

A. Add cyclobenzaprine 5 mg QHS
B. Add ibuprofen 600 mg TID
C. Increase gabapentin to 600 mg TID
D. Increase baclofen to 5 mg TID

Answer: D.

This patient is exhibiting worsening spasticity, with an exam suggestive of Modified Ashworth Scale grade 3 spasticity. Conservative management of spasticity with therapy and range of motion exercises should be the first step. If spasticity remains uncontrolled, oral medication can be considered. Baclofen is a commonly used agent that is indicated for spasticity in patients with SCI, and it is typically administered 1–3 times per day up to 80 mg/day, the Federal Drug Administration approved maximum daily dose (Option D). There is literature supporting titration of baclofen up to 240 mg a day. Other agents such as tizanidine, diazepam, dantrolene, or clonidine can be used also, although baclofen is generally a first-line agent for spasticity in SCI (Options A, B, C).

Dario A, Tomei G. A benefit-risk assessment of baclofen in severe spinal spasticity. Drug Saf. 2004;27(11):799–818. https://doi.org/10.2165/00002018-200427110-00004.

Walker HW, Hon A, Hess MJ. Spasticity management. In: Kirshblum S, Lin VW, editors. Spinal cord medicine. New York: Springer Publishing Company; 2018. p. 472–86.

Aisen ML, Dietz MA, Rossi P, Cedarbaum JM, Kutt H. Clinical and pharmacokinetic aspects of high dose oral baclofen therapy. J Am Paraplegia Soc. 1992;15(4):211–6. https://doi.org/10.1080/01952307.1992.11761520.

3. Which of the following scenarios is necessary to determine that a patient is no longer experiencing post-traumatic amnesia (PTA)?

   A. A score of 76 or higher on the Galveston Orientation and Amnesia Test (GOAT) for two consecutive testing sessions
   B. A score of 23 or higher on the Montreal Cognitive Assessment (MoCA) at least 1 week after initial injury
   C. An improvement of at least five points on the St. Louis University Mental Status Examination (SLUMS) within 3 days of testing
   D. Clinically observed improvement in memory and speech without the need for specific testing

Answer: A.

By definition, a score of 76 or higher on two consecutive testing sessions with the GOAT indicates that the patient is out of PTA (Option A). While clinical observation may suggest ongoing improvement of PTA, testing with GOAT should be completed to objectively assess for changes in cognition (Option D). MoCA and SLUMS are traditionally used to assess for dementia, and not for PTA (Options B and C).

Lombard LA, Kwasnica C, Brooks M. Dual diagnosis: spinal cord injury and traumatic brain injury. In: Kirshblum S, Lin VW, editors. Spinal cord medicine. New York: Springer Publishing Company; 2018. p. 567–76.

4. You are consulted on a 19-year-old man with an incomplete T9 SCI in the setting of a motorcycle accident. His Glasgow coma scale (GCS) has improved from 3 on arrival to 9 on hospital day 3. For the past 24 h, his heart rate has been elevated above 130 bpm with an average blood pressure of 155/85 mmHg, and temperature ranging between 99.4 and 100.1 °F. His respiratory rate is currently 20 breaths/min. His skin is diaphoretic and normal in color. Last bowel movement is reported to be 30 min ago and an indwelling foley is draining clear urine. Given the most likely diagnosis, which pharmacotherapy should be considered?

   A. Nitropaste
   B. Hypertonic saline
   C. Propranolol
   D. Dantrolene

Answer: C.

This patient is most likely experiencing dysautonomia, also known as central storming or paroxysmal sympathetic hyperactivity, given his severe traumatic brain injury (TBI) (initial GCS <8) with sustained hyperactive sympathetic signs. Although there is no clear consensus on pharmacotherapy treatment of this phenomenon, propranolol has been shown to be effective in both aborting and preventing dysautonomia in patients with a TBI (Option C). Presence of a concurrent SCI makes autonomic dysreflexia a possibility but level of injury at T9 (i.e. below T6) makes this less likely (Option A). Hypertonic saline may be considered to mitigate situations with increased intracranial pressures such as spontaneous intracranial bleeding (Option B). Neuroleptic malignant syndrome is less likely in the absence of a history of antipsychotic medication use, marked rigidity, or fever, therefore dantrolene would not be the best choice of pharmacotherapy (Option D).

Baguley IJ, Cameron ID, Green AM, Slewa-Younan S, Marosszeky JE, Gurka JA. Pharmacological management of dysautonomia following traumatic brain injury. Brain Inj. 2004;18(5):409–17. https://doi.org/10.1080/02699050310001645775.

5. Which of the following clinical scenarios is most consistent with post-traumatic syringomyelia (PTS)?

   A. Complaints of new burning sensation in the low back radiating toward abdomen 10 years following a T11 SCI
   B. Complaints of new urinary leakage 3 months after spinal cord injury
   C. Complaints of frequent episodes of "racing heartbeat" 2 weeks after the traumatic event
   D. Complaints of cramping, dull, and achy pain in both shoulders and feet 3 days after the traumatic event

Answer: A.

PTS is the most common cause of progressive myelopathy after a SCI, which is described as a fluid-filled cyst inside the spinal cord's gray matter. The most commonly reported symptom associated with syringomyelia is usually neuropathic pain (i.e. aching, burning, sharp) near the level of injury. Its occurrence tends to be many years after the injury rather than in the immediate acute phase (Option A). Other common signs and symptoms of PTS include, but are not limited to, changes in spasticity, new or changes in autonomic dysreflexia, motor or sensory loss, Horner's syndrome, and temperature dysregulation. While new onset of bladder dysfunction (Option B) is a possible finding in PTS, presentation during the subacute period makes it less likely to be secondary to PTS. Overactive bladder or urinary tract infection are more likely etiologies for new urinary leakage. The remaining options (Options C and D) do not fit the typical description of symptoms for PTS nor the time frame.

Frisbie JH, Aguilera EJ. Chronic pain after spinal cord injury: an expedient diagnostic approach. Paraplegia. 1990;28(7):460–5. https://doi.org/10.1038/sc.1990.62.

Scelza WM, Falci SP, Indeck CS. Posttraumatic syringomyelia and spinal cord tethering. In: Kirshblum S, Lin VW, editors. Spinal cord medicine. New York: Springer Publishing Company; 2019. p. 577–83.

6. Which study is the gold standard for the diagnosis of post-traumatic syringomyelia (PTS)?

A. Cerebrospinal fluid analysis
B. Magnetic resonance imaging (MRI) with contrast
C. Computed tomography (CT) myelogram
D. Nerve conduction study

Answer: B.

MRI with contrast is the gold standard for diagnosing PTS as it allows for analysis of spinal cord tethering, myelomalacia, and cystic cavitation (Option B). Contrast also enhances the ability to determine the etiology of the imaging findings (e.g. infectious, vascular, neoplastic, etc.). CT myelograms can be used as a modality if MRI is not possible, such as in cases of MRI incompatible instrumentation, pacemakers, or bullet fragments (Option C). Nerve conduction studies can be considered but may be more difficult to interpret in the presence of chronic SCI (Option D). MRI with cerebral spinal fluid (CSF) flow studies can show regions of aberrant CSF flow but the CSF analysis does not have a role in diagnosis of PTS (Option A).

Asano M, Fujiwara K, Yonenobu K, Hiroshima K. Post-traumatic syringomyelia. Spine (Phila Pa 1976). 1996;21(12):1446–53. https://doi.org/10.1097/00007632-199606150-00009.

Scelza WM, Falci SP, Indeck CS. Posttraumatic syringomyelia and spinal cord tethering. In: Kirshblum S, Lin VW, editors. Spinal cord medicine. New York: Springer Publishing Company; 2019. p. 577–83.

7. Which of the following interventions is the most appropriate next step for a man with T6 AIS B SCI whose spasticity has been managed with an intrathecal baclofen (ITB) pump for a year but has had difficulties with clean intermittent catheterization (CIC) and pelvic hygiene due to uncontrolled spasticity in bilateral hip adductors despite titration to maximum ITB dose?

A. Suprapubic catheter placement
B. Mitrofanoff procedure
C. Wheelchair modification to promote hip abduction
D. Neurotomy

Answer: D.

The patient's difficulty with CIC is apparently due to the spasticity in the hip adductors that prevent him from easily self-catheterizing, rather than due to urological anatomy dysfunction. Therefore, Options A and B are not directly addressing the problem at this point, although these are surgical options that can be used for patients with detrusor sphincter dyssynergia (DSD), inability to self-catheterize due to impaired hand functioning, or spasticity refractory to conservative management. A suprapubic catheter will address difficulties with CIC but not difficulties with lower body hygiene or dressing that may be present with uncontrolled hip adduction tone. Repositioning of the legs to counteract the spasticity in the hip adduction is only likely to add mechanical stress in the muscles and neurovasculature of the legs (Option C). Obturator neurotomy (Option D) is a surgical procedure for hip adductor spasticity that has been shown to be beneficial, along with other techniques such as tenotomy, tendon lengthening, and tendon transfer procedures.

Walker HW, Hon A, Hess MJ. Spasticity management. In: Kirshblum S, Lin VW, editors. Spinal cord medicine. New York: Springer Publishing Company; 2019. p. 472–86.

8. Which of the following statements below describe the current understanding of hydrocephalus as a complication secondary to an isolated SCI?

   A. It is extremely rare with few cases reported, when it does happen, it is almost always after cervical spinal cord injuries.
   B. It is rare, occurring in about 1 in 100, and presents most commonly with worsening neck and back pain.
   C. It is common, occurring in about 1 in 20, and presents most commonly with seizures, and prophylactic anti-epileptic drugs (AEDs) must be initiated.
   D. It is very common, occurring in 1 in 5, and any early signs of hydrocephalus should prompt immediate placement of ventriculoperitoneal (VP) shunts.

   Answer: A.

   Hydrocephalus secondary to isolated SCI is extremely rare and the existing case reports in current literature are mainly limited to patients who suffered concomitant TBI or iatrogenic insult, with the diagnosis of hydrocephalus often being an incidental finding. The location of the spinal cord involved is invariably in the cervical region. Postulated mechanisms include CSF malabsorption and ascending spinal cord edema, but no exact mechanism has been established thus far. Prevalence of hydrocephalus in general is most common in the pediatric population, with incidence of less than 1 in 1000 live births (Option B). Seizures, altered mental status, vision changes, vomiting, and other signs of elevated intracranial pressure are certainly sequelae of hydrocephalus after an SCI, but a thorough workup to ascertain the etiology of the patient's change in status should be completed prior to initiation of any AEDs or interventions such as VP shunts (Options C and D).

Chrastina J, Novák Z, Feitová V. Is hydrocephalus after spinal cord injury really caused by the injured spinal cord? Two case reports and a literature review. Rozhl Chir. 2016;95(5):203–5 (English).

Joseph G, Johnston RA, Fraser MH, McLean AN. Delayed hydrocephalus as an unusual complication of a stab injury to the spine. Spinal Cord. 2005;43(1):56–8. https://doi.org/10.1038/sj.sc.3101655.

9. Which neuromodulation technique has been shown to be effective in aiding with functional walking after chronic incomplete SCI in both animal and human models?

    A. Transcutaneous electrical nerve stimulation (TENS)
    B. Electrical spinal cord stimulation (ESCS)
    C. Deep brain stimulation (DBS)
    D. Functional electrical stimulation (FES)

Answer: B.

ESCS therapy can be used to recruit spinal neural circuitry as well as muscle in order to evoke locomotor movements in a way that is more coordinated than direct stimulation of muscle as seen in FES (Option D). TENS can be useful for decreasing pain and spasticity via modulation of nociceptive and proprioceptive afferent nerves but has not been shown to be independently beneficial in improving motor function (Option A). DBS is commonly used for conditions such as Parkinson's disease or epilepsy, and not routinely used for locomotor function in SCI patients (Option C).

Huang H, He J, Herman R, Carhart MR. Modulation effects of epidural spinal cord stimulation on muscle activities during walking. IEEE Trans Neural Syst Rehabil Eng. 2006;14(1):14–23. https://doi.org/10.1109/TNSRE.2005.862694.

Lee HJ, Tansey KE. Recent advances in spinal cord research: preclinical spinal cord injury, plasticity, and repair. In: Kirshblum S, Lin VW, editors. Spinal cord medicine. New York: Springer Publishing Company; 2018. p. 870–89.

Wagner FB, Mignardot JB, Le Goff-Mignardot CG, Demesmaeker R, Komi S, Capogrosso M, Rowald A, Seáñez I, Caban M, Pirondini E, Vat M, McCracken LA, Heimgartner R, Fodor I, Watrin A, Seguin P, Paoles E, Van Den Keybus K, Eberle G, Schurch B, Pralong E, Becce F, Prior J, Buse N, Buschman R, Neufeld E, Kuster N, Carda S, von Zitzewitz J, Delattre V, Denison T, Lambert H, Minassian K, Bloch J, Courtine G. Targeted neurotechnology restores walking in humans with spinal cord injury. Nature. 2018;563(7729):65–71. https://doi.org/10.1038/s41586-018-0649-2. Epub 2018 Oct 31.

10. A 40-year-old male patient with a diagnosis T1 AIS A in the SCI unit has two recorded temperatures of 100.8 and 101.1 °F overnight. When seen on rounds, he states that he feels well, denies subjective fevers and chills, and any other complaints. Blood pressure, heart rate, and respiratory status are all within normal limits. Urinalysis and CBC obtained are both within normal limits. Blood cultures are pending. Physical exam is also unremarkable without any open sores on his body. What is the next best step in management?

A. Administer an antipyretic and observe
B. Order troponins and an electrocardiogram
C. Obtain a chest X-ray
D. Order telemetry for close cardiac monitoring and consider cardiology consult

Answer: C.

This patient was noted to be febrile on two different occasions overnight, feeling well this morning without symptoms with an unremarkable preliminary workup. Given the isolated fever in the absence of other obvious abnormalities, the diagnosis of neurogenic fever (NF) becomes more likely at this point. NF has been described in approximately 5% of all SCI patients and likely to be more common in higher (cervical, thoracic) complete (AIS A) injuries. Its pathophysiology is unclear, although it is likely related to the disrupted autonomic system. NF is a diagnosis of exclusion and other potential sources must be evaluated as most fevers in SCI have an identifiable source, such as a UTI or an upper respiratory tract infection (Option C). Preliminary urine studies were already completed in this case. A chest X-ray would be the next diagnostic test of choice. Other causes of fever in SCI patients can be soft tissue injuries, gastrointestinal causes, deep venous thrombosis, pulmonary embolism, heterotopic ossification, and drug fevers. Antipyretic administration is not unreasonable, but a workup should follow to rule out an identifiable cause of the fever (Option A). Cardiac arrest has rarely been reported as the cause of death following a diagnosis of NF, but there is no consensus of preemptively initiating a cardiac workup in SCI patients with NF (Options B and D).

Savage KE, Oleson CV, Schroeder GD, Sidhu GS, Vaccaro AR. Neurogenic fever after acute traumatic spinal cord injury: a qualitative systematic review. Global Spine J. 2016;6(6):607–14. https://doi.org/10.1055/s-0035-1570751. Epub 2016 Jan 30.

11. A 34-year-old male with severe traumatic brain injury (TBI) and C4 AIS D SCI following a mountain biking accident is admitted to the inpatient rehabilitation unit 8 days after his injury. He was managed nonoperatively during the acute period and his course was noted to be unremarkable per report with improving agitation and no witnessed seizures. His medication list includes phenytoin 100 mg every 8 h, which he has received for the past week. What is the most appropriate course of action regarding the medication as he begins rehabilitation?

A. Continue phenytoin 100 mg every 8 h indefinitely given the severity of his TBI
B. Discontinue phenytoin
C. Continue phenytoin for another 3 weeks to complete 1 month of seizure prophylaxis

D. Decrease phenytoin frequency to once a day and continue 100 mg for 1-year post-injury

Answer: B.

In the setting of severe TBI, seizure prophylaxis for the first 7 days is standard of care. Following the 7-day course, however, the prophylactic use of antiepileptic medications (e.g. phenytoin, carbamazepine, valproate) should not be routinely extended beyond this period as there is currently no evidence of benefit for prevention of post-traumatic seizures (Options A, C, D).

Lombard LA, Kwasnica C, Brooks M. Dual diagnosis: spinal cord injury and traumatic brain injury. In: Kirshblum S, Lin VW, editors. Spinal cord medicine. New York: Springer Publishing Company; 2018. p. 567–76.
Chang BS, Lowenstein DH, Quality Standards Subcommittee of the American Academy of Neurology. Practice parameter: antiepileptic drug prophylaxis in severe traumatic brain injury: report of the Quality Standards Subcommittee of the American Academy of Neurology. Neurology. 2003;60(1):10–6. https://doi.org/10.1212/01.wnl.0000031432.05543.14.

12. A 25-year-old male with moderate TBI and C6 AIS D SCI is admitted to the rehab unit 4 weeks after a motor vehicle collision. His medical issues include bilateral clavicular fractures and a right humeral fracture managed nonoperatively, right femoral deep vein thrombosis currently on therapeutic anticoagulation, right internal carotid dissection managed nonoperatively with high dose aspirin, left tibial and fibular fracture managed surgically with open reduction and internal fixation, hypertension on amlodipine, and asthma. In the morning, the nurse reports that he is becoming more difficult to arouse after being alert and oriented for the last few weeks. His temperature is 98.9 °F, blood pressure is 147/78 mmHg, pulse is 68, respiratory rate is 15, with oxygen saturation of 98% on room air. On physical exam, his eyes are closed but open to loud speech, and 8 mm pupils are seen minimally reactive to light bilaterally. He responds to questions with inappropriate words, making non-purposeful movements and flexing his arms to painful pinching. What is the most appropriate next step in management?

A. Naloxone administration
B. Sit the patient up then serial blood pressure checks until patient is normotensive
C. Obtain non-contrast head CT
D. Intubate the patient

Answer: C.

This is a patient with TBI and SCI with multiple orthopedic and vascular injuries who has been doing well in therapy until sudden onset of altered mental status with abnormal pupillary findings. Dilated pupils with abnormal pupillary light reflex are an ominous sign of increased intracranial pressure (e.g. intracranial hemorrhage). This particular patient is at an extremely high risk for potential intracranial hemorrhage given his recent traumatic brain injury, either as a sequela of a new traumatic event (e.g. unwitnessed fall overnight), or due to a spontaneous hemorrhage as he is on therapeutic anticoagulation. This patient needs emergent imaging with a non-contrast CT of his head to evaluate for an acute intracranial process (Option C) as well as a neurosurgery consult. Dilated pupils without signs of respiratory depression make opioid overdose unlikely (Option A). Sitting the patient up and looking for noxious stimuli is a good first step in management of autonomic dysreflexia (Option B). While this patient may require intubation if his mental status continues to deteriorate, he currently has a GCS of 10 (eyes 3, verbal 3, motor 4), protecting his airway, thus urgent imaging should take priority over intubation at this time (Option D).

Chen JW, Gombart ZJ, Rogers S, Gardiner SK, Cecil S, Bullock RM. Pupillary reactivity as an early indicator of increased intracranial pressure: the introduction of the neurological pupil index. Surg Neurol Int. 2011;2:82. https://doi.org/10.4103/2152-7806.82248. Epub 2011 Jun 21.

Levy AS, Salottolo K, Bar-Or R, Offner P, Mains C, Sullivan M, Bar-Or D. Pharmacologic thromboprophylaxis is a risk factor for hemorrhage progression in a subset of patients with traumatic brain injury. J Trauma. 2010;68(4):886–94. https://doi.org/10.1097/TA.0b013e31827dd5.

Cohen DB, Rinker C, Wilberger JE. Traumatic brain injury in anticoagulated patients. J Trauma. 2006;60(3):553–7. https://doi.org/10.1097/01.ta.0000196542.54344.05.

13. Which pharmacotherapy would be appropriate for a patient admitted to inpatient rehabilitation with a severe TBI and incomplete SCI who is unable to participate in therapy due to excessive sleeping throughout the night and multiple times during the day for 2–3 h duration?

    A. Ramelteon
    B. Carbidopa-Levodopa
    C. Propranolol
    D. Modafinil

Answer: D.

Excessive daytime sleepiness (EDS) is common in patients with TBI, up to nearly 40% of patients. The exact etiology is unclear but there is evidence of decreased levels of orexin secretion from the hypothalamus that promotes wakefulness in patients with TBI. Modafinil, a neurostimulant that is widely used for EDS related to various etiologies (obstructive sleep apnea, narcolepsy, shift-work) can be helpful in TBI patients with EDS; it has been shown to improve wakefulness by objective measures such as Fatigue Severity Scale and Epworth Sleepiness Scale (Option D). Ramelteon is a melatonin receptor agonist that can be useful for insomnia, which this patient does not have (Option A). Carbidopa-Levodopa is a dopamine precursor used for Parkinson's disease and potentially beneficial for motor recovery in stroke, but there is no evidence for its use in EDS in TBI patients (Option B). Propranolol is a non-selective beta blocker that can be used for management of paroxysmal sympathetic hyperactivity in TBI (Option C).

Kaiser PR, Valko PO, Werth E, Thomann J, Meier J, Stocker R, Bassetti CL, Baumann CR. Modafinil ameliorates excessive daytime sleepiness after traumatic brain injury. Neurology. 2010;75(20):1780–5. https://doi.org/10.1212/WNL.0b013e3181fd62a2.

14. Which of the following statements is most consistent with the current understanding regarding the relationship between post-traumatic syrinx (PTS) and post-traumatic spinal cord tethering (PTSCT)?

    A. Discrete entities that arise as a result of unrelated pathophysiology in the setting of SCI trauma
    B. PTSCT is a natural progression of PTS that occurs months after initial trauma
    C. PTSCT is a complication after surgical treatment for PTS
    D. PTSCT is a precursor to PTS

Answer: D.

Current understanding of these two conditions is that PTSCT is a necessary precursor to development of progressive myelomalacia with PTS as an end process (Option D). This relationship was first described by Edgar and Quail (1994) after a patient with PTS underwent successful shunting yet continued to have progressive myelopathy. It was subsequently discovered that surgical detethering of the cord arrested progressive myelopathy, further corroborating that post-traumatic scarring of the arachnoid with tethering to the dura is a precursor to PTS and other progressive symptoms related to myelopathy (Option B and C). Therefore, PTSCT and PTS are closely related entities that can manifest concurrently and identically (Option A).

Scelza WM, Falci SP, Indeck CS. Posttraumatic syringomyelia and spinal cord tethering. In: Kirshblum S, Lin VW, editors. Spinal cord medicine. New York: Springer Publishing Company; 2018. p. 577–83.
Falci SP. Surgical treatment of posttraumatic tethered, myelomalacic and cystic spinal cords. Semin Spine Surg. 2005;17(1):40–5.
Edgar R, Quail P. Progressive post-traumatic cystic and non-cystic myelopathy. Br J Neurosurg. 1994;8(1):7–22. https://doi.org/10.3109/02688699409002388.

15. Which of the following statements is true regarding post-traumatic progressive myelomalacic myelopathy (PPMM)?

    A. Meninges tend to appear thin on MRI
    B. There is no established, definitive treatment
    C. The incidence and prevalence are higher than that of post-traumatic syringomyelia (PTS)
    D. Prognosis tends to be much better compared to PTS

Answer: B.

PPMM is a rare, long-term complication of SCI that presents with a wide variety of neurological manifestations. Signs and symptoms include, but are not limited to, pain, paresthesia, weakness, urinary incontinence, and spasticity. Incidence is reported to be anywhere between 0.3% and 3.2% in SCI patients from 2 months to >30 years after injury, thus far less common than other complications such as PTS, which is cited to occur in more than 20% of patients in a relatively similar time frame (Option C). Studies with MRI and histopathological samples of patients with PPMM have revealed meningeal thickening of the pia and arachnoid (Option A). Although surgical intervention may mitigate worsening myelopathy, symptomatic treatment remains the current standard of management (Option B). Prognosis is similar between PTS and PPMM (Option D).

Nehaw S, Lee BS, Benzel EC. Spine complications in patients with chronic spinal cord injury. In: Kirshblum S, Lin VW, editors. Spinal cord medicine. New York: Springer Publishing Company; 2018. p. 559–66.
Falcone S, Quencer RM, Green BA, Patchen SJ, Post MJ. Progressive posttraumatic myelomalacic myelopathy: imaging and clinical features. AJNR Am J Neuroradiol. 1994;15(4):747–54.

16. What is the significance of neurotrophin nerve growth factor (NGF) and its role in SCI?

    A. Alters neuronal excitability and synaptic strength
    B. Increases functional plasticity of cortical neurons
    C. Directly acts as serotonin receptor agonist
    D. Correlates positively with level of calcium gene-related peptide (CGRP+) afferent sprouting

Answer: D.

Overexpression of NGF has shown to increase CGRP+ afferent sprouting following SCI (Option D). The use of intrathecal anti-NGF after SCI has been shown to suppress CGRP+ axonal sprouting in animal models, which in turn led to decreased severity of autonomic dysreflexia secondary to colorectal distension. Brain derived neurotrophic factor (BDNF) is another neurotrophin that has been studied in SCI which increases neuronal excitability and has a potential role in early phrenic nerve activation following cervical SCI (Option A). While NGF is not a direct agonist for serotonin receptors (Option C), treatment with serotonin receptor agonists appears to aid in functional plasticity of cortical neurons to promote somatotopic reorganization (Option B).

Lee HJ, Tansey KE. Recent advances in spinal cord research: preclinical spinal cord injury, plasticity, and repair. In: Kirshblum S, Lin VW, editors. Spinal cord medicine. New York: Springer Publishing Company; 2018. p. 870–89.

Cameron AA, Smith GM, Randall DC, Brown DR, Rabchevsky AG. Genetic manipulation of intraspinal plasticity after spinal cord injury alters the severity of autonomic dysreflexia. J Neurosci. 2006;26(11):2923–32. https://doi.org/10.1523/JNEUROSCI.4390-05.2006.

Krenz NR, Meakin SO, Krassioukov AV, Weaver LC. Neutralizing intraspinal nerve growth factor blocks autonomic dysreflexia caused by spinal cord injury. J Neurosci. 1999;19(17):7405–14. https://doi.org/10.1523/JNEUROSCI.19-17-07405.1999.

17. What is the most appropriate treatment of Kümmell disease?

    A. Surgery
    B. Pain control
    C. Physical therapy
    D. Antibiotics

Answer: A.

Kümmell disease (KD) is a rare complication of SCI leading to osteonecrosis of the vertebral body, resulting in vertebral body collapse. The disease seems to be progressive in nature, usually reported weeks or months after the initial traumatic injury to the spinal cord. Patients are often asymptomatic in the early stages of the disease, then later, they have been noted to report low back pain with structural changes in the spine including kyphosis. The pathophysiology remains unknown. KD is a diagnosis of exclusion, and usually arrived at via serial imaging after having ruled out other causes of avascular necrosis such as steroid use, radiation therapy, or Gaucher disease. On imaging, reported findings consistent with KD include the "vacuum cleft" which can indicate ischemic vertebral collapse on X-ray, and hyperintensity surrounded by a band of hypointensity on a T2 MRI known as the "double line sign", thought to represent sclerosis. Patients in reported cases required surgery (e.g. vertebroplasty, fusion, decompression) for definitive treatment (Options A). KD is not an infectious etiology (Option D).

Nehaw S, Lee BS, Benzel EC. Spine complications in patients with chronic spinal cord injury. In: Kirshblum S, Lin VW, editors. Spinal cord medicine. New York: Springer Publishing Company; 2018. p. 559–66.

Swartz K, Fee D. Kümmell's disease: a case report and literature review. Spine (Phila Pa 1976). 2008;33(5):E152–5. https://doi.org/10.1097/BRS.0b013e3181657f31.

Brower AC, Downey EF Jr. Kümmell disease: report of a case with serial radiographs. Radiology. 1981;141(2):363–4. https://doi.org/10.1148/radiology.141.2.7291557.

18. Which of the following best describes a Charcot spinal arthropathy diagnosis?

    A. Progressive destruction of vertebral body and disc, accompanied by hypertrophic bone formation and crepitus in the spine
    B. Sequela of recurrent autonomic dysreflexia leading to spinal vasculature infarction
    C. Acute neuropathic pain episodes lasting weeks to months following traumatic SCI that is recalcitrant to medication
    D. Post-traumatic scarring of the arachnoid leading to tethering

Answer: A.

Charcot spinal arthropathy is a rare complication, occurring after an average of 17 years following SCI. Patients have been known to manifest worsening back pain (most common in thoracolumbar region), and crepitus with movement of the spine, back pain (even in complete SCI). Radiological findings typically reveal significant disc degeneration with erosion of vertebral body and hypertrophic osteophyte formation. Charcot spinal arthropathy generally does not lead to autonomic dysreflexia (Option B). While pain is a symptom of Charcot spinal arthropathy, it is not the defining characteristic (Option C). Post-traumatic spinal cord tethering (PTSCT) is a different condition and unrelated than Charcot spine (Option D).

Nehaw S, Lee BS, Benzel EC. Spine complications in patients with chronic spinal cord injury. In: Kirshblum S, Lin VW, editors. Spinal cord medicine. New York: Springer Publishing Company; 2018. p. 559–66.

Barrey C, Massourides H, Cotton F, Perrin G, Rode G. Charcot spine: two new case reports and a systematic review of 109 clinical cases from the literature. Ann Phys Rehabil Med. 2010;53(3):200–20 (English, French). https://doi.org/10.1016/j.rehab.2009.11.008. Epub 2009 Dec 31.

Standaert C, Cardenas DD, Anderson P. Charcot spine as a late complication of traumatic spinal cord injury. Arch Phys Med Rehabil. 1997;78(2):221–5. https://doi.org/10.1016/s0003-9993(97)90267-7.

19. What pharmacological agent has been shown to be beneficial for prevention of heterotopic ossification (HO)?

    A. Indomethacin
    B. Warfarin
    C. Etidronate
    D. Calcitonin

Answer: A.

HO is a common complication in SCI that most often occurs in the first 2 months following an SCI which arises due to ectopic bone formation within the soft tissue surrounding the peripheral joints. In SCI patients, the most commonly affected area is the hip. Classic presentation consists of decreased range of motion in the affected joint along with swelling. Other associated findings may be pain, erythema, warmth, low grade fever, or increased spasticity. While pharmacologic prophylaxis of HO has not been robustly studied, there is evidence based on a randomized controlled trial that initiation of daily indomethacin for 3 weeks showed decreased incidence of HO compared to placebo (Option A). Disodium etidronate (EHDP) can be used for treatment once a patient has been diagnosed with HO but has not been shown to be helpful in prevention of HO (Option C). Warfarin and calcitonin have been investigated separately as potential agents for treatment of HO, but the results have not been clinically significant, and their role in HO prevention is yet to be investigated (Option B and D).

van Kuijk AA, Geurts AC, van Kuppevelt HJ. Neurogenic heterotopic ossification in spinal cord injury. Spinal Cord. 2002;40(7):313–26. https://doi.org/10.1038/sj.sc.3101309.

Banovac K, Williams JM, Patrick LD, Haniff YM. Prevention of heterotopic ossification after spinal cord injury with indomethacin. Spinal Cord. 2001;39(7):370–4. https://doi.org/10.1038/sj.sc.3101166.

20. What is an advantage of quantifying spasticity in SCI patients with the Modified Tardieu Scale (MTS) over Modified Ashworth Scale (MAS)?

A. MTS has better interrater reliability than MAS
B. MTS is quicker and easier to complete than MAS
C. MTS involves electromyography (EMG) to ascertain denervation of a muscle
D. MTS incorporates different angles and velocities to activate a stretch reflex

Answer: D.

MTS was originally developed as the Tardieu scale in 1959 and has since undergone several modifications. Its goal is to measure spasticity by incorporating different speeds of movement when testing a muscle group, thereby obtaining a more velocity-dependent measure of spasticity in patients. Grading is typically done from 0 to 4, similar to MAS, with 0 indicating no resistance throughout the course of passive movement, to 4 indicating sustained clonus for more than 10 s occurring at a specific angle. Because it involves more movement and measurements, this scale is not faster or easier to use than the MAS (Option B). Although EMG was used in early studies to understand the pathophysiology of spasticity as a velocity-dependent increase in tone of a muscle, it is not required in MTS nor is denervation of muscle relevant (Option C). The direct comparison of MTS vs. MAS for interrater reliability is inconclusive thus far (Option A).

Walker HW, Hon A, Hess MJ. Spasticity management. In: Kirshblum S, Lin VW, editors. Spinal cord medicine. New York: Springer Publishing Company; 2018. p. 472–86.

Akpinar P, Atici A, Ozkan FU, Aktas I, Kulcu DG, Sarı A, Durmus B. Reliability of the Modified Ashworth Scale and Modified Tardieu Scale in patients with spinal cord injuries. Spinal Cord. 2017;55(10):944–9. https://doi.org/10.1038/sc.2017.48. Epub 2017 May 9.

Haugh AB, Pandyan AD, Johnson GR. A systematic review of the Tardieu scale for the measurement of spasticity. Disabil Rehabil. 2006;28(15):899–907. https://doi. org/10.1080/09638280500404305.

21. A 20-year-old man with T4 complete paraplegia presents to clinic with concerns of excessive facial, upper chest, and axillary sweating that is impacting his social relationships. On review of systems, he denied changes in strength or sensation, but does mention a prolonged history of burning and tingling in bilateral lower extremities that interfere with his ability to concentrate on his college courses. What is the best treatment option for this patient?

    A. Botulinum toxin injections
    B. Nortriptyline
    C. Scopolamine patch
    D. Gabapentin

Answer: B.

Nortriptyline. Hyperhidrosis above the level of injury with minimal sweating below the level of injury is a common clinical pattern that is attributed to reflex activation of the sweat glands in the setting of autonomic dysreflexia. Initial management includes identification of noxious stimuli that may be triggering reflexive sweating. Anticholinergic medications are most frequently used for the management of hyperhidrosis. Nortriptyline would address his neuropathic pain, a potential noxious stimulus, and have anticholinergic effects to treat the hyperhydrosis. A scopolamine patch is a commonly used anticholinergic option, but it does not address the neuropathic pain. Botulinum toxin injections have been used for hyperhidrosis in the general population and would be impractical for the diffuse body parts involved. There is a case report of gabapentin used for hyperhidrosis in pediatric SCI but is not routinely used.

Staas WE Jr, Nemunaitis G. Management of reflex sweating in spinal cord injured patients. Arch Phys Med Rehabil. 1989;70(7):544–6.
Fast A. Reflex sweating in patients with spinal cord injury: a review. Arch Phys Med Rehabil. 1977;58(10):435–7.
Adams BB, Vargus-Adams JN, Franz DN, Kinnett DG. Hyperhidrosis in pediatric spinal cord injury: a case report and gabapentin therapy. J Am Acad Dermatol. 2002;46(3):444–6. https://doi.org/10.1067/mjd.2002.113681.

22. A 53-year-old woman with chronic low back pain that radiates down her left lower extremity reports new onset bilateral lower extremity weakness. An MRI of the lumbar spine revealed nerve root thickening with enhancement, a soft tissue mass within the spinal canal, and a loss of subarachnoid space that is consistent with adhesive arachnoiditis. How would you grade her MRI finding?

A. Grade I
B. Grade II
C. Grade III
D. Grade IV

Answer: C.

MRI findings associated with adhesive arachnoiditis have been described by Delamarter et al. (1990). Grade I is defined by a conglomeration of adherent nerve roots centrally within the thecal sac. Grade II is defined by peripherally adherent nerve roots and "empty thecal sac appearance" with meningeal thickening. Grade III is defined by soft tissue mass within the spinal canal with obliteration of subarachnoid space. There is no Grade IV.

Delamarter RB, Ross JS, Masaryk TJ, Modic MT, Bohlman HH. Diagnosis of lumbar arachnoiditis by magnetic resonance imaging. Spine (Phila Pa 1976). 1990;15(4):304–10. https://doi.org/10.1097/00007632-199004000-00011.

23. A 33-year-old manual wheelchair user has cubital tunnel syndrome. Which of the following may have contributed to this patient's symptoms?

A. The axle of the wheel is lower than indicated
B. The push rims are frequently used as armrests
C. The footrests are too high.
D. The seat dump is angle is greater than indicated

Answer: B.

Cubital tunnel syndrome describes symptoms due to ulnar nerve entrapment at the cubital tunnel during full flexion of the elbow or direct trauma at the elbow. When the axle of the wheel on a manual wheelchair is higher than indicated, the user will have to flex the elbow more to propel. Using the hard surface of a wheelchair's push rim as an armrest can lead to trauma to the ulnar nerve at the elbow because its outer surface is only covered by a ligament sheath. Seat dump helps prevent the wheelchair user from sliding forward and therefore maintain a more optimal distance between the upper limb and the wheels. The footrest height is unlikely to impact cubital tunnel syndrome.

Gellman H, Chandler DR, Petrasek J, Sie I, Adkins R, Waters RL. Carpal tunnel syndrome in paraplegic patients. J Bone Joint Surg Am. 1988;70(4):517–9.
Boninger ML, Baldwin M, Cooper RA, Koontz A, Chan L. Manual wheelchair pushrim biomechanics and axle position. Arch Phys Med Rehabil. 2000;81(5):608–13. https://doi.org/10.1016/s0003-9993(00)90043-1.
van der Woude LH, Bouw A, van Wegen J, van As H, Veeger D, de Groot S. Seat height: effects on submaximal hand rim wheelchair performance during spinal cord injury rehabilitation. J Rehabil Med. 2009;41(3):143–9. https://doi.org/10.2340/16501977-0296.

24. A 34-year-old man with complete paraplegia is followed for long-term intrathecal baclofen pump (ITB) management. He presents to the clinic with worsening spasticity despite being in his usual state of health. He denied new urinary, bowel, or skin complaints. The ITB pump was interrogated without apparent issues, a bolus dose was given without improvement, and the pump reservoir volume was verified. What is the next step in management?

    A. Plain radiography of the abdomen and spine
    B. Increase ITB dose in setting of pharmacologic tolerance
    C. Diagnostic catheter access port aspiration
    D. Diagnostic catheter contrast study

Answer: C.

Catheter access port (CAP) aspiration. The patient's benign history is unremarkable for clinical symptoms suggestive of an infectious etiology for this patient's worsening spasticity. If initial ITB pump troubleshooting is unrevealing after pump interrogation and reservoir volume verification, the CAP should be aspirated to evaluate catheter patency or malfunction. Cerebrospinal fluid should be readily aspirated if the distal end of the catheter lies within the subarachnoid space. Aspiration of 2–3 mL is sufficient to rule out catheter disruption or occlusion. Difficulty with aspiration or minimal fluid obtained from CAP aspiration is suggestive of a catheter occlusion or kink. If the catheter cannot be aspirated, a catheter contrast study is not recommended due to risks of overdose from drug in the catheter.

Saulino M, Anderson DJ, Doble J, Farid R, Gul F, Konrad P, Boster AL. Best practices for intrathecal baclofen therapy: troubleshooting. Neuromodulation. 2016;19(6):632–41. https://doi.org/10.1111/ner.12467. Epub 2016 Jul 19.

25. A 24-year-old with T4 AIS A paraplegia with 3 months of wrist pain is found to have a positive carpal compression test, Tinel's test, and Phalen's test. Which factor is unlikely to have contributed to his current symptoms?

    A. Wrist hyperextension during wheelchair transfers
    B. High compressive and shearing forces at the wrist during wheelchair propulsion
    C. Large ulnar and radial deviation angles at the wrist
    D. Unpadded wheelchair armrests

Answer: D.

Unpadded wheelchair armrests. This is more likely to contribute to ulnar nerve entrapment at the elbow, also known as cubital tunnel syndrome. The patient's level of injury is most consistent with use of a manual wheelchair. The exam findings are suggestive of carpal tunnel syndrome (CTS) which is commonly attributed to wheelchair use in the SCI population. Propulsion of a manual wheelchair is often associated with high compressive and shearing forces, large flexion/extension angles, and large ulnar/radial deviation angles (Choices A and C). Propulsion with increased force and number of strokes was found to be associated with electrodiagnostic findings of CTS. Wrist hyperextension beyond the physiological limit during a wheelchair transfer may increase carpal tunnel pressures and contribute to CTS (Choice B).

Boninger ML, Cooper RA, Robertson RN, Rudy TE. Wrist biomechanics during two speeds of wheelchair propulsion: an analysis using a local coordinate system. Arch Phys Med Rehabil. 1997;78(4):364–72. https://doi.org/10.1016/s0003-9993(97)90227-6.

Boninger ML, Cooper RA, Baldwin MA, Shimada SD, Koontz A. Wheelchair pushrim kinetics: body weight and median nerve function. Arch Phys Med Rehabil. 1999;80(8):910–5. https://doi.org/10.1016/s0003-9993(99)90082-5.

Boninger ML, Impink BG, Cooper RA, Koontz AM. Relation between median and ulnar nerve function and wrist kinematics during wheelchair propulsion. Arch Phys Med Rehabil. 2004;85(7):1141–5. https://doi.org/10.1016/j.apmr.2003.11.016.

Gagnon D, Koontz A, Mulroy S, et al. Biomechanics of sitting pivot transfers among individuals with a spinal cord injury: a review of the current knowledge. Top Spinal Cord Inj Rehabil. 2009;15(2):33–58. https://doi.org/10.1310/sci1502-33.

Werner RA, Andary M. Carpal tunnel syndrome: pathophysiology and clinical neurophysiology. Clin Neurophysiol. 2002;113(9):1373–81. https://doi.org/10.1016/s1388-2457(02)00169-4.

26. A 42-year-old man with C2 complete tetraplegia spent a winter afternoon on his porch watching his children play in the snow. His partner found him cool to touch with a temperature of 96 °F. Which of the following is true regarding hypothermia in SCI?

A. Hyperthermia is more common than hypothermia
B. Hypothermia is not linked to cardiac arrhythmias
C. Gabapentin may induce hypothermia
D. He should not be allowed to go out into cold environments in the future

Answer: A.

Hyperthermia is more common than hyperthermia due to loss of descending sympathetic pathways and subsequent impairments to regulation of blood flow and sweating in the body. Hypothermia can lead to respiratory compromise and cardiac arrhythmias. Gabapentin, oxybutynin, and serotonin-norepinephrine reuptake inhibitors may reduce hypothermia. He can still go out into cold environments if using the appropriate clothing, blankets, etc. to stay warm.

Price MJ. Thermoregulation during exercise in individuals with spinal cord injuries. Sports Med. 2006;36(10):863–79. https://doi.org/10.2165/00007256-200636100-00005.

Khan S, Plummer M, Martinez-Arizala A, Banovac K. Hypothermia in patients with chronic spinal cord injury. J Spinal Cord Med. 2007;30(1):27–30. https://doi.org/10.1080/1079026 8.2007.11753910.

Savage KE, Oleson CV, Schroeder GD, Sidhu GS, Vaccaro AR. Neurogenic fever after acute traumatic spinal cord injury: a qualitative systematic review. Global Spine J. 2016;6(6):607–14. https://doi.org/10.1055/s-0035-1570751. Epub 2016 Jan 30.

27. Which of the following is NOT considered a possible neural mechanism for spasticity?

    A. Decreased excitation of inhibitory interneurons
    B. Increased alpha-motor neuron excitability
    C. Decreased cutaneous reflexes due to abnormal processing in dorsal horn
    D. Exaggeration of stretch reflexes

Answer: C.

Decreased cutaneous reflexes due to abnormal processing in dorsal horn. Choices A, B, and D are true statements in regards to the pathophysiology of spasticity. Spasticity is a clinical manifestation of an exaggeration of the stretch reflex secondary to abnormal intraspinal processing of afferent impulses, loss of descending inhibitory regulation of segmental reflexes, and increased excitability of the motor neurons. The stretch reflex originates in the muscle spindles, located parallel to the muscle fibers, and activated by passive muscle stretch. This activates the Ia afferent neuron to the spinal cord, which synapses with interneurons and alpha-motor neurons. The alpha-motor neurons send an efferent impulse to the agonist muscle with resulting contraction. Spinal reflex activity is influenced by afferent pathways. Enhanced cutaneous reflexes due to abnormal processing in the dorsal horn contributes to increased excitation of motor neurons.

Young RR. Spasticity: a review. Neurology. 1994;44(11 Suppl 9):S12–20.

Thilmann AF, Fellows SJ, Garms E. The mechanism of spastic muscle hypertonus. Variation in reflex gain over the time course of spasticity. Brain. 1991;114(Pt 1A):233–44.

Rothwell J. Control of human voluntary movement. 2nd ed. London: Chapman & Hall; 1994.

28. A 40-year-old man with complete paraplegia of 10 years duration presents with new bilateral triceps weakness. History and physical exam were concerning for spinal cord tethering. A focused electrodiagnostic exam of the upper limbs was completed. Which of the following electrodiagnostic findings would support this diagnosis?

    A. An increased compound motor unit action potential
    B. Enlarged motor units
    C. Increased maximal firing rate of motor units
    D. Absence of positive sharp waves

Answer: B.

Enlarged motor units consistent with compensatory motor unit sprouting in the setting of denervation. A tethered spinal cord would present as progressive myelopathy due to anterior horn cell loss would demonstrate the following electrodiagnostic findings: (1) denervation potentials, (2) reduced compound motor unit action potential, (3) enlarged motor units due to compensatory motor unit sprouting, and (4) reduced maximal firing rate of motor units.

Rossier AB, Foo D, Shillito J, Dyro FM. Posttraumatic cervical syringomyelia. Incidence, clinical presentation, electrophysiological studies, syrinx protein and results of conservative and operative treatment. Brain. 1985;108(Pt 2):439–61. https://doi.org/10.1093/brain/108.2.439.

Little JW, Robinson LR, Goldstein B, Stewart D, Micklesen P. Electrophysiologic findings in post-traumatic syringomyelia: implications for clinical management. J Am Paraplegia Soc. 1992;15(2):44–52. https://doi.org/10.1080/01952307.1992.11735861.

Nogués MA, Stålberg E. Electrodiagnostic findings in syringomyelia. Muscle Nerve. 1999;22(12):1653–9.

Bursell JP, Little JW, Stiens SA. Electrodiagnosis in spinal cord injured persons with new weakness or sensory loss: central and peripheral etiologies. Arch Phys Med Rehabil. 1999;80(8):904–9. https://doi.org/10.1016/s0003-9993(99)90081-3.

29. Which structure is responsible for generating efferent responses to afferent thermal input during thermoregulation?

A. Pons
B. Hypothalamus
C. Midbrain
D. Amygdala

Answer: B.

Hypothalamus. Thermoregulation becomes impaired in persons with spinal cord injuries above T8. This is attributed to multiple factors associated with the loss of hypothalamic control due to a loss of connections from the afferent and efferent spinal circuits. Thermoregulation is defined by three phases, (1) afferent thermal sensing, (2) central regulation, and (3) efferent responses. Afferent thermal sensing occurs at the skin surface and visceral organs. Central regulation occurs in the hypothalamus, where it receives afferent input and triggers efferent responses. Affected efferent responses after SCI include impaired vasomotor reactions, abnormal sweating responses, and impaired shiver responses.

Downey JA, Chiodi HP, Darling RC. Central temperature regulation in the spinal man. J Appl Physiol. 1967;22(1):91–4. https://doi.org/10.1152/jappl.1967.22.1.91.

Khan S, Plummer M, Martinez-Arizala A, Banovac K. Hypothermia in patients with chronic spinal cord injury. J Spinal Cord Med. 2007;30(1):27–30. https://doi.org/10.1080/1079026 8.2007.11753910.

Price MJ. Thermoregulation during exercise in individuals with spinal cord injuries. Sports Med. 2006;36(10):863–79. https://doi.org/10.2165/00007256-200636100-00005.

Blauwet CA, Benjamin-Laing H, Stomphorst J, Van de Vliet P, Pit-Grosheide P, Willick SE. Testing for boosting at the Paralympic games: policies, results and future directions. Br J Sports Med. 2013;47(13):832–7. https://doi.org/10.1136/bjsports-2012-092103. Epub 2013 May 16.
Taguchi A, Kurz A. Thermal management of the patient: where does the patient lose and/or gain temperature? Curr Opin Anaesthesiol. 2005;18(6):632–9. https://doi.org/10.1097/01. aco.0000191890.36691.cc.

30. Surgical decompression after spinal cord injury was associated with improved outcomes with which of the following surgical timing?

    A. Within 24 h
    B. Within 48 h
    C. Within 1 week
    D. Within 1 month

Answer: A.

Within 24 h. Fehlings et al. (2012) reported more people were likely to demonstrate improvements in their AIS score by at least two grades if they received early surgery rather than late surgery in the Surgical Timing in Acute Spinal Cord Injury (STASCIS) trial. 19.8% of persons who received early surgery within 24 h after spinal cord injury had improvements in AIS score by at least two grades compared to 8.8% of persons who received late surgery at 24 h or later. In animal studies, earlier decompression at 6 and 12 h after SCI was associated with less total lesion volume compared to decompression at 24 h, thereby suggesting improved neurologic outcomes.

Fehlings MG, Vaccaro A, Wilson JR, Singh A, W Cadotte D, Harrop JS, Aarabi B, Shaffrey C, Dvorak M, Fisher C, Arnold P, Massicotte EM, Lewis S, Rampersaud R. Early versus delayed decompression for traumatic cervical spinal cord injury: results of the Surgical Timing in Acute Spinal Cord Injury Study (STASCIS). PLoS One. 2012;7(2):e32037. https://doi.org/10.1371/journal.pone.0032037. Epub 2012 Feb 23.
Shields CB, Zhang YP, Shields LB, Han Y, Burke DA, Mayer NW. The therapeutic window for spinal cord decompression in a rat spinal cord injury model. J Neurosurg Spine. 2005;3(4):302–7. https://doi.org/10.3171/spi.2005.3.4.0302.

Pressure Injuries

13

Gianna M. Rodriguez, Maryam Berri,
and Michael Bush-Arnold

1. In regards to the manifestation of a deep tissue injury, which of the following statement is NOT true?

   A. Of the tissue layers, subcutaneous tissue is the most prone to ischemia.
   B. Prolonged sitting in a wheelchair increases mechanical load on the bone soft tissue interface.
   C. Ischemia leads to necrosis of skin, subcutaneous fat, and muscle.
   D. Collapse of capillaries with the rise of localized interstitial pressure results to ischemia that leads to pressure injuries.

   Answer: A.

   Prolonged sitting in a wheelchair has been demonstrated to increase mechanical load and stress primarily at the bone-soft tissue interface as soft tissue is compressed and deformed between the supporting surface and bony prominences; specifically the ischial and sacral areas. This subsequently leads to necrosis of skin, subcutaneous fat, and muscle necrosis. Of these, muscle has been found

G. M. Rodriguez (✉) · M. Berri
Department of Physical Medicine and Rehabilitation, Michigan Medicine,
Ann Arbor, MI, USA
e-mail: giannar@med.umich.edu; mberri@med.umich.edu

M. Bush-Arnold
Spinal Cord Injury Unit, Rehabilitation Institute of Michigan, Detroit, MI, USA
e-mail: MBush-Ar@dmc.org

© The Author(s), under exclusive license to Springer Nature Switzerland AG 2022
B. A. Abramoff et al. (eds.), *The Essential Spinal Cord Injury Medicine Question Bank*, https://doi.org/10.1007/978-3-031-07796-8_13

to be the most prone to ischemia and hypoxia since it is highly vascularized. It is frequently stated that any load greater than 32 mmHg is harmful because it exceeds capillary refill, thus causing occlusion.

Kosiak M. Etiology and pathology of ischemic ulcers. Arch Phys Med Rehabil. 1959;40(2):62–9.

Bouten CV, Knight MM, Lee DA, Bade DL. Compressive deformation and damage of muscle cell subpopulations in a model system. Ann Biomed Eng. 2001;29(2):153–63. https://doi.org/10.1114/1.1349698.

Wywialowski EF. Tissue perfusion as a key underlying concept of pressure ulcer development and treatment. J Vasc Nurs. 1999;17(1):12–6. https://doi.org/10.1016/s1062-0303(99)90003-1.

2. A 68-year-old male with a past medical history of nontraumatic L2 American Spinal Injury Association Impairment Scale (AIS) C SCI, well controlled Type II diabetes mellitus (DM) on Metformin, newly diagnosed prostate cancer, and a 70 pack year history of smoking presents with stage 3 sacral pressure injury which is not healing despite prone positioning and conservative management. Which risk factor contributes most to his tissue ischemia and delayed wound healing?

A. Diabetes Mellitus II
B. Advanced age
C. Smoking
D. L2 AIS C SCI

Answer: C.

Smoking cigarettes have been found to have a multitude of toxic compounds like nicotine, carbon monoxide and hydrogen cyanide which affect skin and soft tissue and impair wound healing. Smoking has been demonstrated to impair skin and soft tissues in two main ways. Firstly, it alters the function of neutrophils and macrophages responsible for the inflammatory phase of wound healing and phagocytosis to decrease bacterial activity. Secondly, it impairs the proliferation of erythrocytes and decreases tissue perfusion, reduces fibroblasts responsible for rebuilding tissue structure, granulation, and epithelialization and interferes with collagen production for strengthening of tissue. Nicotine has been shown to activate the sympathetic nervous system and release of catecholamines stimulating vasoconstriction resulting in hypoxia. Nicotine has also been found to increase coagulability, further decreasing tissue perfusion and contributing to hypoxia. While the others are risk factors, they are likely not leading to delayed healing in this case.

McDaniel JC, Browning KK. Smoking, chronic wound healing, and implications for evidence-based practice. J Wound Ostomy Continence Nurs. 2014;41(5):415–23; quiz E1–2. https://doi.org/10.1097/WON.0000000000000057.

Lane CA, Selleck C, Chen Y, Tang Y. The impact of smoking and smoking cessation on wound healing in spinal cord-injured patients with pressure injuries: a retrospective comparison cohort study. J Wound Ostomy Continence Nurs. 2016;43(5):483–7. https://doi.org/10.1097/WON.0000000000000260.

McNichol L, Watts C, Mackey D, Beitz JM, Gray M. Identifying the right surface for the right patient at the right time: generation and content validation of an algorithm for support surface selection. J Wound Ostomy Continence Nurs. 2015;42(1):19–37. https://doi.org/10.1097/WON.0000000000000103.

3. A 42-year-old obese female with a 10-year history of T2 AIS C SCI, significant bilateral lower extremity edema, and non-healing lower extremity ulcers presents to the wound care clinic. What is true regarding chronic venous insufficiency?

A. Venous insufficiency only occurs in the deep veins.
B. Chronic venous insufficiency leads to unidirectional blood flow.
C. Chronic venous sufficiency often presents with hemosiderin staining.
D. Symptoms of chronic venous insufficiency worsen with leg elevation and improve with compression.

Answer: C.

Venous insufficiency occurs in the superficial, perforator, and deep veins. Chronic venous insufficiency leads to bidirectional blood flow. Chronic venous sufficiency often presents with hemosiderin staining. Symptoms of chronic venous insufficiency improve with leg elevation and improve with compression.

Gloviczki P, Comerota AJ, Dalsing MC, Eklof BG, Gillespie DL, Gloviczki ML, Lohr JM, McLafferty RB, Meissner MH, Murad MH, Padberg FT, Pappas PJ, Passman MA, Raffetto JD, Vasquez MA, Wakefield TW, Society for Vascular Surgery, American Venous Forum. The care of patients with varicose veins and associated chronic venous diseases: clinical practice guidelines of the Society for Vascular Surgery and the American Venous Forum. J Vasc Surg. 2011;53(5 Suppl):2S–48S. https://doi.org/10.1016/j.jvs.2011.01.079.

4. Which of the following factors does NOT increase the risk for sacral pressure injuries?

A. Body mass index (BMI) of <19 kg/m^2
B. Emphysema
C. Indwelling foley catheter
D. Hemoglobin A1c of 9.5

Answer: C.

People who have decreased mobility, prolonged hospital admissions for medical or surgical problems, poor nutrition, systemic conditions, advanced age, vascular problems, diabetes, tobacco and/or alcohol use are at higher risk of developing pressure injuries. People who have malnutrition with inadequate protein and caloric intake, impaired ability to feed appropriately, with low weight and BMI less than 20, intravascular volume deficits increase the risk for pressure injuries. Deficiency in protein has been shown to result to increased skin and soft tissue breakdown. Furthermore, appropriate protein intake contributes to prevention of and improvement of skin breakdown. The recommendation for protein intake for wound healing is 1.25–1.5 g protein/kg/day body weight.

While there can be pressure injuries due to indwelling catheter, they generally will not lead to a sacral pressure injury. Furthermore, reducing moisture due to incontinence may be needed to allow the pressure injury to heal.

Consortium for Spinal Cord Medicine. Pressure ulcer prevention and treatment following spinal cord injury: a clinical practice guideline for health-care professionals. 2nd ed. Washington, DC: Paralyzed Veterans of America; 2014.

Posthauer ME, Banks M, Dorner B, Schols JM. The role of nutrition for pressure ulcer management: National Pressure Ulcer Advisory Panel, European Pressure Ulcer Advisory Panel, and Pan Pacific Pressure Injury Alliance White Paper. Adv Skin Wound Care. 2015;28(4):175–88; quiz 189–90. https://doi.org/10.1097/01.ASW.0000461911.31139.62.

Sprigle S, McNair D, Sonenblum S. Pressure ulcer risk factors in persons with mobility-related disabilities. Adv Skin Wound Care. 2020;33(3):146–54. https://doi.org/10.1097/01.ASW.0000653152.36482.7d.

5. All of the following statements are true EXCEPT:

   A. Support surfaces redistribute pressure from areas of bony prominences which are high risk areas for pressure injuries.
   B. Turning and repositioning are used to reduce the duration of tissue load.
   C. Support surfaces can be used as the primary method for prevention and treatment of pressure injuries.
   D. The choice of support surface must be customized to the patient's risk factors for developing pressure injuries, existing and previous pressure injuries, height, weight, motor and sensory deficits, and patient preference.

Answer: C.

A support surface is defined as a specialized device (i.e., any overlay, mattress, or integrated bed system) for pressure redistribution designed for management of pressure, shear, or friction forces on tissue; microclimate; or other therapeutic functions. Support surfaces are NOT primary method for prevention and treatment of pressure injuries. They are used in addition to appropriate pressure relief, repositioning, good nutrition, incontinence management, and patient and caregiver education. The Wound, Ostomy and Continence Nurses Society

(WOCN) developed an evidence- and consensus-based algorithm for guidance for selecting support surfaces based on specific patient needs. It is recommended that an appropriate pressure-redistribution seating surface or cushion should also be used.

McNichol L, Watts C, Mackey D, Beitz JM, Gray M. Identifying the right surface for the right patient at the right time: generation and content validation of an algorithm for support surface selection. J Wound Ostomy Continence Nurs. 2015;42(1):19–37. https://doi.org/10.1097/WON.0000000000000103.

6. What is the best choice for a patient with multiple full thickness, stage 3–4 pressure injuries?

   A. Mattresses with single-stage alternating pressure (AP) feature
   B. Mattress gel overlay
   C. Mattress foam overlay
   D. Mattresses with multi-stage AP feature

Answer: D.

Mattresses with multistage AP feature. Mattresses with single-stage AP inflate and deflate in one cycle, those with multi-stage AP inflate and deflate in a gradual progressive manner. Treatment of multiple stage 2, or large, multiple stage 3 or stage 4 pressure injuries on the trunk or pelvis should involve the use of a reactive support surface with multi-stage AP with a low air loss or air fluidized feature. Evidence has demonstrated that mattresses with multi- and single-stage AP features were shown to be effective in *preventing* occurrence of and worsening of pressure injuries compared with the overlays with an AP feature or viscoelastic foam mattress when controlling for Braden score and age.

McNichol L, Watts C, Mackey D, Beitz JM, Gray M. Identifying the right surface for the right patient at the right time: generation and content validation of an algorithm for support surface selection. J Wound Ostomy Continence Nurs. 2015;42(1):19–37. https://doi.org/10.1097/WON.0000000000000103.

7. A 62-year-old male with a past medical history of hypertension, diabetes mellitus type II, hyperlipidemia, and a 31-year history of C4 AIS A spinal cord injury presents to your clinic for follow up of a left ischial stage 4 pressure injury s/p debridement. He has an air-fluidized bed and his wound is healing well. What position should he avoid while lying in his air-fluidized bed to protect the wound and prevent other pressure injuries?

   A. Laying supine with no head elevation to relieve pressure on the ischium
   B. Maintaining the head elevation 20°
   C. Sitting upright at a 90° angle to promote anterior pelvic tilt
   D. Laying on lateral sides without head elevation

Answer: C.

Pressure relief by repositioning every 1–2 h while lying in bed is ideal. Sitting at a 90° angle (or any head elevation >30°) puts more pressure directly over the ischium. Maintaining the head elevation at a <30° elevation for supine or side lying can decrease pressure over bony prominences. The prone, not supine, position has a large surface area of low-pressure and a smaller surface area of high pressure, although many patients cannot tolerate this position. Laying on the lateral side increases the risk of pressure injuries to the greater trochanters.

Air fluidized support surfaces provide pressure redistribution by a fluid-like medium by forcing air through beads. These beds reduce pressure while simultaneously reducing shearing forces. Low air loss support surfaces use a series of connected, air-filled cushions or compartments which are inflated to specific pressures to provide a continuous flow which replaces air lost through the surface's pores. Alternating pressure support surfaces provides pressure redistribution by cyclic changes in loading and unloading by changes in frequency, duration, amplitude, and rate of change parameters over the active area of the surface. Pressure is shifted to a different surface contact area by air-filled chambers arranged lengthwise pumped at various intervals.

Peterson M, Schwab W, McCutcheon K, van Oostrom JH, Gravenstein N, Caruso L. Effects of elevating the head of bed on interface pressure in volunteers. Crit Care Med. 2008;36(11):3038–42. https://doi.org/10.1097/CCM.0b013e31818b8dbd.
Baranoski S, et al. Skin: an essential organ. In: Baranoski S, Ayello EA, editors. Wound care essentials, practice principles. Philadelphia: Wolters Kluwer; 2016. p. 408–10.

8. Recommendation for wheelchair seating for a person with C5 AIS A spinal cord injury to prevent and/or heal pressure injuries should include all of the following EXCEPT:

   A. Custom seating to redistribute pressure appropriately
   B. Use of doughnut cushions to off load healing wounds
   C. Power wheelchair with tilt
   D. Pressure relieving cushion—air, gel or foam

   Answer: B.

It is imperative that a patient with significant motor and sensory impairments be evaluated for custom seating and mobility by trained therapists, assistive technology providers (ATPs) and physicians. Seating and wheelchair equipment are essential in optimizing function and health and promoting physical, emotional, and psychological well-being. Custom wheelchair and seating should provide adequate support from head to toe, prevent asymmetries and poor posture, and maximize independence and mobility in the home and community. Wheelchair backrests and cushions should meet the patients' specific needs for pressure relief and redistribution of pressure. Risk of pressure injuries are increased with prolonged wheelchair sitting time. However, the wheelchair enables the patient with physical impairments to engage in daily routines in and outside the home. Therefore, prevention of pressure injuries while seated in the wheelchair is key in allowing the patient to be active in their own lives. Aside from custom seating, PVA Guideline for Pressure Ulcer Prevention and Treatment recommendations include the use of power wheelchairs with tilt to allow individuals to do appropriate pressure relief and the use of pressure relieving support surfaces. There is no literature that supports the use of doughnut cushions to offload healing wounds.

Consortium for Spinal Cord Medicine. Pressure ulcer prevention and treatment following spinal cord injury: a clinical practice guideline for health-care professionals. 2nd ed. Washington, DC: Paralyzed Veterans of America; 2014.

9. A 55-year-old male with a Type B aortic dissection underwent a thrombectomy of the left common and external iliac arteries which led to T10 complete spinal cord injury and acute limb ischemia. Which tissue requires the greatest demand for oxygen and is most sensitive to ischemia and pressure?

A. Subcutaneous tissue
B. Bone
C. Epidermis
D. Muscle

Answer: D.

Muscle has the greatest demand for oxygen of all tissues and is most sensitive to ischemia and pressure damage. Three primary independent predictors for pressure injury development are mobility/activity, perfusion, and skin/pressure injury status.

Pressure injuries form due to cellular distortion and damage due to mechanical loading and deformation of soft tissues overlying bony prominences. Mechanical loading affects tissues based on tissue size, shape, stiffness, strength, and diffusion properties as well as the length of time and amount of pressure applied to tissue. External pressure transmits downward from the epidermis toward the bone as well as by counter-pressure from the bone. This causes deformation of soft tissues such as adipose tissue, connective tissues, and muscle.

Baranoski S, et al. Skin: an essential organ. In: Baranoski S, Ayello EA, editors. Wound care essentials, practice principles. Philadelphia: Wolters Kluwer; 2016. p. 408–10.

10. Repositioning while in bed and while in a chair is critical in prevention and treatment of pressure injuries. Indicate the statement that is FALSE:

A. Side leans and forward leans should last 30 s to be effective
B. Side leans and forward leans are generally the preferred pressure relieving techniques than push-up lifts
C. Tilting back in the wheelchair to greater than 65° is required for appropriate pressure relief
D. Reclining back in a wheelchair can provide pressure relief but must be used with caution because it can also create shear

Answer: A.

Regular pressure relief in a power wheelchair or manual wheelchair is crucial in preventing pressure injuries. Studies have demonstrated that sitting interface pressures are significantly greater than supine support interface pressures due to smaller contact areas. Higher intermittent pressures may be tolerated more than uninterrupted continuous lower pressures as well, therefore, the importance of doing intermittent pressure relief. It is recommended that pressure relief should be held at least 1 min and 51 s to increase tissue oxygenation to normal, off loaded levels. There are various ways of doing pressure relief—side leans, forward leans, push-up lifts. For patients unable to do independent pressure relief techniques, power tilt, recline and standing can be utilized for appropriate pressure relief. Tilting back to greater than 65° and using the full range of tilt in the power wheelchair is required for effective pressure relief and achieving reperfusion of tissues in the ischial and other areas. Side leans and forward leans are preferred over push-up lifts due to repetitive stress on the shoulders and wrists, increasing risk of chronic musculoskeletal issues. Forward lean to 45° and lateral trunk leaning to 15° are recommended for adequate pressure relief.

Consortium for Spinal Cord Medicine. Pressure ulcer prevention and treatment following spinal cord injury: a clinical practice guideline for health-care professionals. 2nd ed. Washington, DC: Paralyzed Veterans of America; 2014

11. The Braden scale evaluates six subscales to determine risk of pressure injuries. Which of the following is NOT an element of the Braden scale.

A. Moisture
B. Nutrition
C. Mobility
D. Age

Answer: D.

The Braden scale is generally useful for predicting which patients are at risk for developing pressure-induced skin and soft tissue injuries. The Braden scale rates patients in six subscales, these include: sensory perception, moisture, activity, mobility, nutrition, and friction and shear. Age is not a component of the Braden scale. The lower the Braden scale, the higher the risk for pressure injury development. A score of 15–18 is mild risk, 13–14 is moderate risk, 10–12 is high risk, and 9 or less is very high risk.

Bergstrom N, Braden BJ, Laguzza A, Holman V. The Braden scale for predicting pressure sore risk. Nurs Res. 1987;36(4):205–10.
Hyun S, Vermillion B, Newton C, Fall M, Li X, Kaewprag P, Moffatt-Bruce S, Lenz ER. Predictive validity of the Braden scale for patients in intensive care units. Am J Crit Care. 2013;22(6):514–20. https://doi.org/10.4037/ajcc2013991.

12. A 71-year-old female with T9 AIS A SCI is concerned about a ruptured serum-filled blister on her heel which she first noticed 2 days ago. What is the next best course of management?

A. Start acyclovir for herpes simplex treatment
B. Begin local wound care with a topical agent
C. Obtain a complete blood count (CBC), erythrocyte sedimentation rate (ESR) and c-reactive protein (CRP) to evaluate for osteomyelitis
D. Pressure mapping of her wheelchair

Answer: B.

According to the National Pressure Ulcer advisory group, a ruptured serum filled blister describes a stage 2 pressure injury. It is further described as a partial-thickness loss of skin with exposed dermis. The wound bed is viable, pink or red, and moist. Herpes Simplex eruption occurs in a dermatomal pattern with a rash containing multiple vesicular blisters. Although C is not entirely unreasonable, the stage of the ulcer is less likely associated with osteomyelitis at this time. Pressure mapping of the wheelchair may be a good option to prevent further skin breakdown but the location on the heel makes pressure mapping less needed. The next best course of management is to promote healing of the current ulcer with local wound care.

Edsberg LE, Black JM, Goldberg M, McNichol L, Moore L, Sieggreen M. Revised national pressure ulcer advisory panel pressure injury staging system: revised pressure injury staging system. J Wound Ostomy Continence Nurs. 2016;43(6):585–97. https://doi.org/10.1097/WON.0000000000000281.

13. A patient with thoracic myelomeningocele developed a deep tissue pressure injury after a prolonged hospitalization. Two weeks after discharging home, the home care RN noticed that it is now a much larger wound with visible muscle and necrotic tissue. This wound is best characterized as a:

A. A deep tissue pressure injury
B. Unstageable deep pressure injury
C. Stage 3 pressure injury
D. Stage 4 pressure injury

Answer: D.

Staging of pressure injuries:
- *Stage 1 pressure injury*: Nonblanchable erythema. There is intact skin with nonblanchable redness of a localized area usually over a bony prominence. Tissue may be painful, firm, soft, warmer, or cooler compared to surrounding tissues.
- *Stage 2 pressure injury*: Partial-thickness skin loss. There is a partial-thickness loss of dermis presenting as a shallow open ulcer with a red-pink wound bed, without slough which can present as an intact or open serum-filled blister. It can also present as a shiny or dry shallow ulcer without slough or bruising.
- *Stage 3 pressure injury*: Full-thickness skin loss. There may be visible subcutaneous fat but bone, tendon, or muscle is not exposed. Slough does not obscure the depth of tissue loss. Undermining and tunneling may be present. The bridge of the nose, ear, occiput, and malleolus do not have subcutaneous tissue and shallow ulcers at these locations are automatically stage 3 pressure injuries.
- *Stage 4 pressure injury*: Full-thickness tissue loss. There is exposed bone, tendon, or muscle. Bone or tendon is visible or directly palpable. Slough or eschar may be present. Tunneling and undermining are often present.
- *Unstageable pressure injury*: Depth unknown. There is full thickness tissue loss in which the base of the ulcer is covered by slough and/or eschar. Stable (dry, adherent, intact without erythema, or fluctuance) eschar on heels is a protective biologic cover and should not be removed.
- *Deep tissue injury*: Depth unknown. There is a purple or maroon localized area of discolored intact skin or blood-filled blister due to underlying soft tissue from pressure or shear. The area may be preceded by tissue that is painful, firm, mushy, or boggy, or warmer or cooler compared to surrounding tissues. The wound may further evolve and develop a thin eschar leading to exposed additional layers of affected tissue.

Edsberg LE, Black JM, Goldberg M, McNichol L, Moore L, Sieggreen M. Revised national pressure ulcer advisory panel pressure injury staging system: revised pressure injury staging system. J Wound Ostomy Continence Nurs. 2016;43(6):585–97. https://doi.org/10.1097/WON.0000000000000281.

Baranoski S, et al. Skin: an essential organ. In: Baranoski S, Ayello EA, editors. Wound care essentials, practice principles. Philadelphia: Wolters Kluwer; 2016. p. 408–10.

National Pressure Ulcer Advisory Panel (NPUAP) announces a change in terminology from pressure ulcer to pressure injury and updates the stages of pressure injury. National Pressure Ulcer Advisory Panel; Apr 2016. Available at http://www.npuap.org/national-pressure-ulcer-advisory-panel-npuap-announces-a-change-in-terminology-from-pressure-ulcer-to-pressure-injury-and-updates-the-stages-of-pressure-injury. Accessed Dec 2020.

14. A left stage 3 lateral malleolus pressure injury has been offloaded over the past 4 months in a patient with T12 AIS B SCI. The patient is concerned that there is plateau in healing. What characteristics are indicative of desired active wound healing?

    A. Biofilm with dusky red tissue underneath
    B. Beefy red granulation tissue that that fills 75% of the wound bed
    C. White perimeter epithelization with surrounding pitting edema
    D. Raspberry ruby red granulation tissue that bleeds easily

    Answer: B.

    Stages of wound healing can be reviewed based on time. From day 0–3, the stage is typically hemostasis and coagulation in which the pathophysiological goals are to clot and vasoconstrict to stop bleeding. Day 1–25 is the inflammatory phase to which growth factors and cytokines are released leading to swelling and erythema. Concurrently, one can also expect proliferation which is characterized by new blood vessel growth and wound closure though increased collagen (Type III) synthesis. The last stage (day 30 onwards) is the stage of maturation and modeling.
        Here scar remodeling transforms collagen from Type III to Type I collagen. According to the Pressure Ulcer Scale for healing, beefy red granulation tissue that fills the wound bed is associated with good healing. Pink or dull dusky red granulation tissue is farther from the desired outcome but better than biofilm or necrotic tissue. Pitting edema is not desired around a wound and can be documented based on the cm surrounding the wound.

    Baranoski S, Ayello EA. Wound care essentials. 3rd ed. Wolters Kluwer; 2015.
    Günes UY. A prospective study evaluating the Pressure Ulcer Scale for Healing (PUSH Tool) to assess stage II, stage III, and stage IV pressure ulcers. Ostomy Wound Manage. 2009;55(5):48–52.

15. A 17-year-old male with a history of T8 AIS A SCI sees you in the wound care clinic after acquiring a stage 3 sacral pressure injury. He is following your orders of pressure relief, calcium alginate, and a protective border. He wants to know how nutrition impacts his wound healing. Which statement has the best evidence for wound healing?

    A. Patients require adequate protein for positive nitrogen balance and wound healing.
    B. Carbohydrates contain the most concentrated energy source needed for cell regeneration.

C. Patients should consume a diet high in fat given need for excess low density lipoproteins.
D. 5–6 grams of protein/kg body weight is the minimum amount of protein to help heal a pressure injury.

Answer: A.

There is level B evidence that patients require adequate protein for positive nitrogen balance. Fat contains the most concentrated energy source of all the food groups. There is level C evidence that early referral to a dietician most improves wound healing. 1.25–1.5 g/kg body weight of protein is the minimum amount of protein recommended for wound healing.

Inadequate intake of proteins and calories is associated with increased pressure injuries. High calorie and high protein foods (e.g. coconut milk, nuts/nut butters, avocados, whole grains, dried fruits, whey protein, and cottage cheese) help accelerate wound healing. Commercial oral supplements range from 1 to 2 kcal/mL, 13–25% of total calories from protein, and contain the recommended amount of vitamins and minerals.

An estimate of the difference in basal energy expenditure between persons with SCI who have severe pressure injuries and those who do not have pressure injuries is approximately 5 kcal/kg of body weight per day likely due to the chronic inflammatory state. The increased protein requirement in persons with pressure injuries ranges from 1.25 to 2 g protein/kg of body weight per day.

Baranoski S, et al. Skin: an essential organ. In: Baranoski S, Ayello EA, editors. Wound care essentials, practice principles. Philadelphia: Wolters Kluwer; 2016. p. 408–10.
Consortium for Spinal Cord Medicine. Pressure ulcer prevention and treatment following spinal cord injury: a clinical practice guideline for health-care professionals. 2nd ed. Washington, DC: Paralyzed Veterans of America; 2014.

16. A 31-year-old male with a history of T4 AIS C SCI, type I diabetes, venous thrombus embolism on long term anticoagulation, and a 9 month history of a right greater trochanter stage 4 decubitus ulcer presents with increased serosanguineous drainage classified as moderate to large amount of drainage, wound base covered by 80% yellowish slough, and slight maceration of peri-wound tissue. There is no surrounding erythema, patient denies symptoms concerning for infection (fatigue, fever, chills), and inflammatory markers are stable. What wound dressing recommendations are most appropriate?

    A. Collagenase combined with wet to dry dressing changes ensuring complete packing of all areas of undermining
    B. Begin negative pressure therapy
    C. Collagenase combined with silver impregnated hydrofiber
    D. Collagenase combined with a calcium alginate dressing

Answer: D.

Collagenase can be used for enzymatic debridement to facilitate break down and removal of necrotic tissue including slough. When using collagenase, practitioners must avoid using additional products with impregnated metals such as silver or iodine as they will de-activate the collagenase rendering it ineffective. In wounds that have moderate to maximal drainage, more absorptive products should be considered to control drainage and avoid macerating the periwound tissue such as dry collagen dressings followed by dry hydrofiber dressing. Wet to dry dressings do not have the same ability to absorb high amounts of drainage.

While negative pressure wound therapy is another alternative, the wound should be mostly debrided of necrotic tissue before beginning this therapy. Additionally, one needs to be mindful of the fact that this patient is on anticoagulation for which one would need to exercise caution with starting this type of therapy.

Adequate moisture balance promotes keratinocyte migration and wound healing. For wounds with heavy exudate, choose an absorbent dressing such as an alginate. For dry wounds, use a moisturizing dressing such as a hydrogel. A dressing that will keep the wound moist but not too wet or too dry should be chosen. The five basic moisture retentive dressings are films, foams, hydrocolloids, alginates, and hydrogels.

Sunn G. Spinal cord injury pressure ulcer treatment: an experience-based approach. Phys Med Rehabil Clin N Am. 2014;25(3):671–80, ix. https://doi.org/10.1016/j.pmr.2014.05.002.
Jones RE, Foster DS, Longaker MT. Management of chronic wounds-2018. JAMA. 2018;320(14):1481–2. https://doi.org/10.1001/jama.2018.12426.
Powers JG, Higham C, Broussard K, Phillips TJ. Wound healing and treating wounds: Chronic wound care and management. J Am Acad Dermatol. 2016;74(4):607–25; quiz 625–6. https://doi.org/10.1016/j.jaad.2015.08.070.

17. A 53-year-old male with T6 AIS B SCI presents to your clinic with a stage 2 pressure injury on his sacrum. The wound is 3.9 × 2.4 cm, has a copious amount of serosanguinous drainage, slough covering <10% of the wound bed, is without necrotic/devitalized tissue, has 90% healthy reddish granulation tissue, and is without warmth, swelling, or induration. What is the best dressing to place on this wound?

A. Transparent film
B. Hydrogel dressing
C. Foam dressing
D. Zinc impregnated gauze

Answer: C.

Foam dressing is the correct answer because it is a primary dressing for absorption and insulation, used in partial and full thickness wounds, and is used in in minimal to heavy exudate. Zinc impregnated gauze is incorrect because of low absorption although can be used in infected wounds, wounds with cavities or dead space, and can also be used in partial or full-thickness wounds. Transparent film is an incorrect answer because they are impermeable to bacteria, used for high-risk intact skin, used for minimal or no exudate, and promotes autolytic debridement. Hydrogel dressing is incorrect because it increases fluid into the wound, is used for deep wounds, is used for dry to minimal exudate, and is used in combination with other dressings.

The role of dressings are to maintain a physiologic local wound bed environment that has an appropriate level of moisture, controls exudate, eliminates dead space, controls odor, eliminates or minimizes pain, protects the wound and periwound skin, removes nonviable tissue, and prevents and manages infection. Excessive exudate can cause maceration of the periwound skin and is associated with prolonged healing.

Other dressings are included below:

- Alginate dressings can absorb up to 20 times its weight, supports debridement in the presence of exudate, and is indicated for superficial wounds with minimal or no exudate. Hydrocolloids provide a moist wound bed allowing clean wounds to granulate and necrotic wounds to debride autolytically, are used for partial and full-thickness wounds, are used for minimal-moderate exudates. Gauze is used in partial and full-thickness wounds, used in exudative wounds, and wounds with cavities, tunneling, or sinus tracts. Composites are impermeable barriers used in partial and shallow thickness wounds, are used for minimal exudate, and used for healthy granulation tissue. Contact layers are placed on the wound base used in as primary dressing in partial and full-thickness wounds with minimal to heavy exudate used in combination with negative pressure wound therapy. Wound pouches are used for highly exudative and malodourous wounds.

- Negative pressure wound therapy is a proven way to decrease wound size and healing time as seen in multiple clinical trials. It also decreases the frequency of dressing changes and improves patient comfort. Enzymatic products with protease-modulating matrices have been shown to decrease healing time compared to wet-to-dry dressings. Antimicrobial dressings have not been shown to improve healing time over standard dressings. Most common antimicrobial dressings include sliver and honey-impregnated dressings. Skin substitutes have been shown to support faster wound healing but evidence is not as robust as moisture retentive dressings or negative pressure wound therapy.

Consortium for Spinal Cord Medicine. Pressure ulcer prevention and treatment following spinal cord injury: a clinical practice guideline for health-care professionals. 2nd ed. Washington, DC: Paralyzed Veterans of America; 2014.

Gupta S, Andersen C, Black J, de Leon J, Fife C, Lantis Ii JC, Niezgoda J, Snyder R, Sumpio B, Tettelbach W, Treadwell T, Weir D, Silverman RP. Management of chronic wounds: diagnosis, preparation, treatment, and follow-up. Wounds. 2017;29(9):S19–36.

18. A 22-year-old female with lumbar spina bifida developed a coccygeal pressure injury after a prolonged hospital stay for a severe COVID-19 infection. Her current wound is 8 cm × 6 cm × 5 cm with areas of undermining. The base has 90% necrotic gray devitalized tissue, large thick yellow foul-smelling drainage, without surrounding edema or erythema. The most appropriate mechanism for removal of the necrotic and devitalized tissue is:

A. Surgical debridement
B. Autolytic debridement
C. Application of collagenase ointment followed by wound vac
D. Application of wound vac without collagenase ointment

Answer: A.

Debridement is utilized to help remove devitalized tissue from the wound bed. The types of debridement include: Autolytic, sharp, mechanical, enzymatic, and surgical. Wound care can utilize one or more methods of debridement at a time. Autolytic debridement utilizes enzymes (proteolytic, collagenolytic) in the setting of patients own white blood cells to accomplish removal of devitalized tissue. This requires a moist wound setting. Sharp debridement utilizes an instrument such as a scalpel, curette, or scissors to remove necrotic tissue. Mechanical debridement can be accomplished though wet to dry dressings although can be non-selective and can remove viable granulated tissue. Other forms of mechanical debridement are high pressure pulsatile lavage. Enzymatic debridement is accomplished though application of a topical biological enzymatic agent. This digests slough and the collagen that stabilizes necrotic tissue to the wound bed. Surgical debridement can be done in clinic or at bedside if removal of necrotic tissue can be done without significant bleeding. Surgical debridement is typically performed under anesthesia for larger and deeper wounds. Given the significant necrotic tissue, fibrosis, and concern for possible infection, sharp debridement is the preferred method in this case.

Consortium for Spinal Cord Medicine. Pressure ulcer prevention and treatment following spinal cord injury: a clinical practice guideline for health-care professionals. 2nd ed. Washington, DC: Paralyzed Veterans of America; 2014.
Gupta S, Andersen C, Black J, de Leon J, Fife C, Lantis Ii JC, Niezgoda J, Snyder R, Sumpio B, Tettelbach W, Treadwell T, Weir D, Silverman RP. Management of chronic wounds: diagnosis, preparation, treatment, and follow-up. Wounds. 2017;29(9):S19–36.

19. A 24-year-old female with a 6 year history of C7 AIS A SCI has had multiple pressure injuries since her injury. Currently she has a stage 4 non-healing sacral pressure injury. ESR and CRP were elevated and MRI pelvis showed decreased T1 signal and increased T2 signal due to marrow edema suggestive of acute osteomyelitis. She is started on IV antibiotics for 6 weeks and is referred to a plastic surgeon. The surgeon is most likely to recommend which type of surgery?

A. Free flap
B. Skin graft
C. Musculocutaneous flap
D. Skin flap

Answer: C.

All patients with stage 3 or 4 pressure injuries should be evaluated for surgical treatment. In debilitated patients, surgical debridement without subsequent reconstruction may be an optimal treatment. Reconstruction of stage 3 or 4 pressure injuries with myocutaneous flaps is indicated in SCI patients who are not expected to regain sensation.

Skin grafting is not effective in eliminating a deep defect such as in this stage 4 pressure injury. Split-thickness grafts are indicated in large, shallow, and well-granulated pressure injuries where high mechanical forces are not a factor. A full thickness skin graft has better mechanical properties than a split-thickness graft.

There are multiple different types of flaps including fasciocutaneous flaps and myocutaneous (aka musculocutaneous) flaps. Fasciocutaneous flaps have a better blood supply than most cutaneous flaps. However, the subcutaneous tissue is of limited value in pressure injury treatment because of its low resistance to pressure and tear. Fasciocutaneous flaps are suitable for select stage 3 and 4 pressure injuries without underlying osteomyelitis and without nonphysiological loading. Myocutaneous flaps are the preferred treatment in deep pressure injuries because they provide sufficient bulk with excellent blood supply. However, these flaps have a low tolerance for ischemic injury. 80% of flaps are myocutaneous flaps.

Myocutaneous flaps have become the coverage of choice for SCI patients who require surgical closure of pressure injuries. Because of their blood supply, these flaps are better able to withstand pressure and shear. They can also be useful in osteomyelitis by bringing highly vascularized muscle tissue into the area of infection. Free flaps, skin flaps, and skin grafts are rarely used because they do not tolerate future pressure or shear.

Sørensen JL, Jørgensen B, Gottrup F. Surgical treatment of pressure ulcers. Am J Surg. 2004;188(1A Suppl):42–51. https://doi.org/10.1016/S0002-9610(03)00290-3.

20. A 44-year-old female with T2 AIS A SCI with a non-healing stage 4 sacral pressure injury undergoes a musculocutaneous flap procedure. Which is NOT a sign of flap failure?

    A. Wound separation
    B. Cyanosis
    C. Hematoma
    D. Hyperemia

Answer: C.

Many complications can follow surgical operation of a wound. Sliding or direct pressure can cause separation from its vascular bed leading to seroma, hematoma, fibrin, or purulence formation. These are not signs of flap failure. Pressure-bearing areas need at least 6 weeks of wound closure before reaching 60% tensile strength. Wounds separation, cyanosis, and hyperemia are all cardinal signs of wound flap failure. However, hematoma formation is a post-op complication but not a sign of failure.

Simman R. Wound closure and the reconstructive ladder in plastic surgery. J Am Col Certif Wound Spec. 2009;1(1):6–11. https://doi.org/10.1016/j.jcws.2008.10.003.

21. A 66-year-old male with a history of C5 AIS B tetraplegia presents back to your clinic with a worsening left ischial tuberosity stage 3 pressure injury which demonstrates healthy periwound tissue, minimal undermining, no tunneling, moderate sanguineous drainage, and covered 80% necrotic tissue characterized primarily by loose slough. The decision is made to utilize hydrotherapy to facilitate mechanical debridement. What recommendations would be most appropriate?

A. Hydrotherapy in the pool with gentle oscillation of water
B. Hydrotherapy in the pool to moisten the wound tissue followed by sharp debridement
C. 4–15 pounds per square inch (psi) pulsatile lavage irrigation with suction
D. 15–24 psi pulsatile lavage irrigation with suction

Answer: C.

Pulsatile lavage therapy provides direct, localized hydrotherapy to pressure injuries by pressurized normal saline. Pulsatile lavage allows for the precise removal of necrotic tissue and is a type of mechanical debridement. Suction permits the user to hold and cut the targeted tissue while aspirating debris from the wound at the same time. Irrigation streams higher than 15 psi can cause trauma to healthy tissue thus negatively impacting wound healing. The optimal hydrotherapy pressure is 4–15 psi.

The immersion of large body surface areas into a whirlpool may lead to cross contamination for both the patient and operator. Transfer to whirlpool is difficult for SCI patient population and does not target specific areas like pulsatile lavage does.

Bogie KM, Ho CH. Pulsatile lavage for pressure ulcer management in spinal cord injury: a retrospective clinical safety review. Ostomy Wound Manage. 2013;59(3):35–8.
Ho CH, Bensitel T, Wang X, Bogie KM. Pulsatile lavage for the enhancement of pressure ulcer healing: a randomized controlled trial. Phys Ther. 2012;92(1):38–48. https://doi.org/10.2522/ptj.20100349. Epub 2011 Sept 23.
Consortium for Spinal Cord Medicine. Pressure ulcer prevention and treatment following spinal cord injury: a clinical practice guideline for health-care professionals. 2nd ed. Washington, DC: Paralyzed Veterans of America; 2014.

22. The spouse of a patient with T2 AIS A SCI is concerned about an area of skin with markedly increasing redness with clearly demarcated swelling near the antecubital fossa on the left upper extremity that has worsened over the past 24 h. She notes odd behaviors and depression in the patient as of late as well. The patient dismisses her concerns and says she is paranoid and that the rash is from pressure on his elbow from his wheelchair. You suspect IV drug abuse, and patient admits to current use. What is the next best step of management?

A. MRI of the left elbow to evaluate for osteomyelitis
B. Urine toxicology screen, CBC, ESR CRP and starting a course of oral antibiotics
C. CBC and bone scan
D. MRI of the elbow region, urine tox screen, CBC, ESR, CRP and course of oral antibiotics

Answer: B.

This patient's case is consistent with cellulitis. Both present clinically as areas of skin erythema, edema, and warmth that developed as a response to bacteria breaching the skin barrier. Cellulitis is nearly always unilateral. Cellulitis involves the dermis and subcutaneous fat. This patient is presenting with cellulitis in a region associated with intravenous drug administration—a skin barrier disruption risk. The most common cause of cellulitis is beta-hemolytic streptococci, most commonly group A *Streptococcus* or *Streptococcus pyogenes* or *Staphylococcus aureus* which includes methicillin-resistant strains. An MRI of the elbow is not currently indicated because the rash developed over the course of 2–3 days and is currently clinically consistent cellulitis. MRI can help distinguish between cellulitis from osteomyelitis. Osteomyelitis may underlie an area of cellulitis but that is more typical in the setting of a chronic soft tissue infection that fails to improve with appropriate antibiotic therapy.

Raff AB, Kroshinsky D. Cellulitis: a review. JAMA. 2016;316(3):325–37. https://doi.org/10.1001/jama.2016.8825.
Stevens DL, Bisno AL, Chambers HF, Dellinger EP, Goldstein EJ, Gorbach SL, Hirschmann JV, Kaplan SL, Montoya JG, Wade JC. Practice guidelines for the diagnosis and management of skin and soft tissue infections: 2014 update by the infectious diseases society of America. Clin Infect Dis. 2014;59(2):147–59. https://doi.org/10.1093/cid/ciu296. Epub 2014 Jun 18.

23. A patient with history of C6 AIS B SCI presents with an increasing exudate volume, foul smelling odor and new undermining in a chronic right ischial wound. Which laboratory tests are indicated?

A. Zinc level, CBC with differential
B. ESR, CRP, pre-albumin, CBC with differential

C. Complete metabolic panel (CMP), pre-albumin
D. CRP, CMP, zinc level

Answer: B.

It is prudent to monitor for changes in the clinical characteristics of chronic pressure injuries. Bacterial overgrowth on the surface of the wound known as biofilm, accumulation of devitalized tissue, hyperkerotic tissue and increased or change in exudate are signs of worsening of suboptimal wound healing. Laboratory results can help assess for acute infection and can be used to trend response to treatment. These include ESR, CRP, CBC with differential. Of note though, in the setting of chronic osteomyelitis leukocytosis is uncommon. Pre-albumin can be useful to help assess for adequate nutritional status.

Ross R, Everett NB, Tyler R. Wound healing and collagen formation. VI. The origin of the wound fibroblast studied in parabiosis. J Cell Biol. 1970;44(3):645–54. https://doi.org/10.1083/jcb.44.3.645.
Perry M. Erythrocyte sedimentation rate and C reactive protein in the assessment of suspected bone infection—are they reliable indices? J R Coll Surg Edinb. 1996;41(2):116–8.

24. A patient with T3 myelopathy due to transverse myelitis developed a right greater trochanteric infection due to a sub-optimally fitted lightweight manual wheelchair. There is high clinical suspicion of osteomyelitis in this patient secondary to increased tone, new autonomic dysreflexia, and elevated WBC with left-shift. What is the next best step in confirming the suspected organism causing the osteomyelitis?

A. Bone scan
B. Bone biopsy
C. Deep tissue biopsy
D. Wound tissue swab

Answer: B.

Osteomyelitis is an infection involving the bone. Osteomyelitis may be classified based on the mechanism of infection (hematogenous versus nonhematogenous) and the duration of illness (acute versus chronic). Risk factors for nonhematogenous osteomyelitis include poorly healing soft tissue wounds— such as pressure injuries, which is the most common cause of osteomyelitis in patients with spinal cord injuries. Bone biopsy is the best method to make the diagnosis of osteomyelitis. 25% of non-healing pressure injuries have underlying osteomyelitis. Bone scans are associated with high false positives due to the underlying inflammatory characteristics of a wound. The microbiologic yield of bone biopsy remains quite sensitive ranging around greater than 50%. Deep tissue biopsy and wound tissues swabs are non-specific given high levels of bacterial colonization in chronic wounds.

Wu JS, Gorbachova T, Morrison WB, Haims AH. Imaging-guided bone biopsy for osteomyelitis: are there factors associated with positive or negative cultures? AJR Am J Roentgenol. 2007;188(6):1529–34. https://doi.org/10.2214/AJR.06.1286.

25. For wounds to heal, good circulation, nutrition, immune response, and pressure relief are necessary. Wound healing occurs in phases. The normal process of wound healing takes place in the following order:

    A. Remodeling, inflammation, and proliferation
    B. Remodeling, proliferation, and inflammation
    C. Proliferation, inflammation, and remodeling
    D. Inflammation, proliferation, and remodeling

Answer: D.

Wound healing is initiated by the inflammatory phase during which bacteria and debris are cleared by neutrophils, macrophages, and phagocytes. A sufficient supply of growth factors and a healthy immune system are required for this phase of wound healing. The proliferative phase follows when fibroblasts create a collagen matrix, new blood vessels grow, and granulation tissue develops. Epidermal cells appose and migrate along the wound surface to bring the borders together. In the remodeling phase, fibroblasts reconstruct the collagen matrix and begin to form myofibroblasts which complete the composition of connective tissue and facilitate wound contraction. Tissue typically regains 20% of its strength in the first few weeks of wound formation. Protein deficiency, necrotic tissue, and poor perfusion are some factors that can delay and compromise any phase of the wound healing process.

Powers JG, Higham C, Broussard K, Phillips TJ. Wound healing and treating wounds: chronic wound care and management. J Am Acad Dermatol. 2016;74(4):607–25; quiz 625–6. https://doi.org/10.1016/j.jaad.2015.08.070.

Pain and Spinal Cord Injury

14

Reuben Horace, Christopher Woolley, Danielle Zheng, and Joel Castellanos

---

Questions

1. A 42-year-old man with a T10 level spinal cord injury who is wheelchair dependent complains of numbness and tingling in his hands. His thumb and index fingers are most affected, and his little finger is not affected. When you tap over his volar wrist, you reproduce his symptoms. According to the International Spinal Cord Injury Pain (ISCIP) classification, his pain would be classified as:

   A. Above-level pain
   B. Below-level pain
   C. Nociceptive pain
   D. Neuropathic pain

   Answer: D.

   The patient has carpal tunnel syndrome from wheelchair use. The ISCIP classification was designed to be comprehensive, including pains that are directly related to SCI as well as pains that are not pathologically and causally related to the injury itself. Tier 1 covers pain types: nociceptive, neuropathic, other, and unknown. Tier 2 covers pain subtypes, while Tier 3 further sub-categorizes by primary pain source and/or pathology. Carpal tunnel syndrome is a type of

R. Horace
New York Institute of Technology COM, Old Westbury, NY, USA

C. Woolley · D. Zheng
Pain Medicine, Department of Anesthesiology, UC San Diego, San Diego, CA, USA

J. Castellanos (✉)
Inpatient Rehabilitation, Department of Anesthesiology, UC San Diego Health,
San Diego, CA, USA
e-mail: jcastellanos@health.ucsd.edu

© The Author(s), under exclusive license to Springer Nature Switzerland AG 2022
B. A. Abramoff et al. (eds.), *The Essential Spinal Cord Injury Medicine Question Bank*, https://doi.org/10.1007/978-3-031-07796-8_14

neuropathic (nerve-related) pain, not a nociceptive pain. While carpal tunnel syndrome is technically an above-level pain, the ISCIP classification does not recognize this in their new tier classification. Below-level pain is a subtype of neuropathic pain, but carpal tunnel syndrome is not below the level of the patient's injury.

Bryce TN, Biering-Sørensen F, Finnerup NB, Cardenas DD, Defrin R, Ivan E, Lundeberg T, Norrbrink C, Richards JS, Siddall P, Stripling T, Treede RD, Waxman SG, Widerström-Noga E, Yezierski RP, Dijkers M. International Spinal Cord Injury Pain (ISCIP) classification: part 2. Initial validation using vignettes. Spinal Cord. 2012;50(6):404–12.
Asheghan M, Hollisaz MT, Taheri T, Kazemi H, Agoda AK. The prevalence of carpal tunnel syndrome among long-term manual wheelchair users with spinal cord injury: a cross-sectional study. J Spinal Cord Med. 2016;39(3):265–71.

2. A patient with spinal cord injury at T6 complains of chronic neck pain. On physical examination, taut bands are identified in the trapezius. Palpation of the region causes referred pain throughout the shoulder girdle bilaterally. The patient has not tried anything for the pain. For treatment, you suggest:

A. Oxycodone
B. Gabapentin
C. Acetaminophen
D. Trigger point injection with corticosteroid

Answer: C.

The patient is suffering from myofascial pain in the neck and upper back. According to the World Health Organization (WHO) analgesic ladder, mild pain should be treated with non-opioid analgesics such as non-steroidal anti-inflammatory drugs (NSAID)s or acetaminophen. Non-pharmacologic approaches such as physical therapy should also be attempted. Oxycodone is considered a potent opioid and would be the third and final step of the WHO analgesic ladder. There is insufficient evidence to determine whether pain relief is sustained and whether function or quality of life improves with long-term opioid therapy. While gabapentin is a useful treatment for neuropathic pain, it is not first line for myofascial (nociceptive) pain. Trigger point injection could be considered, but the patient has not tried more conservative measures. Furthermore, corticosteroids are not recommended as a first line therapy for trigger points given the potential for additional adverse effects.

Dowell D, Haegerich TM, Chou R. CDC Guideline for prescribing opioids for chronic pain—United States, 2016. MMWR Recomm Rep. 2016;65(1):1–49. https://doi.org/10.15585/mmwr.rr6501e1. Erratum in: MMWR Recomm Rep. 2016;65(11):295.
Anekar AA, Cascella M. WHO analgesic ladder. 18 May 2021. In: StatPearls, editor. Treasure Island, FL: StatPearls Publishing; 2022.
Lavelle ED, Lavelle W, Smith HS. Myofascial trigger points. Anesthesiol Clin. 2007;25(4):841–51, vii–iii. https://doi.org/10.1016/j.anclin.2007.07.003.

3. A patient reports burning and shooting pain with occasional pins and needles in his lower extremities 6 months after spinal cord injury. This is associated with increased sensitivity of his lower extremities. For treatment, you suggest:

A. Oxycodone
B. Gabapentin
C. Acetaminophen
D. Epidural steroid injection

Answer: B.

This patient is experiencing classical symptoms of neuropathic pain after spinal cord injury. Although this can be very difficult to treat, the best evidence is for gabapentin. While analgesics such as NSAIDs and acetaminophen can be trialed, they have not been found to be as effective in relieving neuropathic pain. Opioids have also not been found to be as helpful, and are associated with adverse side effects including constipation, respiratory depression, sedation, dependency, and increased abuse potential. Epidural steroid injections can be effective for radiculopathy but would not be effective in treating neuropathic pain from spinal cord injury.

Cardenas DD, Jensen MP. Treatments for chronic pain in persons with spinal cord injury: a survey study. J Spinal Cord Med. 2006;29(2):109–17. https://doi.org/10.1080/1079026 8.2006.11753864.
Finnerup NB. Pain in patients with spinal cord injury. Pain. 2013;154(Suppl 1):S71–6. https://doi.org/10.1016/j.pain.2012.12.007. Epub 2012 Dec 22.
Teasell RW, Mehta S, Aubut JA, Foulon B, Wolfe DL, Hsieh JT, Townson AF, Short C, Spinal Cord Injury Rehabilitation Evidence Research Team. A systematic review of pharmacologic treatments of pain after spinal cord injury. Arch Phys Med Rehabil. 2010;91(5):816–31. https://doi.org/10.1016/j.apmr.2010.01.022.

4. There is evidence for the effectiveness of all the following medications in treating neuropathic pain following spinal cord injury EXCEPT:

A. Gabapentin
B. Intravenous (IV) lidocaine
C. Cannabinoids
D. Amitriptyline

Answer: C.

Cannabinoids show conflicting evidence in improving neuropathic pain following spinal cord injury. Gabapentin has strong evidence (multiple randomized controlled trials) supporting its treatment for post-SCI neuropathic pain. IV lidocaine has been shown to be effective, but typically only leads to short-term benefit. Amitriptyline and other tricyclic antidepressants show benefit for neuropathic pain in depressed persons.

Cardenas DD, Jensen MP. Treatments for chronic pain in persons with spinal cord injury: a survey study. J Spinal Cord Med. 2006;29(2):109–17. https://doi.org/10.1080/1079026 8.2006.11753864.

Finnerup NB. Pain in patients with spinal cord injury. Pain. 2013;154(Suppl 1):S71–6. https://doi.org/10.1016/j.pain.2012.12.007. Epub 2012 Dec 22.

Teasell RW, Mehta S, Aubut JA, Foulon B, Wolfe DL, Hsieh JT, Townson AF, Short C; Spinal Cord Injury Rehabilitation Evidence Research Team. A systematic review of pharmacologic treatments of pain after spinal cord injury. Arch Phys Med Rehabil. 2010;91(5):816–31. https://doi.org/10.1016/j.apmr.2010.01.022.

5. Spasticity following SCI can lead to significant pain. The following treatments are all effective in spasticity reduction EXCEPT:

    A. Stretching/range of motion exercises
    B. Hot/cold packs
    C. Baclofen
    D. Botulinum toxin

Answer: B.

Hot/cold packs should be used carefully on body areas that have impaired sensation as prolonged exposure can result in burn or frostbite. In some cases, they can also trigger spasms. Stretching/range of motion exercises, baclofen, and botulinum toxin injection have all been demonstrated to reduce spasticity.

Elbasiouny SM, Moroz D, Bakr MM, Mushahwar VK. Management of spasticity after spinal cord injury: current techniques and future directions. Neurorehabil Neural Repair. 2010;24(1):23–33. https://doi.org/10.1177/1545968309343213. Epub 2009 Sept 1.

6. Which antispasmodic is correctly paired with its mechanism of action?

    A. Baclofen—gamma-aminobutyric acid (GABA)-B agonist
    B. Diazepam—alpha-2 agonist
    C. Tizanidine—ryanodine receptor 1 antagonist
    D. Dantrolene—GABA-A agonist

Answer: A.

Baclofen is a GABA-B agonist which leads to inhibition of mono- and polysynaptic spinal reflexes. Diazepam facilitates the activity of GABA by allosterically binding at GABA-A receptors. This leads to an increased frequency of chloride channel opening and subsequent hyperpolarization/reduced excitability of neurons. Tizanidine is an alpha-2 receptor agonist which causes a decrease in the release of excitatory neurotransmitters from spinal interneurons. Dantrolene is a ryanodine receptor 1 antagonist within the sarcoplasmic reticulum which inhibits the release of calcium necessary for muscle contraction.

Dhaliwal JS, Rosani A, Saadabadi A. Diazepam. 14 Sept 2021. In: StatPearls, editor. Treasure Island, FL: StatPearls Publishing; 2022.
Ghanavatian S, Derian A. Baclofen. 17 Dec 2021. In: StatPearls, editor. Treasure Island, FL: StatPearls Publishing; 2022.
Ghanavatian S, Derian A. Tizanidine. 13 Aug 2021. In: StatPearls, editor. Treasure Island, FL: StatPearls Publishing; 2022.
Ratto D, Joyner RW. Dantrolene. 26 Jul 2021. In: StatPearls, editor. Treasure Island, FL: StatPearls Publishing; 2022.

7. Which of the following statements about visceral pain related to SCI is true?

   A. It is the most common type of pain experienced after SCI
   B. It is easy to treat
   C. It can manifest as increased spasticity
   D. It is most associated with diarrhea

Answer: C.

In patients with increased spasticity, it is important to rule out increased visceral pain. Visceral pain has a low (5%) incidence following SCI. Musculoskeletal pain followed by neuropathic pain are the most common pain types following SCI. Patients with visceral pain are more likely to report their pain as severe or excruciating, and it is very difficult to treat. Visceral pain is more often associated with constipation rather than diarrhea.

Finnerup NB. Pain in patients with spinal cord injury. Pain. 2013;154(Suppl 1):S71–6. https://doi.org/10.1016/j.pain.2012.12.007. Epub 2012 Dec 22.
Siddall PJ, McClelland JM, Rutkowski SB, Cousins MJ. A longitudinal study of the prevalence and characteristics of pain in the first 5 years following spinal cord injury. Pain. 2003;103(3):249–57. https://doi.org/10.1016/S0304-3959(02)00452-9.

8. All of the following mechanisms are thought to be involved in central sensitization after spinal cord injury EXCEPT:

   A. Production of nitric oxide
   B. Upregulation of TNF-alpha
   C. Decrease in intracellular calcium
   D. Increase in reactive oxygen species

Answer: C.

There is a significant increase in intracellular calcium after spinal cord injury. Calcium is directly involved in multiple intracellular signaling pathways, including pain sensitization. Production of nitric oxide, upregulation of TNF-alpha, and an increase in reactive oxygen species are all seen after SCI and are thought to be involved in the process of central sensitization.

Benzon H, Raja SN, Liu S, Fishman S, Cohen S. Central Pain States. Chapter 28. In: Essentials of pain medicine. Philadephia, PA: Elsevier; 2011.

9. A patient who has HIV presents to the ED describing "lightning pain" and ataxia of bilateral lower extremities and urinary retention. On physical examination, he has areflexia at L4, L5, and S1 reflexes bilaterally, loss of vibratory sensation and proprioception in his lower extremities, and pupils that react to accommodation but not light. A thoracic and lumbar magnetic resonance imaging (MRI) study is performed. The MRI is most likely to show which of the following?

A. A central T2 hyperintense spinal cord lesion at the T10–T11 level that involves most of the cross-sectional area of the cord.
B. T2 hyperintensities along the dorsal columns of the spinal cord.
C. Obliteration of perineural and epidural fat as well as compression of the lateral recess of the spinal canal.
D. Normal MRI findings

Answer: B.

This patient presents with late neurosyphilis, specifically tabes dorsalis. 60% of patients who present with tabes dorsalis also have Argyll Robertson pupil as seen in this patient. The pain associated with tabes dorsalis is often characterized as a "lightning pain" that radiates down both extremities. Symptoms and physical exam signs, as well as lesions on imaging, are typically localized to the posterior elements of the spinal cord. Choice A describes the typical MRI findings in transverse myelitis. Choice C correlates to the MRI findings of severe spinal stenosis. With this correlation of upper motor neuron symptoms (neurogenic bladder, ataxia, and loss of vibratory sense), a negative MRI would be highly unlikely.

Merritt HH, Adams RD, Solomon HC. Neurosyphilis. New York, NY: Oxford University Press; 1946.
Holmes G. A British Medical Association lecture on some clinical manifestations of tabes dorsalis: delivered to the Harrogate Branch, October 7, 1922. BMJ. 1923;1(3237):47–51.
Romberg E. Pupillary disturbances in tabes. Arch Psychiatr Nervenkr Z Gesamte Neurol Psychiatr. 1939;165:369–72.
Schaller WF. Early diagnosis of tabes dorsalis. JAMA. 1917;LXVIII(3):190–4.
Choi K, Lee K, Chung S. Idiopathic transverse myelitis: MR characteristics. AJNR Am J Neuroradiol. 1996;17:1151–60.

10. A patient with T10 spinal cord injury has decreased, but non-painful, sensation to light touch over his central abdomen. Which of the following terms would best describe this sensation?

A. Allodynia
B. Hypoesthesia
C. Paresthesia
D. Dysesthesia

Answer: B.

Hypoesthesia is defined as an abnormally decreased sensitivity to stimuli such as touch. The other terms are defined as: allodynia = painful sensation caused by a stimuli that would not typically invoke pain, such as touch; paresthesia = an abnormal sensation, whether spontaneous or evoked; dysesthesia = an unpleasant, abnormal sensation whether spontaneous or evoked.

Backonja MM. Defining neuropathic pain. Anesth Analg. 2003;97(3):785–90. https://doi.org/10.1213/01.ANE.0000062826.70846.8D. Erratum in: Anesth Analg. 2004;98(1):67.

11. Gabapentin is thought to have its effect through which of the following?

A. GABA-A antagonist
B. GABA-B antagonist
C. Alpha-2-Delta-1 ligand
D. Alpha 2 antagonist

Answer: C.

Gabapentin is named due to its chemical structure being a derivative of gamma-aminobutyric acid (GABA). However, it does not have any activity on GABA receptors nor influences its synthesis or uptake. Instead, it is a ligand of the alpha-2-delta-1 subunit of voltage-gated calcium channels. Binding to the subunit leads to reduced activation of the calcium channels and inhibition of the release of excitatory neurotransmitters. The full mechanism action remains incompletely understood. Diazepam is a GABA-A positive allosteric modulator. Baclofen is a GABA-B agonist. Tizanidine is an alpha-2 receptor agonist.

Yasaei R, Katta S, Saadabadi A. Gabapentin. 27 Dec 2021. In: StatPearls, editor. Treasure Island, FL: StatPearls Publishing; 2022.
Patel R, Dickenson AH. Mechanisms of the gabapentinoids and $\alpha 2 \delta$-1 calcium channel subunit in neuropathic pain. Pharmacol Res Perspect. 2016;4(2):e00205.

12. A patient with a spinal cord injury presents to the emergency department with tachycardia, mydriasis, and hyperhidrosis. He is confused, restless and agitated. No spasticity is noted, and the patient reports 0/10 pain. His medication list includes gabapentin, tramadol, metformin, and lisinopril. What other medication is this patient likely taking?

   A. Baclofen
   B. Sertraline
   C. Clonidine
   D. Ibuprofen

   Answer: B.

   Based on clinical description, this patient is likely presenting with serotonin syndrome, a condition characterized by altered mental status, tachycardia, mydriasis, hyperhidrosis, nausea, or muscle rigidity. Serious cases can result in seizures, rhabdomyolysis, and even respiratory failure. Serotonin syndrome is caused by excessive levels of serotonin and is often iatrogenic in nature. Due to its action as a serotonin-norepinephrine reuptake inhibitor, the use of tramadol is contraindicated in individuals who are also taking a serotonin reuptake inhibitor (SSRI) such as sertraline. Baclofen overdose would present with hypotension, bradycardia, hyporeflexia and hypoventilation. While baclofen withdrawal may also present with confusion, agitation, and hyperthermia, you would not expect to see mydriasis. Furthermore, rebound spasticity or severe pain may also be seen in baclofen withdrawal. Clonidine and Ibuprofen are not SSRI's and would not likely contribute to the constellation of symptoms seen in this case.

   Lipscomb DJ, Meredith TJ. Baclofen overdose. Postgrad Med J. 1980;56(652):108–9. https://doi.org/10.1136/pgmj.56.652.108.
   Shakoor M, Ayub S, Ahad A, Ayub Z. Transient serotonin syndrome caused by concurrent use of tramadol and selective serotonin reuptake inhibitor. Am J Case Rep. 2014;15:562–4.

13. A 35-year-old male with paraplegia following an L3 spinal cord injury presents with complaints of bilateral shoulder pain. He lives alone and uses a wheelchair for mobility. His exam is pertinent for positive Neers and positive Hawkins-Kennedy test. What intervention would most likely be diagnostic and therapeutic?

   A. Subacromial bursa steroid injection
   B. Biceps tendon steroid injection

C. Acromioclavicular joint steroid injection
D. Glenohumeral joint steroid injection

Answer: A.

Overuse injuries of the upper extremities are very common amongst independently functioning paraplegic patients. Neer impingement test is designed to reproduce subacromial impingement. It is performed by stabilizing the patient's scapula with one hand while passively flexing the shoulder while it is internally rotated. Hawkin's-Kennedy test is performed with the patient's arm in 90° of shoulder and elbow flexion. The examiner then internally rotates the arm repetitively while moving the arm across the midline of the patient's body. Pain reported during these tests is indicative for subacromial impingement. While multiple areas are often targeted in interventional therapy for rotator cuff injury, the other injections listed are less likely to be this patient's primary source of pain based on exam findings.

Somerville L, Bryant D, Willits K, Johnson A. Protocol for determining the diagnostic validity of physical examination maneuvers for shoulder pathology. BMC Musculoskelet Disord. 2013;14:60.
Nazari G, MacDermid JC, Bryant D, Athwal GS. The effectiveness of surgical vs conservative interventions on pain and function in patients with shoulder impingement syndrome. A systematic review and meta-analysis. PLoS One. 2019;14(5):e0216961.

14. Following a spinal cord injury, a patient endorses band like pain extending from both hips into his groin. What is the most likely level of injury?

A. T10
B. L1
C. L3
D. L5

Answer: B.

The L1 dermatome is described with pain extending from both hips into the groin. See Fig. 14.1 demonstrating the different dermatome locations.

Bouwense SA, Olesen SS, Drewes AM, Poley JW, van Goor H, Wilder-Smith OH. Effects of pregabalin on central sensitization in patients with chronic pancreatitis in a randomized, controlled trial. PLoS One. 2012;7(8):e42096.
This is an open-access article distributed under the terms of the Creative Commons Attribution License, which permits unrestricted use, distribution, and reproduction in any medium, provided the original author and source are properly credited.

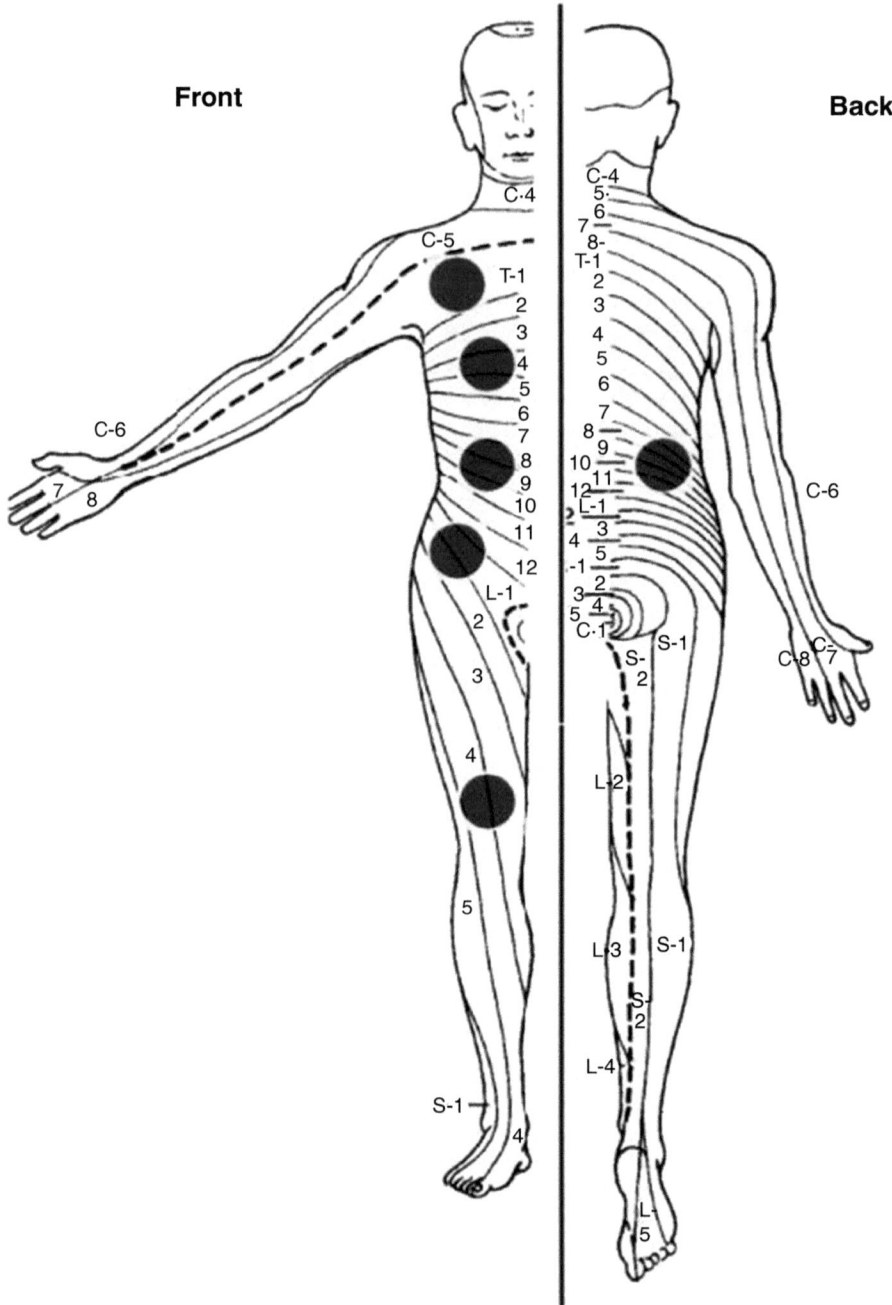

Fig. 14.1 Different dermatome locations. (Copyright © 2012 Bouwense et al.)

15. All of the following describe "below-level" spinal cord injury pain EXCEPT:

    A. "Below-level" pain is characterized as centrally mediated pain
    B. Patients often complain of burning, stabbing, electric-like pain
    C. Limiting ischemia after traumatic SCI may decrease the extent of "below-level" pain
    D. It is mediated by a shift in microglia from activated to inactive state

Answer: D.

"Below-level" spinal cord injury pain is characterized as centrally mediated pain that is often described as burning, stabbing, and electric-like pain. Limiting post-injury ischemia may decrease the incidence and severity of "below-level" pain. Microglia have been demonstrated to be activated both acutely after spinal cord injury and chronically.

Hulsebosch CE, Hains BC, Crown ED, Carlton SM. Mechanisms of chronic central neuropathic pain after spinal cord injury. Brain Res Rev. 2009;60(1):202–13. https://doi.org/10.1016/j.brainresrev.2008.12.010. Epub 2008 Dec 25.

16. All of the following regarding spinal cord stimulation (SCS) and treatment of SCI pain are true EXCEPT:

    A. SCS is most effective in patients with incomplete lesions
    B. SCS is most effective at treating pain that exists in transition zones between dermatomes with normal sensation and dermatomes with complete analgesia
    C. The therapeutic effect of SCS usually declines over time
    D. SCS is most effective at treating central dysesthetic "below-level" pain

Answer: D.

In a study of 35 patients who suffered a spinal cord injury and received SCS, an analysis based on the level and severity of injury showed that conventional SCS may be more effective for reducing pain in patients with incomplete SCI and transitional zone pain. Another study demonstrated that incomplete SCI at the thoracic level, and paraplegic pain from spasm or contracture are positive prognostic factors for conventional SCS treatment.

Tasker RR, DeCarvalho GT, Dolan EJ. Intractable pain of spinal cord origin: clinical features and implications for surgery. J Neurosurg. 1992;77(3):373–8. https://doi.org/10.3171/jns.1992.77.3.0373.
Cioni B, Meglio M, Pentimalli L, Visocchi M. Spinal cord stimulation in the treatment of paraplegic pain. J Neurosurg. 1995;82(1):35–9. https://doi.org/10.3171/jns.1995.82.1.0035.

17. Disruption of which tract is likely related to the development of "below-level" spinal cord injury pain?

    A. Corticospinal tract
    B. Spinothalamic tract
    C. Dorsal column tract
    D. Vestibulospinal tract

Answer: B.

In patients with spinal cord injury, greater damage to the spinothalamic tract has been correlated with increased "below level" pain.

Garcia-Larrea L, Convers P, Magnin M, et al. Laser-evoked potential abnormalities in central pain patients: the influence of spontaneous and provoked pain. Brain. 2002;125:2766–81.
Zeilig G, Enosh S, Rubin-Asher D, Lehr B, Defrin R. The nature and course of sensory changes following spinal cord injury: predictive properties and implications on the mechanism of central pain. Brain. 2012;135(Pt 2):418–30. https://doi.org/10.1093/brain/awr270. Epub 2011 Nov 16.
Wasner G, Lee BB, Engel S, McLachlan E. Residual spinothalamic tract pathways predict development of central pain after spinal cord injury. Brain. 2008;131:2387–400.

18. A patient with a history of chronic T1 ASIA A spinal cord injury presents to the rehabilitation clinic complaining of severe neck pain, worsening burning pain in his hands and difficulty propelling his manual wheelchair. Physical exam demonstrates normal vital signs, increased weakness compared to previous exam of bilateral finger abduction, grip, and elbow extension and normal strength in his shoulders. Which of the following is the best next step in management?

    A. MRI cervical spine
    B. Nerve conduction studies of upper extremities
    C. Somatosensory evoked potentials
    D. Close monitoring

Answer: A.

Post-traumatic cystic syringomyelia is the most likely cause of worsening pain and function in this patient. It occurs in approximately 1–4% of cases of SCI and can occur as early as 3 months after spinal cord trauma or as late as several decades after initial injury. It is diagnosed with MRI and early intervention with surgical decompression can help reverse or prevent further neurological deterioration. Although radiculopathies and peripheral neuropathies may lead to similar symptoms, the bilateral nature and elbow weakness would not be common. Thus, nerve conduction studies should come after MRI imaging. Somatosensory evoked potentials would not be appropriate prior to MRI imaging. Given the patient's increased weakness and severe pain, close monitoring would not be appropriate.

Holly LT, Johnson JP, Masciopinto JE, Batzdorf U. Treatment of posttraumatic syringomyelia with extradural decompressive surgery. Neurosurg Focus. 2000;8(3):E8. https://doi.org/10.3171/foc.2000.8.3.8.

19. Which of the following factors correlates the most with increased incidence of chronic pain after spinal cord injury?

    A. Decreased coping or acceptance of injury and disability
    B. Veteran status
    C. Significant surgical intervention during acute injury
    D. Complete injury

Answer: A.

Summers et al. (1991) identified several psychosocial factors associated with pain after spinal cord injury. These include: high levels of emotional distress, perception that a significant other has expressed a negative or punishing response to pain complaints, and poor acceptance of the injury. Overall psychosocial factors were more closely associated with the experience of pain compared to physiological factors, demonstrating the importance of a good social support system. Level of injury, completeness of injury, surgical interventions, and veteran status were not associated with pain severity after spinal cord injury.

Summers JD, Rapoff MA, Varghese G, Porter K, Palmer RE. Psychosocial factors in chronic spinal cord injury pain. Pain. 1991;47(2):183–9. https://doi.org/10.1016/0304-3959(91)90203-a.

20. Which of the following is associated with an increased risk of lower extremity fractures?

    A. African American race
    B. Opioid use
    C. Tetraplegia
    D. Thiazide diuretic use

Answer: B.

A retrospective cohort study of the Veterans Affairs Healthcare System looked at over 7000 male patients with a history of traumatic spinal cord injury to determine associations with lower extremity fractures. It found that opioid use was associated with increased lower extremity fractures. White race, paraplegia, complete injuries, chronicity (greater than 10 years), and use of osteoporosis therapies were also positively correlated with lower extremity fractures. Use of a thiazide diuretic correlated negatively with fractures.

Carbone LD, Chin AS, Lee TA, et al. The association of opioid use with incident lower extremity fractures in spinal cord injury. J Spinal Cord Med. 2013;36(2):91–6. https://doi.org/10.1179/2045772312Y.0000000060.

21. A 38-year-old who suffered a T5 ASIA A spinal cord injury denies any at-level or below-level pain. This is likely due to:

    A. Increased glutamatergic metabolism in the anterior cingulate cortex
    B. Decreased glial activation
    C. Level of Injury
    D. Complete injury of spinothalamic tract

    Answer: D.

    Post-SCI neuropathic pain has been shown to be correlated with both decreased glutamatergic metabolism in the anterior cingulate cortex and increased glial activation. Incomplete injury of the spinothalamic tract may also contribute to development of neuropathic pain after SCI. The secondary inflammatory process may amplify the residually damaged spinothalamic tract signals and lead to at-level or below-level pain.

    Widerström-Noga E, Cruz-Almeida Y, Felix ER, Pattany PM. Somatosensory phenotype is associated with thalamic metabolites and pain intensity after spinal cord injury. Pain. 2015;156(1):166–74. https://doi.org/10.1016/j.pain.0000000000000019.

22. Which of the following is not a first-line pharmacologic treatment of neuropathic pain?

    A. Pregabalin
    B. Gabapentin
    C. Amitriptyline
    D. Lamotrigine

    Answer: D.

    First-line therapies include pregabalin, gabapentin, and amitriptyline. Gabapentinoids (pregabalin and gabapentin) likely influence pain by reducing activation of voltage gated calcium channels in the spinal cord through their binding to the alpha-2-delta subunit. Tricyclic antidepressants affect pain perception through inhibition of noradrenaline reuptake. Lamotrigine is a second line neuropathic pain medication for spinal cord injury and has a primary mechanism of inhibiting voltage-sensitive sodium channels.

    Widerström-Noga E. Neuropathic pain and spinal cord injury: phenotypes and pharmacological management. Drugs. 2017;77(9):967–84. https://doi.org/10.1007/s40265-017-0747-8.

23. What is defined as the perception of pain from a non-painful stimulus?

    A. Hyperalgesia
    B. Hypoethesia
    C. Allodynia
    D. Dysesthesia

Answer: C.

Allodynia is defined as a painful sensation caused by a stimulus that would not typically invoke pain, such as touch. Hyperalgesia is increased perception of pain from an already painful stimulus. Hypoesthesia is an abnormally decreased sensitivity to stimuli such as touch. Dysesthesia describes unpleasant abnormal sensation, whether spontaneous or evoked.

Backonja MM. Defining neuropathic pain. Anesth Analg. 2003;97(3):785–90. https://doi.org/10.1213/01.ANE.0000062826.70846.8D. Erratum in: Anesth Analg. 2004;98(1):67.

24. Pain after spinal cord injury occurs in approximately what percent of patients?

    A. 25%
    B. 50%
    C. 66%
    D. 80%

Answer: C.

Approximately two-thirds of patients with spinal cord injury develop post-injury pain related to their spinal cord injury. This is categorized as nociceptive (mostly secondary to overuse of the arms and back) and neuropathic pain.

Siddall PJ, McClelland JM, Rutkowski SB, Cousins MJ. A longitudinal study of the prevalence and characteristics of pain in the first 5 years following spinal cord injury. Pain. 2003;103(3):249–57.
Finnerup NB, Johannesen IL, Sindrup SH, Bach FW, Jensen TS. Pain and dysesthesia in patients with spinal cord injury: a postal survey. Spinal Cord. 2001;39(5):256–62.

25. A patient with a T3 spinal cord injury who lives alone presents with pain in bilateral wrists and numbness of the second and third digits. What is the likely cause?

    A. Median nerve injury
    B. Ulnar nerve injury
    C. Cervicogenic claudication
    D. Central neuropathic pain

Answer: A.

Secondary peripheral nerve injury is common in patients who live alone and function independently. Upper extremity peripheral nerves can become injured by overuse due to transferring or using a wheelchair. This patient has neuropathic symptoms in the median nerve distribution, most consistent with a median nerve injury (most commonly carpal tunnel syndrome). A patient with ulnar neuropathy would more likely have symptoms in the fourth and fifth digits. Central pathologies such as cervicogenic claudication or central neuropathic pain are less likely given the patient's complaints are limited to his hands.

Barr C, Suarez P, Ota D, Curtin CM. Is carpal tunnel release under-utilized in veterans with spinal cord injury? J Spinal Cord Med. 2011;34(6):563–8. https://doi.org/10.1179/2045772311Y.0000000031.

Nutrition, Endocrine, and Immune Function

15

Elisabeth K. Acker

Questions

1. High levels of which of the following vitamins or minerals may impair wound healing, phagocytosis, and copper metabolism?

   A. Vitamin A
   B. B vitamins
   C. Calcium
   D. Zinc

   Answer: D.

   Zinc is a co-factor with a role in collagen formation. Zinc deficiency is associated with impaired wound healing and immune function. However, high levels of zinc can also impair wound healing, phagocytosis, and copper metabolism; copper is also used for collagen cross-linking. Vitamin A plays a role in cellular differentiation and proliferation, collagen synthesis, and immune function. Vitamin A deficiency is associated with delayed wound healing and increased susceptibility to infections. The B vitamins serve as coenzymes or cofactors for enzymes needed in carbohydrate, protein, and fat breakdown. Calcium has a role in supporting skeletal structural integrity and smooth and skeletal muscle contraction.

E. K. Acker (✉)
Spinal Cord Injury and Disorders Service, Central Virginia VA Health Care System, Richmond, VA, USA

Department of Physical Medicine and Rehabilitation, Virginia Commonwealth University, Richmond, VA, USA
e-mail: elisabeth.acker@va.gov

© The Author(s), under exclusive license to Springer Nature Switzerland AG 2022
B. A. Abramoff et al. (eds.), *The Essential Spinal Cord Injury Medicine Question Bank*, https://doi.org/10.1007/978-3-031-07796-8_15

NPUAP, EPUAP, Pan Pacific Pressure Injury Alliance. Prevention and treatment of pressure ulcers: quick reference guide. In: Haesler E, editor. Osborne Park, Western Australia: Cambridge Media; 2014.

Asthagiri H, Wilson J, Frost F. Nutrition in spinal cord injury. In: Kirshblum S, Lin VS, editors. Spinal cord medicine. 3rd ed. New York City: Springer Publishing Company; 2019. p. 318–31.

2. Due to its short half-life, which of the following is the preferred marker for laboratory assessment of malnutrition?

    A. Albumin
    B. Prealbumin
    C. Transferrin
    D. Retinol-binding protein

    Answer: B.

    Prealbumin has a short half-life of 2 days, making it a good indicator of protein and nutrition status. Albumin has a half-life of 20 days, so it is less sensitive to changes in nutritional status. Transferrin has a half-life of 8–10 days but lacks specificity to nutritional status. Retinol-binding protein levels in the liver rise, while serum levels fall, in vitamin A deficiency.

    Beck FK, Rosenthal TC. Prealbumin: a marker for nutritional evaluation. Am Fam Physician. 2002;65(8):1575–8. Erratum in: Am Fam Physician. 2002;66(12):2208.

    Matarese LE, Gottschlich MM. Contemporary nutrition support practice: a clinical guide. 2nd ed. Philadelphia, PA: Saunders; 2003.

3. In spinal cord injury, increased fat mass correlates with all of the following EXCEPT:

    A. Higher HDL-C
    B. Higher level of injury
    C. Older age
    D. Longer duration of injury

    Answer: A.

    The works of Nuhlicek et al. (1988) demonstrated that individuals with higher spinal cord lesions had diminished total body water, intracellular water, lean body mass, and body cell mass; and increased fat mass. The works of Manns et al. (2005) found that individuals with paraplegia older age and longer duration of injury were associated with greater amounts of total body fat, as measured by Dual-energy X-ray absorptiometry (DEXA) scans, and that greater amounts of total body fat were strongly associated with higher fasting and 2-h post-load insulin levels, lower HDL-C, higher triglycerides, and higher C-reactive protein levels.

Nuhlicek DN, Spurr GB, Barboriak JJ, Rooney CB, el Ghatit AZ, Bongard RD. Body composition of patients with spinal cord injury. Eur J Clin Nutr. 1988;42(9):765–73.

Manns PJ, McCubbin JA, Williams DP. Fitness, inflammation, and the metabolic syndrome in men with paraplegia. Arch Phys Med Rehabil. 2005;86(6):1176–81. https://doi.org/10.1016/j.apmr.2004.11.020.

4. In considering the loss of lean body mass and increased fat mass in chronic spinal cord injury, body mass index (BMI) greater than what value may indicate increased risk for obesity and obesity-related chronic diseases?

   A. 18 kg/m^2
   B. 22 kg/m^2
   C. 26 kg/m^2
   D. 30 kg/m^2

Answer: B.

The work of Laughton et al. (2009) explored the sensitivity and specificity of the general population BMI cutoff for obesity (30 kg/m^2) in a representative sample of individuals with spinal cord injury. These individuals underwent anthropometric measures (including measurement of percent fat mass by bioelectrical impedance analysis, length, weight, and BMI), and had their serum C-Reactive Protein (CRP) levels measured. The study found that a BMI cutoff of 30 kg/m^2 failed to identify 73.9% of obese participants. BMI cutoffs based on percent fat mass and CRP considered together ranged from 22.1 to 26.5 kg/m^2. As such, the team suggest that individuals with chronic spinal cord injury and BMI values >22 kg/m^2 should be considered as being at risk for obesity and obesity-related chronic diseases.

Laughton GE, Buchholz AC, Martin Ginis KA, Goy RE, SHAPE SCI Research Group. Lowering body mass index cutoffs better identifies obese persons with spinal cord injury. Spinal Cord. 2009;47(10):757–62. https://doi.org/10.1038/sc.2009.33. Epub 2009 Apr 7.

5. Regarding weight loss in acute spinal cord injury, all of the following are true EXCEPT:

   A. 10% reduction of pre-injury weight within the first month is typical
   B. Individuals with tetraplegia and paraplegia sustain similar weight loss
   C. Most early weight loss is related to loss of lean body mass from denervation atrophy of muscles below the level of the lesion
   D. Protein nutritional status may be monitored with serial prealbumin levels

Answer: B.

The work of Kearns et al. (1992) prospectively studied the metabolic response to complete spinal cord injury in 10 individuals and found that initial resting energy expenditures were 10% below what was predicted, and body weight decreased by 10%. They suggest that during acute spinal cord injury, the major cause of nitrogen loss (which paralleled weight loss) is muscle atrophy related to disuse and denervation. The work of Cloninger (1980) found that individuals with tetraplegia sustain greater weight loss (30–50 lb) than those with paraplegia (10–35 lb). Prealbumin has a short half-life of 2 days, making it a good indicator of protein and nutrition status.

Kearns PJ, Thompson JD, Werner PC, Pipp TL, Wilmot CB. Nutritional and metabolic response to acute spinal-cord injury. J Parenter Enteral Nutr. 1992;16(1):11–5. https://doi.org/10.1177/014860719201600111.

Cloninger MC. Nutritional management of patients with spinal injury: paraplegia versus quadriplegia. Arch Phys Med Rehabil. 1980;61:489.

Beck FK, Rosenthal TC. Prealbumin: a marker for nutritional evaluation. Am Fam Physician. 2002;65(8):1575–8. Erratum in: Am Fam Physician 2002;66(12):2208.

6. Risk factors for the development of dysphagia in acute spinal cord injury include all of the following EXCEPT:

A. Cervical immobilization with orthoses
B. Impaired consciousness
C. Posterior spine stabilization
D. Tracheostomy placement

Answer: C.

The work of Wolf et al. (2003) found that in patients with acute cervical spinal cord injury, dysphagia is related to structural disturbances of the larynx and hypolarynx. Anterior spinal surgery is associated with development of postoperative dysphagia. It has been estimated that 45–60% of those who have undergone anterior cervical fusion or discectomy sustain voice and swallowing impairment. Cervical orthoses can impair normal swallow mechanics as well as limit compensatory swallowing techniques. Tracheostomy tubes may interfere with normal swallowing by disrupting normal breathing-swallowing pattern, tethering the pharynx, removing subglottal pressure, changing airway sensitivity.

Wolf C, Meiners TH. Dysphagia in patients with acute cervical spinal cord injury. Spinal Cord. 2003;41(6):347–53. https://doi.org/10.1038/sj.sc.3101440.

Gross RD, Mahlmann J, Grayhack JP. Physiologic effects of open and closed tracheostomy tubes on the pharyngeal swallow. Ann Otol Rhinol Laryngol. 2003;112(2):143–52. https://doi.org/10.1177/000348940311200207.

7. Which form of mobility is associated with the greatest energy expenditure?

A. Ambulation without use of an assistive device in an individual without a spinal cord injury
B. Ambulation with braces and crutches in an individual with a spinal cord injury
C. Manual wheelchair propulsion
D. Power wheelchair navigation

Answer: B.

Energy costs of different methods of mobility and ambulation were evaluated in the work of Fisher and Gullickson (1978). Compared to walking at 5 km/h in individuals without spinal cord injury, cal/m expended by individuals with paraplegia during manual wheelchair propulsion were 9% greater, whereas cal/m expended via ambulation with braces and crutches at a much slower rate were over five times greater. As such, in individuals with paraplegia, manual wheelchair use is often preferred over ambulation with braces and crutches, as the former is associated with less energy expenditure and faster mobility speed. Use of a power wheelchair typically requires minimal energy expenditure.

Fisher SV, Gullickson G Jr. Energy cost of ambulation in health and disability: a literature review. Arch Phys Med Rehabil. 1978;59(3):124–33.

8. For healing of advanced pressure injuries in spinal cord injury, how much calorie and protein intake/day is recommended?

A. 30–35 cal/kg/day; 0.5–1 g protein/kg/day
B. 30–35 cal/kg/day; 1.25–2 g protein/kg/day
C. 60–80 cal/kg/day; 0.5–1 g protein/kg/day
D. 60–80 cal/kg/day; 1.25–2 g protein/kg/day

Answer: B.

A risk factor for the development of pressure injuries in spinal cord injury is malnutrition. Adequate oral protein, calorie, and fluid intake is essential for the healing of pressure injuries; 30–35 cal/kg/day and 1.25–2 g protein/kg/day is recommended. Given the large losses of protein and fluids occurring at the wound site, protein and fluid intake helps to replace such and facilitate a positive nitrogen balance.

Bergstrom N, Bennett MA, Carlson CE, et al. Clinical practice guideline no. 15: treatment of pressure ulcers. Rockville, MD: US Department of Health and Human Services, Agency for Health Care Policy and Research; 1994.
Breslow RA, Hallfrisch J, Guy DG, Crawley B, Goldberg AP. The importance of dietary protein in healing pressure ulcers. J Am Geriatr Soc. 1993;41(4):357–62. https://doi.org/10.1111/j.1532-5415.1993.tb06940.x.

9. All of the following are components of metabolic syndrome EXCEPT:

   A. Increased abdominal obesity
   B. Increased blood pressure
   C. Increased low-density lipoprotein cholesterol (LDL-C)
   D. Increased triglycerides

Answer: C.

Metabolic syndrome is characterized by the following components: decreased levels of high-density lipoprotein cholesterol (HDL-C) and elevated levels of triglycerides, fasting glucose, abdominal obesity, and blood pressure. The work of Manns et al. (2005) showed that individuals with spinal cord injury are at risk of developing metabolic syndrome given their lower physical activity levels relative to able-bodied individuals. Moreover, individuals with spinal cord injury were found to have greater levels of the inflammatory marker C-reactive protein (CRP).

Manns PJ, McCubbin JA, Williams DP. Fitness, inflammation, and the metabolic syndrome in men with paraplegia. Arch Phys Med Rehabil. 2005;86(6):1176–81. https://doi.org/10.1016/j.apmr.2004.11.020.

10. The gold standard for determining resting energy expenditure and caloric needs of an individual with spinal cord injury is:

   A. The Cunningham equation
   B. The Harris Benedict equation
   C. The Spanier and Shizgal equation
   D. Indirect calorimetry

Answer: D.

Individuals with spinal cord injury experience body composition changes over time. Changes are characterized by increased muscle atrophy and fat mass which results in decreases in resting energy expenditure (REE).

Indirect calorimetry is the most reliable means to determine REE and caloric needs of an individual with spinal cord injury. Through indirect calorimetry, a patient's respiratory gas exchange and rate of oxygen utilization is determined. In turn, the known caloric yield from 1 L of oxygen based on differences in oxygen consumption and carbon dioxide production is calculated; providing an estimate of energy expenditure. Equations that predict REE, often derived from uninjured populations, overestimate REE in individuals with spinal cord injury.

Hadley MN, Walters BC, Grabb PA, Oyesiku NM, Przybylski GJ, Resnick DK, Ryken TC. Nutritional support after spinal cord injury. Neurosurgery. 2002;50(3 Suppl):S81–4. https://doi.org/10.1097/00006123-200203001-00015.

Nevin AN, Steenson J, Vivanti A, Hickman IJ. Investigation of measured and predicted resting energy needs in adults after spinal cord injury: a systematic review. Spinal Cord. 2016;54(4):248–53. https://doi.org/10.1038/sc.2015.193. Epub 2015 Dec 22.

11. The most common dyslipidemia after spinal cord injury is:

    A. Elevated triglycerides
    B. Elevated serum low-density lipoprotein (LDL) cholesterol
    C. Depressed serum high-density lipoprotein (HDL) cholesterol
    D. Elevated total cholesterol (TC)

Answer: C.

The most common dyslipidemia after spinal cord injury is an isolated, depressed fasting serum HDL cholesterol concentration. The work of Zlotolow et al. (1992) compared the serum lipid levels of veterans with paraplegia with age-matched controls. Individuals with paraplegia had significantly lower serum HDL cholesterol as compared to the age-matched controls. However, between these two groups, there were no significant differences in serum levels of total cholesterol, LDL cholesterol, or triglycerides. Contributors to decreased serum HDL cholesterol following spinal cord injury include a sedentary lifestyle and low levels of fitness.

Zlotolow SP, Levy E, Bauman WA. The serum lipoprotein profile in veterans with paraplegia: the relationship to nutritional factors and body mass index. J Am Paraplegia Soc. 1992;15(3):158–62. https://doi.org/10.1080/01952307.1992.11735869.
Bauman WA, Spungen AM, Zhong YG, Rothstein JL, Petry C, Gordon SK. Depressed serum high density lipoprotein cholesterol levels in veterans with spinal cord injury. Paraplegia. 1992;30(10):697–703. https://doi.org/10.1038/sc.1992.136.

12. A patient comes to your clinic after spinal cord injury with a recent lab test revealing a hemoglobin A1c level of 8.5%. He was placed on metformin by his primary care physician. Of note, metformin may cause:

    A. Hypertension and constipation
    B. Hypertension and diarrhea
    C. Hypotension and constipation
    D. Hypotension and diarrhea

Answer: D.

Individuals with spinal cord injury are at increased risk of developing disorders of oral carbohydrate tolerance. The work of Duckworth et al. (1980) found that diabetes mellitus and insulin resistance were more prevalent in individuals with a longer duration of spinal cord injury.

   Metformin is widely used as a first-line agent for treatment of diabetes mellitus; however, metformin monotherapy is associated with volume depletion and gastrointestinal complications. Specifically, there is increased risk of supine and postural hypotension, particularly in those with higher levels of injury. Moreover, loose bowel movements may complicate neurogenic bowel programs.

Duckworth WC, Solomon SS, Jallepalli P, Heckemeyer C, Finnern J, Powers A. Glucose intolerance due to insulin resistance in patients with spinal cord injuries. Diabetes. 1980;29(11):906–10. https://doi.org/10.2337/diab.29.11.906.
McCreight LJ, Bailey CJ, Pearson ER. Metformin and the gastrointestinal tract. Diabetologia. 2016;59(3):426–35. https://doi.org/10.1007/s00125-015-3844-9. Epub 2016 Jan 16.

13. Risk factors for hypercalcemia after acute spinal cord injury include all of the following EXCEPT:

   A. High cervical injury
   B. Prolonged immobilization
   C. Male gender
   D. Older adult

Answer: D.

Hypercalcemia may occur following acute spinal cord injury. As a result of immobilization, osteoblastic activity in weight-bearing bones decreases, while the rate of osteoclastic bone resorption increases. Osteoporosis and hypercalciuria results in this setting of imbalanced osteoblastic and osteoclastic activity. Normally, excess calcium is excreted by the kidneys, thereby maintaining normal serum calcium levels. Rate of bone turnover is greater in children and young adults, thus following a SCI, calcium load may exceed the normal regulatory mechanisms of the body resulting in hypercalcemia. Other risk factors for development of hypercalcemia include complete injury, high cervical injury, dehydration, prolonged immobilization, and male gender.

Maynard FM. Immobilization hypercalcemia following spinal cord injury. Arch Phys Med Rehabil. 1986;67(1):41–4.

14. Treatment of hypercalcemia after acute spinal cord injury may include all of the following approaches EXCEPT:

   A. Bisphosphonates
   B. Calcitonin
   C. Fluid restriction
   D. Furosemide

Answer: C.

Hydration, such as with intravenous fluids, will induce diuresis, promoting calciuria and thereby helping to lower serum calcium. Fluids should NOT be restricted, as low fluid intake or relative dehydration will not facilitate the kidneys' excretion of large amounts of calcium. Furosemide enhances calcium excretion, however fluid balance should be closely monitored so that a negative fluid balance does not occur. Calcitonin inhibits osteoclast activity to reduce bone breakdown and acts on the kidneys directly to decrease calcium resorption. Bisphosphonates also inhibit bone resorption through their action on osteoclasts or osteoclast precursors through a separate mechanism.

Maynard FM. Immobilization hypercalcemia following spinal cord injury. Arch Phys Med Rehabil. 1986;67(1):41–4.

15. Which of the following statements is true regarding loss of bone mineral density (BMD) in long bones after spinal cord injury?

   A. BMD at both the epiphyses and diaphysis is lost at a rate approaching 1% per week
   B. BMD at the epiphyses is lost at a rate approaching 1% per week, whereas BMD loss at the diaphysis is insidious and progressive over the course of several years
   C. BMD at the diaphysis is lost at a rate approaching 1% per week, whereas BMD loss at the epiphyses is insidious and progressive over the course of several years
   D. BMD at both the epiphyses and diaphysis is insidious and progressive over the course of several years

Answer: B.

The work of Zehnder et al. (2004) showed a cross-sectional study that evaluated long term changes in bone metabolism and bone mineral density after spinal cord injury. Their study showed that early and rapid demineralization, leveling off within the first 3 years after injury, was seen in the tibial epiphysis, which contains a notable amount of trabecular bone. A slow, continuous demineralization, continuing even beyond 10 years post-injury, was seen in the tibial diaphysis, which contains a significant amount of cortical bone.

Zehnder Y, Lüthi M, Michel D, Knecht H, Perrelet R, Neto I, Kraenzlin M, Zäch G, Lippuner K. Long-term changes in bone metabolism, bone mineral density, quantitative ultrasound parameters, and fracture incidence after spinal cord injury: a cross-sectional observational study in 100 paraplegic men. Osteoporos Int. 2004;15(3):180–9. https://doi.org/10.1007/s00198-003-1529-6. Epub 2004 Jan 13.

16. Which two sites are particularly at increased risk for low-energy fracture?

    A. Proximal femur and distal femur
    B. Distal femur and proximal tibia
    C. Proximal tibia and distal fibula
    D. Distal tibia and talus

Answer: B.

Increased epiphyseal bone loss and the anatomical location of the distal femur and proximal tibia place these two sites at increased risk of low-energy fractures. When transferring from a wheelchair, there is greater torsional stress occurring in the lower extremity long bones and there is also a risk for low-velocity falls, both of which can lead to fractures.

Akhigbe T, Chin AS, Svircev JN, Hoenig H, Burns SP, Weaver FM, Bailey L, Carbone L. A retrospective review of lower extremity fracture care in patients with spinal cord injury. J Spinal Cord Med. 2015;38(1):2–9. https://doi.org/10.1179/2045772313Y.0000000156. Epub 2013 Nov 7.
Zehnder Y, Lüthi M, Michel D, Knecht H, Perrelet R, Neto I, Kraenzlin M, Zäch G, Lippuner K. Long-term changes in bone metabolism, bone mineral density, quantitative ultrasound parameters, and fracture incidence after spinal cord injury: a cross-sectional observational study in 100 paraplegic men. Osteoporos Int. 2004;15(3):180–9. https://doi.org/10.1007/s00198-003-1529-6. Epub 2004 Jan 13.

17. Risk factors for development of fractures after spinal cord injury include all of the following EXCEPT:

    A. Tetraplegia
    B. Motor complete spinal cord injury
    C. Longer duration of injury
    D. Female gender

Answer: A.

Fractures occur more in patients with paraplegia as compared to tetraplegia, given the increased activity level of the former. The work of Morse et al. (2009) examined fractures in veterans with spinal cord injury and found that low-impact fractures were more commonly seen in motor complete spinal cord injury compared to motor incomplete. The work of Vestergaard et al. (1998) studied fracture rates and risk factors for fractures in individuals with spinal cord injury. Their study noted that fracture rate increased after spinal cord injury to a constant level from the third year and beyond. Fractures were more common in female patients than male patients. Male patients with a family history of fractures were also at a greater risk of fractures.

Ragnarsson KT, Sell GH. Lower extremity fractures after spinal cord injury: a retrospective study. Arch Phys Med Rehabil. 1981;62(9):418–23.

Morse LR, Battaglino RA, Stolzmann KL, Hallett LD, Waddimba A, Gagnon D, Lazzari AA, Garshick E. Osteoporotic fractures and hospitalization risk in chronic spinal cord injury. Osteoporos Int. 2009;20(3):385–92. https://doi.org/10.1007/s00198-008-0671-6. Epub 2008 Jun 26.

Vestergaard P, Krogh K, Rejnmark L, Mosekilde L. Fracture rates and risk factors for fractures in patients with spinal cord injury. Spinal Cord. 1998;36(11):790–6. https://doi.org/10.1038/sj.sc.3100648.

18. Regarding bone metabolism after acute spinal cord injury, all of the following laboratory findings can be expected EXCEPT:

    A. Increased serum ionized calcium levels
    B. Increased calciuria
    C. Increased parathyroid hormone
    D. Increased sclerostin

Answer: C.

Acute spinal cord injury is associated with rapid bone resorption, leading to increased serum ionized calcium levels and increased calcium excretion in urine. As a result of increased serum ionized calcium levels, there is suppression of parathyroid hormone (PTH) levels. Serum PTH normally suppresses sclerostin, a potent inhibitor in Wnt/beta-catenin signaling in osteocytes; sclerostin will be increased due to suppression of PTH by elevated serum ionized calcium levels.

Stewart AF, Adler M, Byers CM, Segre GV, Broadus AE. Calcium homeostasis in immobilization: an example of resorptive hypercalciuria. N Engl J Med. 1982;306(19):1136–40. https://doi.org/10.1056/NEJM198205133061903.

Bellido T, Saini V, Pajevic PD. Effects of PTH on osteocyte function. Bone. 2013;54(2):250–7. https://doi.org/10.1016/j.bone.2012.09.016. Epub 2012 Sept 24.

Mirza FS, Padhi ID, Raisz LG, Lorenzo JA. Serum sclerostin levels negatively correlate with parathyroid hormone levels and free estrogen index in postmenopausal women. J Clin Endocrinol Metab. 2010;95(4):1991–7. https://doi.org/10.1210/jc.2009-2283. Epub 2010 Feb 15.

19. Heterotopic ossification (HO) most frequently develops around which joint in an individual with SCI?

    A. Shoulder
    B. Elbow
    C. Hip
    D. Knee

Answer: C.

HO is a complication of spinal cord injury, refers to extra-osseous, ectopic bone formation in soft tissue surrounding joints below the level of the spinal cord injury. Following a SCI, HO most commonly develops around the hip, followed by the knee, shoulder, and elbow, in that order.

van Kuijk AA, Geurts AC, van Kuppevelt HJ. Neurogenic heterotopic ossification in spinal cord injury. Spinal Cord. 2002;40(7):313–26. https://doi.org/10.1038/sj.sc.3101309.

20. How long after a spinal cord injury does heterotopic ossification (HO) typically develop?

    A. 0–2 weeks
    B. 1–6 months
    C. 1–3 years
    D. 5–10 years

Answer B.

HO typically develops 1–6 months after a SCI, with a peak incidence of 2 months after injury. Clinical presentation of HO includes decreased joint range of motion, joint swelling and erythema, low-grade fever, and increased spasticity.

van Kuijk AA, Geurts AC, van Kuppevelt HJ. Neurogenic heterotopic ossification in spinal cord injury. Spinal Cord. 2002;40(7):313–26. https://doi.org/10.1038/sj.sc.3101309.

21. Which of the following statements is true regarding diagnosis of heterotopic ossification (HO)?

    A. Alkaline phosphatase is a marker specific for HO
    B. Creatine phosphokinase levels do not predict HO
    C. Triple phase bone scans are not sensitive in identifying early HO
    D. X-rays lag behind triple phase bone scans in detecting HO

Answer: D.

While alkaline phosphatase (ALP) may be elevated in cases of HO, it is non-specific and cannot reliably predict HO. ALP levels also do not indicate maturity or re-occurrence of HO. Singh et al. (2003) found that creatine phosphokinase (CPK) levels may predict HO formation in individuals with SCI; there is also a correlation between CPK levels and HO grade. Triple phase bone scans are considered the most sensitive method in identifying early HO. X-rays and Computed Tomography (CT) scans are able to detect HO only after osseous calcifications have occurred whereas triple phase bone scans can detect HO weeks earlier.

Singh RS, Craig MC, Katholi CR, Jackson AB, Mountz JM. The predictive value of creatine phosphokinase and alkaline phosphatase in identification of heterotopic ossification in patients after spinal cord injury. Arch Phys Med Rehabil. 2003;84(11):1584–8. https://doi.org/10.1053/s0003-9993(03)00347-2.

Shehab D, Elgazzar AH, Collier BD. Heterotopic ossification. J Nucl Med. 2002;43(3):346–53.

22. All of the following are possible treatments for heterotopic ossification (HO) EXCEPT?

    A. Aggressive joint range of motion
    B. Medications including bisphosphonates and nonsteroidal anti-inflammatories
    C. Radiation therapy
    D. Surgical excision

Answer: A.

Gentle joint mobilization prevents further loss of range of motion (ROM), likely without leading to HO. Aggressive joint ROM may induce tissue micro-trauma and subsequent increased formation of HO. Bisphosphonates block the late mineralization phase of bone formation, therefore decreasing the rate of new bone formation; however, it cannot reverse HO once formed. Nonsteroidal anti-inflammatories inhibit mesenchymal cells' differentiation into osteogenic cells. Radiation therapy is also thought to disrupt pluripotent mesenchymal cells' differentiation into osteoblasts. While radiation therapy has been used as HO treatment, it is generally not the primary treatment given risk of long-term complications such as osteonecrosis and radiation-induced sarcoma. Severe forms of HO may warrant surgical excision, which is not advised until ectopic bone is mature.

van Kuijk AA, Geurts AC, van Kuppevelt HJ. Neurogenic heterotopic ossification in spinal cord injury. Spinal Cord. 2002;40(7):313–26. https://doi.org/10.1038/sj.sc.3101309.

23. In patients with spinal cord injury and testosterone deficiency, testosterone replacement therapy is associated with all of the following adverse effects EXCEPT:

    A. Worsened sleep apnea
    B. Increased non-cancerous growth of the prostate, or increased growth of existing prostate cancer
    C. Increased risk of blood clot formation
    D. Decreased bone density

Answer: D.

Testosterone replacement poses a risk of testicular atrophy or infertility, particularly in young men; this may be reversed with cessation of treatment. Sleep apnea may be exacerbated by testosterone replacement via central mechanisms; replacement is also associated with the development of sleep apnea. Testosterone replacement may increase prostate volume and could be associated with prostate cancer. Testosterone replacement may stimulate erythropoiesis. As this may benefit a patient with anemia, increased hematocrit above the normal range may increase blood viscosity and theoretically increase risk for thromboembolic events. Improving bone density is a potential therapeutic effect of testosterone therapy.

Rhoden EL, Morgentaler A. Risks of testosterone-replacement therapy and recommendations for monitoring. N Engl J Med. 2004;350(5):482–92. https://doi.org/10.1056/NEJMra022251.

24. The two most common causes of death in patients with spinal cord injury are:

    A. Pneumonia and septicemia
    B. Septicemia and cancer
    C. Cancer and heart disease
    D. Pulmonary embolism and urinary diseases

Answer: A.

In individuals with spinal cord injury enrolled in the National Spinal Cord Injury Database, who have been followed up to 45 years after their injury, pneumonia and septicemia are the two most common causes of death.

National Spinal Cord Injury Statistical Center. Facts and figures at a glance. Birmingham, AL: University of Alabama at Birmingham; 2020.

25. Regarding infection in spinal cord injury, _____ is/are the leading cause for rehospitalization after spinal cord injury; _____ has/have the highest infection-related mortality.

    A. Infections of pressure injuries and underlying bone; diseases of the genitourinary system
    B. Pneumonia; infections of pressure injuries and underlying bone
    C. Diseases of the genitourinary system; pneumonia
    D. Pneumonia; pneumonia

Answer: C.

In individuals with spinal cord injury enrolled in the National Spinal Cord Injury Database, who have been followed up to 45 years after their injury, diseases of the genitourinary system, followed by disease of the skin, are the leading causes of re-hospitalization. Pneumonia and septicemia are the two causes of death found to have the greatest impact on reduced life expectancy in the spinal cord injury population.

National Spinal Cord Injury Statistical Center. Facts and figures at a glance. Birmingham, AL: University of Alabama at Birmingham; 2020.

26. The three most common bacterial etiologies of community-acquired pneumonia after spinal cord injury in non-ventilated individuals include all of the following EXCEPT:

    A. *Acinetobacter baumannii*
    B. *Branhamella catarrhalis*
    C. *Haemophilus influenzae*
    D. *Streptococcus pneumoniae*

Answer: A.

Spinal cord injury may lead to respiratory muscle weakness, ineffective cough, and difficulty with bronchial secretion clearance, increasing an injured patient's risk of developing pneumonia. The most common bacterial etiologies of community-acquired pneumonia in spinal cord injury are *Streptococcus pneumoniae*, *Haemophilus influenzae*, and *Branhamella catarralis*.

The most frequently isolated micro-organisms producing ventilator-associated pneumonia include *Pseudomonas aeruginosa*, methicillin-resistant *Staphyloccus aureus*, and *Acinetobacter baumannii*. In injured patients, administration of both the pneumococcal and influenza vaccinations should be considered.

Evans CT, Weaver FM, Rogers TJ, Rapacki L, Miskevics S, Hahm B, Smith B, Lavela SL, Goldstein B, Burns SP. Guideline-recommended management of community-acquired pneumonia in veterans with spinal cord injury. Top Spinal Cord Inj Rehabil. 2012;18(4):300–5. https://doi.org/10.1310/sci1804-300.

García-Leoni ME, Moreno S, García-Garrote F, Cercenado E. Ventilator-associated pneumonia in long-term ventilator-assisted individuals. Spinal Cord. 2010;48(12):876–80. https://doi.org/10.1038/sc.2010.43. Epub 2010 Apr 20.

27. The three most common bacterial etiologies of ventilator-associated pneumonia in spinal cord injury include all of the following EXCEPT:

    A. *Acinetobacter baumannii*
    B. *Branhamella catarrhalis*
    C. Methicillin-resistant *Staphylococcus aureus*
    D. *Pseudomonas aeruginosa*

Answer: B.

Patients who sustain a cervical level acute spinal cord injury may have resultant respiratory dysfunction and associated inability to sustain spontaneous breathing, thereby increasing their risk of respiratory complications and respiratory failure. Ventilator-associated pneumonia (VAP) is a frequent complication in those requiring mechanical ventilation. In the spinal cord injury population, risk factors associated with VAP include longer duration of mechanical ventilation, use of antacids (increasing the frequency of gastric colonization by enteric Gram-negative bacilli), and hypoalbuminemia. The most frequently isolated micro-organisms producing VAP include *Pseudomonas aeruginosa*, methicillin-resistant *Staphylococcus aureus*, and *Acinetobacter baumannii*. *Branhamella catarrhalis* is one of the most common bacterial etiologies of community-acquired pneumonia in spinal cord injury.

García-Leoni ME, Moreno S, García-Garrote F, Cercenado E. Ventilator-associated pneumonia in long-term ventilator-assisted individuals. Spinal Cord. 2010;48(12):876–80. https://doi.org/10.1038/sc.2010.43. Epub 2010 Apr 20.
Evans CT, Weaver FM, Rogers TJ, Rapacki L, Miskevics S, Hahm B, Smith B, Lavela SL, Goldstein B, Burns SP. Guideline-recommended management of community-acquired pneumonia in veterans with spinal cord injury. Top Spinal Cord Inj Rehabil. 2012;18(4):300–5. https://doi.org/10.1310/sci1804-300.

28. All of the following are true about the influenza vaccine and spinal cord injury EXCEPT:

    A. In patients with spinal cord injury, the incidence of death from pneumonia and influenza is higher than in the general population
    B. Influenza vaccination decreases the risk of hospitalization for pneumonia or influenza
    C. Injured individuals with quadriplegia have similar influenza vaccine antibody responses compared to individuals with paraplegia
    D. Antibody responses of individuals with spinal cord injury to the inactivated influenza vaccine was less than that of able-bodied individuals

Answer: D.

The work of Trautner et al. (2004) studied the inactivated influenza vaccination in individuals with spinal cord injury. Their study found that a cohort of individuals with spinal cord injury have a response similar to that of an able-bodied cohort to the inactivated influenza vaccination. The two groups demonstrated similar serum antibody responses to each vaccine antigen: specifically, the two groups demonstrated a similar percentage of individuals achieving a four-fold rise in antibody titers, as well as a similar percentage of individuals achieving post-vaccination antibody titers of 1:32 or more. As such, individuals with spinal cord injury would be expected to benefit from an annual influenza vaccination. Furthermore, in the spinal cord injury cohort, there were no effects of level of injury (quadriplegia vs. paraplegia), nor time since injury (≤1 year vs. >1 year since injury), on the vaccine antibody responses.

Trautner BW, Atmar RL, Hulstrom A, Darouiche RO. Inactivated influenza vaccination for people with spinal cord injury. Arch Phys Med Rehabil. 2004;85(11):1886–9. https://doi.org/10.1016/j.apmr.2004.03.022.

29. Infection of a pressure injury in spinal cord injury is most reliably determined by:

    A. Swab culture of a pressure injury
    B. Swab culture of a sinus tract
    C. Culture of a needle aspiration
    D. Deep tissue biopsy

Answer: D.

Pressure injuries may be complicated by bacterial colonization or bacterial superinfection of the surrounding soft tissue and bone. Superficial swabs of the pressure injury may not differentiate between a true bacterial infection vs. colonization by microbial flora from the external environment, contiguous skin, gastrointestinal tract, or genitourinary tract.

Culture of material obtained via needle aspiration may overestimate the number of bacterial isolates. Bacterial cultures of deep tissue biopsies are considered the reference standard for a microbiological diagnosis. The work of Tedeschi et al. (2017) found a very low grade of concordance between superficial swab cultures and deep samples and as such, discourages the practice of collecting superficial pressure injury swabs as it can promote inappropriate antibiotic usage.

Tedeschi S, Negosanti L, Sgarzani R, Trapani F, Pignanelli S, Battilana M, Capirossi R, Brillanti Ventura D, Giannella M, Bartoletti M, Tumietto F, Cristini F, Viale P. Superficial swab versus deep-tissue biopsy for the microbiological diagnosis of local infection in advanced-stage pressure ulcers of spinal-cord-injured patients: a prospective study. Clin Microbiol Infect. 2017;23(12):943–7. https://doi.org/10.1016/j.cmi.2017.04.015. Epub 2017 Apr 19.

30. The presence of osteomyelitis beneath non-healing deep pressure injuries is best diagnosed by:

    A. Bone biopsy
    B. Computed tomography
    C. Magnetic resonance imaging
    D. Technetium bone scintiscan

Answer: A.

Standard diagnostic tools, including laboratory findings (hemoglobin, erythrocyte sedimentation rates, white blood cells, C-reactive protein), computed tomography, and bone scintigraphy are neither sensitive nor specific in diagnosing osteomyelitis. These techniques are often unable to discriminate osteomyelitis from pressure-related changes in bone. MRI may also be unable to distinguish areas of healed osteomyelitis from active infection. Bone biopsy remains the reference standard to diagnose osteomyelitis.

Brunel AS, Lamy B, Cyteval C, Perrochia H, Téot L, Masson R, Bertet H, Bourdon A, Morquin D, Reynes J, Le Moing V, OSTEAR Study Group. Diagnosing pelvic osteomyelitis beneath pressure ulcers in spinal cord injured patients: a prospective study. Clin Microbiol Infect. 2016;22(3):267.e1–8. https://doi.org/10.1016/j.cmi.2015.11.005. Epub 2015 Nov 24.

31. Allergic reactions to latex have been identified in children with myelomeningocele and spinal cord injury, and are considered what type of allergic reaction?

    A. Type I reaction
    B. Type II reaction
    C. Type III reaction
    D. Type IV reaction

Answer: A.

Allergic reactions to latex are considered immediate reactions, or type I reactions (immunoglobulin IgE-mediated hypersensitivity). Delayed reactions include type II, type III, and type IV reactions. Children with myelomeningocele and spinal cord injury are frequently exposed to medical equipment containing latex, which sensitizes these individuals. Latex allergic reactions may manifest as localized or generalized urticaria, wheezing, angioedema, or anaphylaxis. Of note, allergic reactions to latex that occur intraoperatively may be challenging to diagnose due to surgical drapes covering the patient's skin, which may mask the presence of urticaria.

Rendeli C, Nucera E, Ausili E, Tabacco F, Roncallo C, Pollastrini E, Scorzoni M, Schiavino D, Caldarelli M, Pietrini D, Patriarca G. Latex sensitisation and allergy in children with myelomeningocele. Childs Nerv Syst. 2006;22(1):28–32. https://doi.org/10.1007/s00381-004-1110-4. Epub 2005 Feb 10.

Vogel LC, Schrader T, Lubicky JP. Latex allergy in children and adolescents with spinal cord injuries. J Pediatr Orthop. 1995;15(4):517–20. https://doi.org/10.1097/01241398-199507000-00021.

32. Strategies to mitigate risk from potential latex allergies in children with myelomeningocele and spinal cord injury include all of the following EXCEPT:

    A. Avoiding latex-containing products
    B. Wearing a medical alert identification

C. Carrying auto-injectable epinephrine

D. Eating diet rich with kiwis, bananas, and avocados

Answer: D.

In children with myelomeningocele and spinal cord injury, latex allergy should be suspected in those who have unexplained intraoperative allergic reactions, or with allergies to kiwi, bananas, avocados, or chestnuts. These children, their families, and caregivers should receive education about the potential for latex allergy and the need to avoid all latex-containing products. Children with latex allergies would benefit from wearing a medical alert identification and carrying auto-injectable epinephrine.

Fisher AA. Association of latex and food allergy. Cutis. 1993;52(2):70–1.

Vogel LC, Schrader T, Lubicky JP. Latex allergy in children and adolescents with spinal cord injuries. J Pediatr Orthop. 1995;15(4):517–20. https://doi.org/10.1097/01241 398-199507000-00021.

33. Patients with spinal cord injury and an average risk for colorectal cancer should be endoscopically screened for colorectal cancer starting at what age and at what interval?

    A. Starting at age 40 and every 10 years thereafter
    B. Starting at age 40 and every 5 years thereafter
    C. Starting at age 50 and every 10 years thereafter
    D. Starting at age 50 and every 5 years thereafter

Answer: C.

To date, evidence does not suggest that patients with spinal cord injury are at increased risk of developing colorectal cancer. Accordingly, screening for colorectal cancer in patients with spinal cord injury should take place as recommended for the general population. The US Preventative Services Task Force recommends screening for colorectal cancer in average-risk, asymptomatic adults aged 50–75 years. Initial endoscopic screening should take place at age 50, and every 10 years thereafter. One should consider a patient's overall health and prior screening history when deciding to screen for colorectal cancer in adults aged 76–85 years. Patients with spinal cord injury may need a modified prep for colonoscopy, including potentially admission to the hospital.

Hayman AV, Guihan M, Fisher MJ, Murphy D, Anaya BC, Parachuri R, Rogers TJ, Bentrem DJ. Colonoscopy is high yield in spinal cord injury. J Spinal Cord Med. 2013;36(5):436–42. https://doi.org/10.1179/2045772313Y.0000000091.

US Preventive Services Task Force, Bibbins-Domingo K, Grossman DC, Curry SJ, Davidson KW, Epling JW Jr, García FAR, Gillman MW, Harper DM, Kemper AR, Krist AH, Kurth AE, Landefeld CS, Mangione CM, Owens DK, Phillips WR, Phipps MG, Pignone MP,

Siu AL. Screening for colorectal cancer: US Preventive Services Task Force recommendation statement. JAMA. 2016;315(23):2564–75. https://doi.org/10.1001/jama.2016.5989. Erratum in: JAMA. 2016;316(5):545. Erratum in: JAMA. 2017;317(21):2239.

34. Regarding the development of bladder cancer in patients with spinal cord injury, all of the following statements are true EXCEPT:

    A. Use of chronic indwelling catheters is a risk factor for cancer development
    B. Cigarette smoking has no significant association with bladder cancer
    C. Hematuria may indicate the presence of bladder cancer
    D. Bladder tumors are commonly metastatic and invasive at the time of diagnosis

Answer: B.

Several studies to date have demonstrated that the relative risk of bladder cancer in patients with spinal cord injury is higher than in the general population. In fact, it is the third leading cause of cancer-related death in individuals with spinal cord injury compared to tenth in the general population. In patients with spinal cord injury, use of chronic indwelling catheters and recurrent urinary tract infections are notable risk factors. Other risk factors for the development of bladder cancer include smoking, toxic chemical exposure, and prolonged cyclophosphamide therapy. Bladder cancer may be detected with the aid of urinalysis, urine cytology, cystoscopy, and bladder biopsies. Common histologic findings include squamous cell carcinoma and transitional cell carcinoma; prevalence of these types in the spinal cord injury population varies by study. Bladder tumors are commonly metastatic and invasive at the time of diagnosis.

Gui-Zhong L, Li-Bo M. Bladder cancer in individuals with spinal cord injuries: a meta-analysis. Spinal Cord. 2017;55(4):341–5. https://doi.org/10.1038/sc.2016.151. Epub 2016 Nov 8.
Ho CH, Sung KC, Lim SW, Liao CH, Liang FW, Wang JJ, Wu CC. Chronic indwelling urinary catheter increase the risk of bladder cancer, even in patients without spinal cord injury. Medicine (Baltimore). 2015;94(43):e1736. https://doi.org/10.1097/MD.0000000000001736.

35. All of the following are true regarding cancer screening in women with spinal cord injury EXCEPT:

    A. Starting screening mammography prior to age 50 in women with a first-degree relative with breast cancer
    B. Annual screening mammography for women with average risk for breast cancer at ages 40–74
    C. Cytology screening in women with average risk for cervical cancer every 3 years at ages 21–75
    D. Extending cytology screening to every 5 years in women ages 30–65, assuming that HPV testing is performed alongside cytological analysis

Answer: B.

Regarding breast cancer screening: The USPSTF recommends biennial screening mammography for average-risk women ages 50–74. The USPSTF recommends against routine screening mammography in women ages 40–49; however, women with a first-degree relative with breast cancer may start screening prior to age 50.

Regarding cervical cancer screening: The USPSTF recommends screening for cervical cancer every 3 years with cervical cytology alone in women ages 21–29. The USPSTF recommends screening every 3 years with cytology alone, every 5 years with HPV testing alone, or every 5 years with HPV testing in combination with cytology (co-testing) in women ages 30–65.

Screening for Breast Cancer: US Preventive Services Task Force recommendation statement. Ann Intern Med.2009;151:716–26. [Epub ahead of print 2009 Nov 17]. https://doi.org/10.7326/0003-4819-151-10-200911170-00008.

US Preventive Services Task Force, Curry SJ, Krist AH, Owens DK, Barry MJ, Caughey AB, Davidson KW, Doubeni CA, Epling JW Jr, Kemper AR, Kubik M, Landefeld CS, Mangione CM, Phipps MG, Silverstein M, Simon MA, Tseng CW, Wong JB. Screening for cervical cancer: US Preventive Services Task Force recommendation statement. JAMA. 2018;320(7):674–86. https://doi.org/10.1001/jama.2018.10897.

Psychological Disorders for Individuals with Spinal Cord Injuries

16

Audrey Leung, Kendl Sankary, and Carolyn Campbell

Questions

1. In a patient with a suspected functional neurological disorder leading to lower extremity paralysis, which of the following would most likely be abnormal?

   A. Motor evoked potentials
   B. Interference pattern on electromyography (EMG) in affected muscles
   C. Electroencephalogram (EEG)
   D. Deep tendon reflexes

   Answer: B.

   Electromyography in patients with functional neurological disorders with motor symptoms shows a decreased interference pattern. This finding is non-specific and can be seen in patients either with poor effort or with a lesion involving the corticospinal tract. Motor evoked potentials, EEG, and deep tendon reflexes would likely be normal in the absence of other pathology.

   O'Neal MA, Baslet G. Treatment for patients with a functional neurological disorder (conversion disorder): an integrated approach. Am J Psychiatry. 2018;175(4):307–14. https://doi.org/10.1176/appi.ajp.2017.17040450.

2. A 33-year-old female is admitted to the hospital with acute onset lower extremity weakness, limiting her ability to walk unassisted. After a thorough multidisciplinary evaluation she is diagnosed with a functional neurological disorder.

A. Leung (✉) · K. Sankary · C. Campbell
Department of Physical Medicine and Rehabilitation, University of Washington Hospitals and Clinics, Harborview Medical Center, Seattle, WA, USA
e-mail: asleung3@uw.edu; ksankary@uw.edu; Carolyn.Campbell2@va.gov

© The Author(s), under exclusive license to Springer Nature Switzerland AG 2022
B. A. Abramoff et al. (eds.), *The Essential Spinal Cord Injury Medicine Question Bank*, https://doi.org/10.1007/978-3-031-07796-8_16

Which of the following interventions is most likely to provide lasting benefit to this patient?

A. Admission to acute rehabilitation facility
B. Admission to inpatient psychiatric unit
C. Prescription of a placebo that will help improve their weakness
D. Prescription of a manual wheelchair

Answer: A.

In a randomized controlled crossover study of 60 patients with a functional gait disorder who were randomly assigned to receive immediate treatment with inpatient physical therapy or delayed treatment after 4 weeks (control group), the benefit of the 3-week inpatient course of physical therapy was substantial and was maintained even a year after completion. The role of placebo in the treatment of functional movement disorders is unclear and controversial. Manual wheelchairs are generally a secondary option to a comprehensive rehabilitation program focused on functional gains. Admission to a comprehensive inpatient rehabilitation that includes a physical therapy program is generally indicated over the admission to an inpatient psychiatric unit.

Jordbru AA, Smedstad LM, Klungsøyr O, Martinsen EW. Psychogenic gait disorder: a randomized controlled trial of physical rehabilitation with one-year follow-up. J Rehabil Med. 2014;46(2):181–7. https://doi.org/10.2340/16501977-1246.
Kaas BM, Humbyrd CJ, Pantelyat A. Functional movement disorders and placebo: a brief review of the placebo effect in movement disorders and ethical considerations for placebo therapy. Mov Disord Clin Pract. 2018;5(5):471–8. https://doi.org/10.1002/mdc3.12641.

3. A 63-year-old obese female with C8 American Spinal Injury Association impairment scale (AIS) A spinal cord injury (SCI) is found to have mild ongoing symptoms of depression two months after sustaining her spinal cord injury. She is taking duloxetine, which has relieved her neuropathic pain symptoms, but she still reports a depressed mood that is interfering with her ability to focus at work. She is currently using a manual wheelchair, and performing transfers independently, but requires assistance for bowel/bladder care. She reports sleeping 8 h a night without interruption. Which of the following would be the best addition to her current regimen?

A. Venlafaxine
B. Gabapentin
C. Mirtazapine
D. Cognitive behavioral therapy

Answer: D.

Cognitive behavioral therapy has been found to be an effective treatment of depression in individuals with spinal cord injury. The patient denies any significant neuropathic pain so gabapentin is unlikely to be helpful for this patient. Due to concerns about adverse drug interactions, multiple antidepressants should be used with caution and generally as a second line therapy. In this particular case, there is concern that mirtazapine may lead to weight gain which would be undesirable as the patient is currently performing her own transfers and using a manual wheelchair. Venlafaxine would not be indicated as it is in the same class as duloxetine. When combination therapy is considered, the use of different classes is recommended.

Perkes SJ, Bowman J, Penkala S. Psychological therapies for the management of co-morbid depression following a spinal cord injury: a systematic review. J Health Psychol. 2014;19(12):1597–612. https://doi.org/10.1177/1359105313496445. Epub 2013 Aug 29.

Bauer M, Pfennig A, Severus E, Whybrow PC, Angst J, Möller HJ, World Federation of Societies of Biological Psychiatry, Task Force on Unipolar Depressive Disorders. World Federation of Societies of Biological Psychiatry (WFSBP) guidelines for biological treatment of unipolar depressive disorders, part 1: update 2013 on the acute and continuation treatment of unipolar depressive disorders. World J Biol Psychiatry. 2013;14(5):334–85. https://doi.org/10.3109/15622975.2013.804195. Epub 2013 Jul 3.

4. Which of the following patients is at highest risk of delirium in the acute phase following spinal cord injury?

   A. 24-year-old male with C4 AIS A injury
   B. 70-year-old male with T8 AIS D injury
   C. 70-year-old male with C4 AIS A injury
   D. 24-year-old male with T8 AIS D injury

Answer: C.

Older age and initial International Standards for Neurological Classification of Spinal Cord Injury (ISNCSCI) motor score below 50 (indicating impairment to both upper and lower limbs) are correlated with increased incidence of delirium.

Cheung A, Thorogood NP, Noonan VK, Zhong Y, Fisher CG, Dvorak MF, Street J. Onset, risk factors, and impact of delirium in patients with traumatic spinal cord injury. J Neurotrauma. 2013;30(21):1824–9. https://doi.org/10.1089/neu.2013.2975. Epub 2013 Sept 28.

5. All of the following factors have been shown to increase the risk of post-traumatic stress disorder (PTSD) after spinal cord injury EXCEPT:

   A. Female gender
   B. Anxiety
   C. Disinclination toward expressing emotions
   D. More severe injury

Answer: D.

Severity of spinal cord injury has not been found to impact risk of developing PTSD.

Quale AJ, Schanke AK, Frøslie KF, Røise O. Severity of injury does not have any impact on posttraumatic stress symptoms in severely injured patients. Injury. 2009;40(5):498–505. https://doi.org/10.1016/j.injury.2008.11.006. Epub 2009 Mar 29.

6. Your patient has dry mouth, confusion, orthostasis, sedation. You obtain an EKG which shows new QT-interval prolongation. Of the medications listed below, which is most likely to have contributed?

   A. Tricyclic antidepressant
   B. Duloxetine
   C. Trazodone
   D. Citalopram

Answer: A.

This describes potential anticholinergic side effects of tricyclic antidepressants (TCAs). Anticholinergic side effects include blurred vision, constipation, dry mouth, sedation, confusion, urinary retention, and constipation. QT-interval prolongation is also a possible side effect of TCAs.

Kirshblum S, Lin VW, Sabharwal S. Psychosocial issues and life participation after SCI. In: Kirshblum S, Lin VS, editors. Spinal cord medicine. 3rd ed. New York City: Springer Publishing Company; 2019. p. 394–404.

7. After ruling out other diagnoses, you suspect your patient may have functional neurological disorder. Which physical examination findings would support this diagnosis of exclusion?

   A. The examiner positions the patient's limbs such that the feet are flat on table with knees in a passively flexed position. The examiner then removes the support, and the patient maintains the flexed position.
   B. With the patient supine with heels on table, the examiner places hand under heel of the reported weak leg. The patient is asked to flex the hip of nonaffected leg against resistance, and the examiner feel does not feel increased pressure on the contralateral "unaffected side."
   C. There are abnormal muscle stretch reflexes and superficial reflexes throughout.
   D. There is absent rectal tone on sacral testing.

Answer: A.

This describes a positive Spinal Injuries Center (SIC) test. The examiner positions the patient's limbs such that the feet are flat on table with knees in a passively flexed position. This test is positive because after examiner support is withdrawn, patient maintains the knees in the flexed position, consistent with hysterical paralysis (functional neurological disorder). Answer choice B describes Hoover's test which is useful in cases presenting with paralysis of one leg. Due to synergistic contraction, a patient with functional neurological disorder would be expected to exert pressure from the reportedly paralyzed limb on the examiner's hand while lifting the unaffected limb. However, this patient did not (Hoover's negative), which would make a functional disorder less likely. C and D are both incorrect. In functional neurological disorder rectal tone, muscle stretch reflexes, and superficial reflexes are typically preserved.

Kirshblum S, Lin VW, Sabharwal S. Psychosocial issues and life participation after SCI. In: Kirshblum S, Lin VS, editors. Spinal cord medicine. 3rd ed. New York City: Springer Publishing Company; 2019. p. 394–404.

Smith HE, Rynning RE, Okafor C, Zaslavsky J, Tracy JI, Ratliff J, et al. Clinical Notes: Evaluation of neurologic deficit without apparent cause: the importance of a multidisciplinary approach. J Spinal Cord Med. 2007;30:509.

8. Which of the following is true regarding the project to improve symptoms and mood after SCI (PRISMS) trial?

   A. It found that venlafaxine hydrochloride extended release (XR) was poorly tolerated in spinal cord injured patients
   B. Although well tolerated, venlafaxine XR resulted in no improvements in core depressive symptoms using the Maier subscale
   C. It was a case series
   D. Blurred vision was the only significantly more common new or worsening adverse effect in the venlafaxine XR group compared with the placebo group over 12 weeks.

Answer: D.

The PRISMS trial is one of the few multisite randomized, double-blind placebo-controlled studies specific to treatment of depression in SCI. This study investigated the efficacy and tolerability of venlafaxine XR for major depressive disorder (MDD) or dysthymic disorder in persons with chronic SCI and found it to be well tolerated by most patients and an effective antidepressant for decreasing core symptoms of depression and improving SCI-related disability. Blurred vision was the only significant adverse effect in the venlafaxine XR group compared with the placebo group over 12 weeks.

Fann JR, Bombardier CH, Richards JS, Wilson CS, Heinemann AW, Warren AM, Brooks L, McCullumsmith CB, Temkin NR, Warms C, Tate DG, PRISMS Investigators. Venlafaxine extended-release for depression following spinal cord injury: a randomized clinical trial. JAMA Psychiatry. 2015;72(3):247–58. https://doi.org/10.1001/jamapsychiatry.2014.2482.

9. According to the 2020 Paralyzed Veterans of America Clinical Practice Guideline for Health Care Providers titled "Management of Mental Health Disorders, Substance Use Disorders, and Suicide in Adults with Spinal Cord Injury", which of the following is NOT a recommendation that is supported by Level I scientific evidence, category A, with strong panel agreement?

   A. Treat major depression by using pharmacological and/or nonpharmacological approaches on the basis of clinical presentation (e.g., comorbid conditions), treatment efficacy, and patient preferences.
   B. Consider pharmacological treatments for major depression.
   C. Consider nonpharmacological treatments for major depression.
   D. Admit the patient to a psychiatric unit for major depression.

Answer: D.

Choices A–C are all supported by Level I scientific evidence, category A, with strong panel agreement with the recommendation. Option D is not a recommendation by the panel particularly given access to staff trained to provide SCI care may be limited in a secure psychiatric unit. In some cases, alternative arrangements may need to be considered when an inpatient admission might otherwise be recommended for a spinal cord injured patient.

Bombardier CH, Azuero CB, Fann JR, Kautz DD, Richards JS, Sabharwal S. Management of mental health disorders, substance use disorders, and suicide in adults with spinal cord injury: clinical practice guideline for healthcare providers. Top Spinal Cord Inj Rehabil. 2021;27(2):152–224. https://doi.org/10.46292/sci2702-152.

10. Nonmodifiable risk factors for depression following spinal cord injury include all of the following EXCEPT:

    A. History of depression
    B. Family history of depression or suicide
    C. Coexisting traumatic brain injury (TBI)
    D. Greater than 5 years post injury

Answer: D.

Nonmodifiable risk factors for depression following spinal cord injury include a prior history of depression, family history of depression or suicide, preinjury family fragmentation with poor support structure, being less than (not greater than) 5 years postinjury, and TBI.

Kirshblum S, Lin VW, Sabharwal S. Psychosocial issues and life participation after SCI. In: Kirshblum S, Lin VS, editors. Spinal cord medicine. 3rd ed. New York City: Springer Publishing Company; 2019. p. 394–404.

11. Which of the following is true regarding substance use in young adults who have sustained pediatric-onset SCI?

A. Prevalence rate of substance use is higher compared to the age-matched general population
B. Tetraplegia was associated with higher prevalence of substance use compared to paraplegia
C. Incidence of substance use is higher in those who live independently compared to those who live with a parent or guardian
D. Substance use is not associated with higher incidence of medical complications

Answer: D.

Substance use is associated with increased incidence of pressure injuries, hospitalizations, and pain, substance use in adult-onset SCI populations. In contrast, pediatric-onset SCI is not associated with increased risk of medical complications. Furthermore, the prevalence rate of substance use is lower in the pediatric SCI population compared to the age-matched general population. There were no significant differences in substance use in children who had tetraplegia vs. paraplegia or those who live independently vs. those who live with a parent or guardian.

Hwang M, Chlan KM, Vogel LC, Zebraki K. Substance use in young adults with pediatric-onset spinal cord injury. Spinal Cord. 2012;50(7):497–501.

12. Substance use after traumatic spinal cord injury is associated with all the following demographic factors EXCEPT:

A. Gender
B. Education level
C. Ethnicity
D. Marital status

Answer: C.

Substance use is associated with gender, marital status, and education level. Male gender, single status, and persons with lower level of education (high school level or lower) had higher prevalence rates of substance use. No differences were observed along racial and ethnic lines.

Tate DG, Forschheimer MB, Krauser JS, Meade MA, Bombardier CH. Patterns of alcohol and substance use and abuse in persons with spinal cord injury: risk factors and correlates. Arch Phys Med Rehabil. 2004;85(11):1837–47.

13. Individuals with SCI due to which mechanism of injury are more likely to be at-risk drinkers based on the National Institute of Alcohol Abuse and Alcoholism classification?

   A. Sports-related injuries
   B. Violence
   C. Motor vehicle collision
   D. Falls

Answer: A.

Individuals with sports-related injuries are more likely to be at-risk drinkers (27.1%) in comparison to those who sustained injuries from violence (13.2%), motor vehicle collisions (17.2%) and falls (14.3%). They were also more likely to score positive (score of 2 or more) on the CAGE questionnaire compared to other groups.

Tate DG, Forschheimer MB, Krauser JS, Meade MA, Bombardier CH. Patterns of alcohol and substance use and abuse in persons with spinal cord injury: risk factors and correlates. Arch Phys Med Rehabil. 2004;85(11):1837–47.

14. Which of the following is considered first line treatment for pharmacological management of generalized anxiety disorder (GAD) after SCI?

   A. Amitriptyline
   B. Mirtazapine
   C. Duloxetine
   D. Diazepam

Answer: C.

Currently there is limited evidence for treatment of generalized anxiety disorder in the SCI population. Current recommendations are based on evidence from other populations. Selective serotonin reuptake inhibitors (SSRIs) and serotonin-norepinephrine reuptake inhibitors (SNRIs) are considered first line treatments due to their safer side effect profiles compared to TCAs and benzodiazepines. Mirtazapine is not Food and Drug Administration approved for treatment of GAD and there is insufficient clinical evidence of efficacy.

Bombardier CH, Azuero CB, Fann JR, Kautz DD, Richards JS, Sabharwal S. Management of mental health disorders, substance use disorders, and suicide in adults with spinal cord injury: clinical practice guideline for healthcare providers. Top Spinal Cord Inj Rehabil. 2021;27(2):152–224. https://doi.org/10.46292/sci2702-152.

15. Which of the following demographic factors is associated with higher risk of death by suicide after SCI?

A. Tetraplegia
B. History of drug abuse
C. AIS D
D. SCI secondary to motor vehicle collision

Answer: B.

SCI increases the risk of suicide 3–5 times compared to the general population. Higher risk of death by suicide after SCI has been associated with certain injury characteristics (paraplegia, T1-S3 level with AIS scale A, B or C), history of drug abuse or current alcohol abuse, and individuals whose SCI is caused by attempted suicide.

Bombardier CH, Azuero CB, Fann JR, Kautz DD, Richards JS, Sabharwal S. Management of mental health disorders, substance use disorders, and suicide in adults with spinal cord injury: clinical practice guideline for healthcare providers. Top Spinal Cord Inj Rehabil. 2021;27(2):152–224. https://doi.org/10.46292/sci2702-152.

16. Which of the following is false regarding cognitive function after spinal cord injury?

A. Higher level of injury is associated with cognitive decline
B. Excluding individuals with TBI, incidence of cognitive impairment in individuals with SCI is between 10% and 40%
C. There is a greater prevalence of SCI-associated cognitive impairment with increasing age
D. Individuals with tetraplegia and severe sleep apnea demonstrate worse attention, information processing and immediate recall compared to those with mild/moderate sleep apnea

Answer: A.

According to a recent review article, the majority of studies thus far show no correlation between injury level and cognitive decline or extent of cognitive impairment. Choices B–D are all true statements.

Sachdeva R, Gao F, Chan CCH, Krassioukov AV. Cognitive function after spinal cord injury: a systematic review. Neurology. 2018;91(13):611–21. https://doi.org/10.1212/WNL.0000000000006244. Epub 2018 Aug 29.

17. When performing a Stroop color test to evaluate for attention and processing speed, individuals with spinal cord injury will demonstrate _____ cerebrovascular resistance and _____ cerebral blood flow during the task compared to controls without SCI.

    A. Decreased, decreased
    B. Decreased, increased
    C. Increased, decreased
    D. Increased, increased

    Answer: C.

    In one study, individuals with SCI showed increased cerebrovascular resistance and decreased cerebral blood flow while performing the Stroop color test compared to controls without SCI. This suggests abnormal cerebral hemodynamics and impaired neurovascular coupling after SCI, which is thought to contribute to subsequent cognitive impairment.

    Sachdeva R, Gao F, Chan CCH, Krassioukov AV. Cognitive function after spinal cord injury: a systematic review. Neurology. 2018;91(13):611–21. https://doi.org/10.1212/WNL.0000000000006244. Epub 2018 Aug 29.

18. A 45-year-old male with history of chronic depression and C4 AIS D spinal cord injury from a suicide attempt 8 years ago presents to your clinic after rotator cuff repair 7 days ago. In clinic, he endorses new worsening tremor, diarrhea, diaphoresis, and worsened anxiety. His vitals are significant for a heart rate of 102 and blood pressure of 142/80 (baseline 120/80). His medications include tramadol, oxybutynin, baclofen, dantrolene, phenelzine, acetaminophen and trazodone. What condition are you most concerned of?

    A. Autonomic dysreflexia
    B. Malignant neuroleptic syndrome
    C. Panic disorder
    D. Serotonin syndrome

    Answer: D.

    A combination of phenelzine, trazodone, and tramadol greatly increases this patient's risk of serotonin syndrome. MAOIs, such as phenelzine, are strongly associated with severe cases of serotonin syndrome. Mild cases of serotonin syndrome may present as tachycardia, shivering, diaphoresis or mydriasis with neurological examination revealing intermittent tremor or myoclonus as well as hyperreflexia. More severe cases can present with tachycardia, hypertension, hyperthermia, muscle rigidity, hypertonicity and may deteriorate into shock. It can be hard to differentiate from neuroleptic malignant syndrome (NMS), although in this particular case the patient is not on medications that would put him at risk for NMS. Vital sign changes can also mimic autonomic dysreflexia (AD), although diarrhea and tremor are not commonly seen with AD.

Boyer EW, Shannon M. The serotonin syndrome. N Engl J Med. 2005;352(11):1112–20. https://doi.org/10.1056/NEJMra041867. Erratum in: N Engl J Med. 2007;356(23):2437. Erratum in: N Engl J Med. 2009;361(17):1714.

19. Which of the following is NOT included in DSM-5 criteria for the diagnosis of conversion disorder?

    A. One or more symptoms of altered voluntary motor or sensory function
    B. Initiation or exacerbation of the symptom or deficit is preceded by conflicts or other stressors
    C. Clinical findings provide evidence of incompatibility between the symptom and recognized neurological or medical conditions
    D. The symptom or deficit causes clinically significant distress or impairment in social, occupational or other important areas of functioning or warrants medical evaluation

Answer: B.

The DSM-5 has removed the requirement of "recent psychological stressors" as well as the exclusion of feigning, both of which were previously in the DSM-IV criteria for conversion disorder. Answers A, C, and D are all criteria for functional neurological disorder in the current DSM-5. Another criterion in DSM-5 is that the symptom or deficit is not better explained by another medical or mental disorder.

American Psychiatric Association. Diagnostic and statistical manual of mental disorders (DSM-5). 5th ed. Washington, DC: American Psychiatric Association; 2013.
Lehn A, Gelauff J, Hoeritzauer I, Ludwig L, McWhirter L, Williams S, Gardiner P, Carson A, Stone J. Functional neurological disorders: mechanisms and treatment. J Neurol. 2016;263(3):611–20. https://doi.org/10.1007/s00415-015-7893-2. Epub 2015 Sept 26.

20. Which of the following is true regarding postpartum depression (PPD) and postpartum anxiety (PPA) in women with SCI?

    A. PPA and PPD are most prevalent in women with SCI at the level T7 and below compared to cervical and upper thoracic SCI
    B. Higher prevalence of PPA and PPD are seen in women with SCI compared to the general population
    C. The majority of women with SCI self-report both PPD and PPA after birth
    D. PPD is likely over diagnosed in women with SCI

Answer: B.

Prevalence of PPD (25–37%) and PPA (18–33%) is higher in women with SCI compared to the general population (13% and 18% respectively). In one study, PPA and PPD were more prevalent in women with cervical SCI, followed by upper thoracic (T1–T6) and lower SCI. In this study, 16% of all participants had self-reported both PPA and PPD. Compared to clinically diagnosed PPD, self-reported PPD was 3.6–4.1 times higher in women with SCI, suggesting that PPD may be underdiagnosed in this population.

Lee AHX, Wen B, Walter M, Hocaloski S, Hodge K, Sandholdt N, Hultling C, Elliott S, Krassioukov AV. Prevalence of postpartum depression and anxiety among women with spinal cord injury. J Spinal Cord Med. 2021;44(2):247–52. https://doi.org/10.1080/1079026 8.2019.1666239. Epub 2019 Sept 24.

Rehabilitation of Spinal Cord Injuries

17

Shelly Hsieh, John Lopez, Jeremiah Nieves, and Steven Kirshblum

Questions

1. Early discharge to specialized acute spinal cord injury rehabilitation has been shown to lead to the following outcomes EXCEPT:

   A. Improved motor scores at discharge from rehabilitation
   B. Increased physical independence at 1 year
   C. Reduced risk of rehospitalization
   D. Improved quality of life

   Answer: C.

   Clinical practice guidelines have a weak recommendation in favor of early over late rehabilitation for individuals with acute or subacute spinal cord injury at the point they are medically stable and can tolerate the intensity of rehabilitation.

S. Hsieh (✉)
Department of Physical Medicine and Rehabilitation, Albert Einstein College of Medicine, Bronx, NY, USA

Burke Rehabilitation Hospital, Montefiore Health System, White Plains, NY, USA

Department of Physical Medicine and Rehabilitation, Rutgers New Jersey Medical School, Newark, NJ, USA

Kessler Institute for Rehabilitation, West Orange, NJ, USA
e-mail: shehsieh@burke.org

J. Lopez · J. Nieves · S. Kirshblum
Department of Physical Medicine and Rehabilitation, Rutgers New Jersey Medical School, Newark, NJ, USA

Kessler Institute for Rehabilitation, West Orange, NJ, USA
e-mail: jlopez2@kessler-rehab.com; jdnieves@kessler-rehab.com; skirshblum@selectmedical.com

© The Author(s), under exclusive license to Springer Nature Switzerland AG 2022
B. A. Abramoff et al. (eds.), *The Essential Spinal Cord Injury Medicine Question Bank*, https://doi.org/10.1007/978-3-031-07796-8_17

While there are no studies that directly compare the effect of timing on the effectiveness of rehabilitation, literature demonstrates several benefits to early discharge to specialized acute spinal cord injury rehabilitation. These include improved quality of life, improved performance of activities of daily living, higher Functional Independence Measure motor score at discharge from acute rehabilitation and a higher CHART physical independence score at 1-year post-injury. There have been mixed results regarding timing of rehabilitation and the risk of pressure ulcers and rehospitalization.

Fehlings MG, Tetreault LA, Aarabi B, Anderson P, Arnold PM, Brodke DS, Chiba K, Dettori JR, Furlan JC, Harrop JS, Hawryluk G, Holly LT, Howley S, Jeji T, Kalsi-Ryan S, Kotter M, Kurpad S, Kwon BK, Marino RJ, Martin AR, Massicotte E, Merli G, Middleton JW, Nakashima H, Nagoshi N, Palmieri K, Singh A, Skelly AC, Tsai EC, Vaccaro A, Wilson JR, Yee A, Burns AS. A clinical practice guideline for the management of patients with acute spinal cord injury: recommendations on the type and timing of rehabilitation. Global Spine J. 2017;7(3 Suppl):231S–8S.
Herzer KR, Chen Y, Heinemann AW, González-Fernández M. Association between time to rehabilitation and outcomes after traumatic spinal cord injury. Arch Phys Med Rehabil. 2016;97(10):1620–7.e4.

2. A person having which of the following motor levels would you expect to be at a modified-independent for feeding after set-up?

   A. C4 motor level
   B. C5 motor level
   C. C7 motor level
   D. T1 motor level

   Answer: B.

   A person with a C5 motor level is generally able to achieve a modified independent level after set-up for feeding. Adaptive tools such as a universal cuff, adaptive utensils, plate guard, and Dycem may be used. The C4 motor level is dependent for feeding. The C7 motor level is usually modified independent or independent for feeding. The T1 motor level allows for feeding at an independent level given improved hand and finger function.

Consortium for Spinal Cord Medicine. Outcomes following traumatic spinal cord injury: clinical practice guidelines for health-care professionals. J Spinal Cord Med. 2000;23(4):289–316. https://doi.org/10.1080/10790268.2000.11753539.

3. A 32-year-old woman with C5 motor complete tetraplegia presents to your outpatient clinic for 1-year follow-up post-injury. She reports she came with her husband using medical transportation today and asks if she can become independent in driving herself. She uses a power wheelchair as her primary means of mobility. How should you advise the patient?

A. Continue medical transportation.
B. Explain that she can obtain an adaptive van so that her husband can drive her, which would provide increased convenience as compared to medical transportation.
C. Refer to driver's rehabilitation, with the expectation that she can potentially become independent with driving a highly specialized modified van.
D. Explain that she should transition to a manual wheelchair prior to considering driver's rehabilitation referral.

Answer: C.

An individual with C5 motor complete tetraplegia can become independent with driving using a highly specialized modified van. The patient should be referred to driver's rehabilitation to evaluate for safety and the potential to drive. The driver's rehabilitation specialist will also help plan, develop, coordinate, and implement the necessary services.

An individual with C6 motor complete tetraplegia can become independent with driving in a modified van with sensitized hand controls. An individual with C7 motor complete tetraplegia can become independent in driving a modified van from a captain's seat; or independent in a modified vehicle with hand controls (if independent with transfers and wheelchair loading/unloading).

Patopea M, Asanza JL. Driver training after spinal cord injury. In: Kirshblum S, Lin VS, editors. Spinal cord medicine. 3rd ed. New York City: Springer Publishing Company; 2019. p. 799–805.

Sherman AL, Dalal KL, Taylor J. Activities of daily living and upper limb orthotics. In: Kirshblum S, Lin VS, editors. Spinal cord medicine. 3rd ed. New York City: Springer Publishing Company; 2019. p. 709–27.

4. On your acute inpatient rehabilitation service, a 62-year-old man with T3 American Spinal Injury Association Impairment Scale (AIS) A paraplegia, heart failure, and obesity who sustained his injury 4 weeks ago states that he would rather work on ambulation training rather than wheelchair skills in physical therapy. He states that his roommate with paraplegia has been ambulating in therapy and is being prescribed braces for short distance ambulation at home. You are also caring for the roommate, so you know that the roommate has T12 AIS B paraplegia and has completed 4 weeks in rehabilitation. How should you advise the patient?

A. Explain that it is still early in his rehabilitation course, and you believe he will achieve the same goals as his roommate with time.
B. Explain that you agree ambulation training should be integrated into his physical therapy regimen, and that you will speak to the physical therapist regarding his therapy goals.

C. Explain that you anticipate he will be modified independent at the wheel-chair level on discharge, and it will be important to focus on those skills for now.

D. Explain that you anticipate he will be modified independent at the wheel-chair level upon discharge and in 1-year post-injury. Therefore, it would be a waste of his time to focus on ambulation training in therapy now and in the future.

Answer: C.

Despite full upper extremity strength, there are differences in functional outcomes for people with high versus low motor complete paraplegia due to differences in truncal stability (from abdominal and paraspinal muscle innervation), transfer strength, balance, respiratory capacity, and potential autonomic dysreflexia.

Factors to consider when determining the timing of ambulation training include projected functional outcomes, gait efficiency, upper body strength, weight-bearing precautions, wounds on weight-bearing surfaces or bracing surfaces, unstable cardiovascular disease, osteoporosis, orthostasis, dysreflexia, severe spasticity, contractures and other medical comorbidities.

Those with complete high- to mid-thoracic paraplegia can consider therapeutic gait training with bracing (bilateral Hip-Knee-Ankle-Foot Orthoses (HKAFOs) or Knee-Ankle-Foot Orthoses (KAFOs) with forearm crutches or a walker) or exoskeletons in therapy only. Household and community ambulation is not a functional goal; thus, a wheelchair would be used for primary mobility. KAFOs are indicated for individuals with paraplegia who lack antigravity strength in the lower limbs and have sufficient upper body strength to utilize crutches or a walker.

Individuals with complete T10-L2 paraplegia can consider gait training with bilateral lower limb orthoses for therapy and short distance household ambulation (typically bilateral KAFOs with forearm crutches). A wheelchair will be required for community mobility. Individuals with L3 paraplegia and below can potentially achieve community ambulation. Community ambulation requires bilateral hip flexion strength $\geq 3/5$ and unilateral knee extension strength $\geq 3/5$ with the maximal bracing of one KAFO and one Ankle-Foot Orthosis (AFO).

Due to the progressively shorter rehabilitation length of stays over the past several decades, it is important to consider the pros and cons of initiating gait training during inpatient rehabilitation. If a person is expected to walk at discharge, there are significant benefits. If a person is not expected to walk within the first year, then the focus should be on achieving maximal independence at the wheelchair level.

Donovan J, Snider B, Miller A, Kirshblum S. Walking after spinal cord injury: current clinical approaches and future directions. Curr Phys Med Rehabil. 2020;8:149–58.

Rigot S, Worobey L, Boninger ML. Gait training in acute spinal cord injury rehabilitation-utilization and outcomes among nonambulatory individuals: findings from the SCIRehab project. Arch Phys Med Rehabil. 2018;99(8):1591–8.

Donovan J, Kirshblum S, Didesch M, McNiece M. Spinal cord rehabilitation. In: Kirshblum S, Lin VS, editors. Spinal cord medicine. 3rd ed. New York City: Springer Publishing Company; 2019. p. 690–708.

Sherman AL, Dalal KL, Taylor J. Activities of daily living and upper limb orthotics. In: Kirshblum S, Lin VS, editors. Spinal cord medicine. 3rd ed. New York City: Springer Publishing Company; 2019. p. 709–27.

5. Which level of complete tetraplegia is the most accurately matched to the adaptive equipment one would use with that level of SCI?

   A. C4; balance forearm orthosis
   B. C5; suppository inserter
   C. C6; mouth stylus
   D. C8; universal cuff

   Answer: A.

   A person with C4 complete tetraplegia may potentially benefit from use of a balance forearm orthosis. This allows movement of the elbow flexors in a gravity-eliminated plane, while working to strengthen the proximal shoulder muscles. It can be used to assist with feeding, grooming, and hygiene. Once the biceps and deltoid have $\geq$3/5 strength (e.g., C5 complete tetraplegia with good endurance), a balance forearm orthosis is no longer needed.

   A mouth stylus is helpful for people with impaired hand function, typically C1–C4 complete tetraplegia. At the C5–C6 level, a universal cuff can be utilized to assist with many activities. A pen, stylus, writing utensil, toothbrush, and other items can be inserted into the cuff. At the C5 level of injury, a wrist extension splint can be utilized with a universal cuff. It is unlikely that an individual at the C5 level would have the wrist/hand control to be able to use a suppository inserter. At the C6 level of injury, a wrist extension splint is not needed as a person would have $\geq$3/5 strength of the wrist flexors. A rocker knife is considered at the C6 level of injury given wrist extension, and some wrist flexion and pronation. This allows a person to cut food with one hand using the rocker knife, instead of using two hands for food stabilization with a fork and knife. A person with C8 level of injury will have 3/5 finger flexion that will likely make it unnecessary to use a universal cuff.

   Donovan J, Kirshblum S, Didesch M, McNiece M. Spinal cord rehabilitation. In: Kirshblum S, Lin VS, editors. Spinal cord medicine. 3rd ed. New York City: Springer Publishing Company; 2019. p. 690–708.

6. Range of motion (ROM) exercises are important for people living with spinal cord injury to prevent spasticity and contractures. ROM exercises should be performed daily beginning in the acute care hospital. Care should be taken to avoid over-stretching which of the following pairs of muscles?

A. Elbow flexors; finger flexors
B. Supinators; elbow flexors
C. Knee extensors; dorsiflexors
D. Lumbar paraspinals; finger flexors

Answer: D.

Spasticity or tightness of the lumbar paraspinals provides postural stability in the short and long sitting positions. Stretching of these muscles are typically avoided unless it interferes with function. "Selective tightening" of the finger flexors is helpful to allow for a natural tenodesis grip, thus over-stretching of the finger flexors is avoided. Individuals with C5–C6 motor levels are susceptible to developing elbow flexor and supinator spasticity due to lack of opposing muscle action from the triceps and pronator muscles. An elbow extension splint should be considered. Knee range of motion should be maintained at a 120° arc. Ankle range of motion should be in all planes, with increased focus on preventing plantarflexor spasticity and contractures. Knee and ankle range of motion is important for ADLs, transfers, ambulation, and proper positioning in a wheelchair.

Bergmann M, Zahharova A, Reinvee M, Asser T, Gapeyeva H, Vahtrik D. The effect of functional electrical stimulation and therapeutic exercises on trunk muscle tone and dynamic sitting balance in persons with chronic spinal cord injury: a crossover trial. Medicina. 2019;55(10):619.

Donovan J, Kirshblum S, Didesch M, McNiece M. Spinal cord rehabilitation. In: Kirshblum S, Lin VS, editors. Spinal cord medicine. 3rd ed. New York City: Springer Publishing Company; 2019. p. 609–708.

Masani K, Sin VW, Vette AH, Thrasher TA, Kawashima N, Morris A, Preuss R, Popovic MR. Postural reactions of the trunk muscles to multi-directional perturbations in sitting. Clin Biomech. 2009;24(2):176–82.

7. Your patient with C6 AIS B tetraplegia and a right ischial tuberosity stage 2 pressure injury is working on weight shift techniques during his physical therapy session. Which of the following is an effective weight shift technique for the patient?

   A. Push-up pressure relief
   B. Lateral weight shift
   C. Tipping back the wheelchair to 65°
   D. Leaning forward with the elbows or chest on the thighs

Answer: D.

A weight shift should be performed for 1–2 min every 30 min to provide adequate pressure relief and return of blood flow to areas under pressure when seated. The anterior forward weight shift is ideal for the patient as it unloads both ischial tuberosities. The proper technique is leaning forward with the elbows or chest on thighs with an angle greater than 45° from the wheelchair backrest. Loops can be added to the back of the wheelchair to help the individual return to a seated position. Leaning forward with hands on knees does not provide adequate pressure relief. The anterior forward lean is more effective in offloading pressure than a posterior tilt by tipping the wheelchair back to 65°.

The lateral weight shift unloads one ischial tuberosity (IT), while temporarily increasing pressure on the other IT. The individual hooks their arm over the back of the wheelchair or an attached loop for truncal stability and to help in returning to the seated position. This method is easier to perform because it requires less truncal stability than an anterior forward weight shift. However, this is not ideal as he has already developed a pressure injury on his right IT.

The push-up pressure relief requires triceps function and is a potential technique for individuals with C7 tetraplegia. It should be used in conjunction with other pressure relief techniques to avoid excessive repeated pressure on the shoulder.

Henderson JL, Price SH, Brandstater ME, Mandac BR. Efficacy of three measures to relieve pressure in seated persons with spinal cord injury. Arch Phys Med Rehabil. 1994;75(5):535–9.
Sonenblum SE, Vonk TE, Janssen TW, Sprigle SH. Effects of wheelchair cushions and pressure relief maneuvers on ischial interface pressure and blood flow in people with spinal cord injury. Arch Phys Med Rehabil. 2014;95(7):1350–7.

8. Which of the following cases does NOT include a contraindication for electrical stimulation?

   A. A man with chronic T8 AIS B paraplegia interested in the functional electrical stimulation bike with a right peroneal deep vein thrombosis diagnosed 2 weeks ago
   B. A pregnant woman with chronic T2 paraplegia with lumbar paraspinal spasticity with electrode placement on the low back
   C. A man with chronic tetraplegia s/p cervical posterior decompression and fusion 2 years ago with neck pain
   D. A woman with chronic tetraplegia interested in using electrical stimulation to stimulate wound healing for a stage 4 pressure injury with suspected osteomyelitis and a pending bone biopsy

Answer: C.

Electrical stimulation is safe on intact, well-healed skin overlying implants containing metal, plastic, or cement. Electrical stimulation is contraindicated on the low back/abdomen of pregnant women, areas of known or suspected malignancy, active deep vein thrombosis, actively bleeding tissue, infected tissues, wounds with underlying untreated osteomyelitis, carotid sinus, or the neck/head of a person with seizures.

Martin R, Sadowsky C, Obst K, Meyer B, McDonald J. Functional electrical stimulation in spinal cord injury: from theory to practice. Top Spinal Cord Inj Rehabil. 2012;18(1):28–33.

Rennie S. Electrophysical agents—contraindications and precautions: an evidence-based approach to clinical decision making in physical therapy. Physiother Can. 2010;62(5):1–80.

9. A 62-year-old woman with C1 AIS C tetraplegia is being evaluated for environmental control systems (ECS) during her occupational therapy session. You explain the opportunities and costs of ECS to the patient. Which of the following is NOT a benefit of ECS?

   A. Relatively short time to learn
   B. Promotes positive self-perception
   C. Decreases workload on caregivers
   D. Promotes independence

Answer: A.

Assistive technology needs should be assessed during rehabilitation to maximize a person's independence in communication, mobility and environmental access. Environmental control systems (ECS) allow an individual to control appliances like hospital beds, call buttons, lights, televisions, phones, computers, thermostats, door locks, etc. ECS have associated opportunities and costs. Opportunities include improved independence, decreased workload on caregivers, choice, effective resource use, control over technological functions and applications. Costs included financial resources, technical limitations, and time and frustration associated with learning the ECS. For people with high levels of tetraplegia, ECS use objectively provided "little" change in activity, however it subjectively meant a "lot" to the person in helping them gain independence, providing a sense of security, and promoting positive self-perception.

An individual's readiness for ECS influenced its perception of value and convenience. The medical and rehabilitation team should prepare the individual regarding ECS opportunities and costs to establish expectations, improve user training, and provide support throughout the learning process to maximize its potential benefits. Many of the features of traditional ECS have been supplanted by widely commercially available smart home assistant devices.

Hooper B, Verdonck M, Amsters D, Myburg M, Allan E. Smart-device environmental control systems: experiences of people with cervical spinal cord injuries. Disabil Rehabil Assist Technol. 2018;13(8):724–30.

Martinez RN, Etingen B, French DD, Vallette MA, Bidassie B, Cozart HT, Weaver FM. An ecological perspective on implementing environmental control units for veterans with spinal cord injuries and disorders. Disabil Rehabil Assist Technol. 2020;15(1):67–75.

Myburg M, Allan E, Nalder E, Schuurs S, Amsters D. Environmental control systems—the experiences of people with spinal cord injury and the implications for prescribers. Disabil Rehabil Assist Technol. 2017;12(2):128–36.

Verdonck M, Nolan M, Chard G. Taking back a little of what you have lost: the meaning of using an Environmental Control System (ECS) for people with high cervical spinal cord injury. Disabil Rehabil Assist Technol. 2018;13(8):785–90.

10. You just completed your admission International Standards for Neurological Classification of Spinal Cord Injury (ISNCSCI) exam on a patient with tetraplegia and no prior medical comorbidities. The patient asks you if they will require help for all activities in the future. What is the expected functional outcome for an individual with C7 AIS A tetraplegia at 1-year post-injury?

    A. Independent/mod-I for upper body dressing, independent/mod-I for grooming, some to total assistance for lower body bathing
    B. Independent/mod-I for feeding, some to total assistance for grooming, total assistance for bathing
    C. Independent/mod-I for feeding, independent/mod-I for level transfers, independent/mod-I for manual wheelchair propulsion on even and uneven terrain
    D. Independent/mod-I for feeding, independent/mod-I for level transfers, assistance for manual wheelchair propulsion on uneven terrain

Answer: D.

C7 AIS A tetraplegia is the most common key level for independence with most activities at the manual wheelchair level. Expected functional outcomes include independence or modified independence for feeding, grooming, upper body dressing, weight shifts, and transfers between level surfaces. Some assistance may be required for lower body dressing, bathing, and wheelchair negotiation on uneven surfaces. The individual should be independent with driving in an adapted van, or in a car with hand controls (if independent with transfers and wheelchair loading/unloading).

Answer A: C6 complete tetraplegia. Answer B: C5 complete tetraplegia. Answer C: T1 complete tetraplegia.

Consortium for Spinal Cord Medicine. Outcomes following traumatic spinal cord injury: clinical practice guidelines for health-care professionals. J Spinal Cord Med. 2000;23(4):289–316. https://doi.org/10.1080/10790268.2000.11753539.

Sherman AL, Dalal KL, Taylor J. Activities of daily living and upper limb orthotics. In: Kirshblum S, Lin VS, editors. Spinal cord medicine. 3rd ed. New York City: Springer Publishing Company; 2019. p. 709–27.

11. A man with T2 AIS C paraplegia who uses his ultra-lightweight manual wheelchair as his primary means of mobility inquires about how he will cook for himself upon discharge home. Which modification or adaptive equipment do you recommend?

    A. Rocker knife
    B. Lowering the sink to 46 in.
    C. Over-stove mirror
    D. Cutting board with corner guard

Answer: C.

Instrumental ADLs (IADLs) are activities of daily living that are expanded beyond the basics of self-care. IADLs include cooking, cleaning, laundry, shopping, use of assistive technology, leisure activities, and interpersonal activities. It is essential to include IADLs as a rehabilitation goal. Kitchen management is one of the most important IADLs. After achieving self-feeding and mobility, an individual would need to prepare food. Kitchen modifications are unfortunately often unrealistic for individuals with SCI due to the high associated costs.

Considerations include a sink/countertop height of 32 in., lower-reaching storage areas, accessible stove, accessible sinks with space underneath for the wheelchair, ingredients within reach, stabilizing large pots and mixing bowls, adaptive utensils, and transporting the meal from the countertop to the eating area with the use of a cart. An over-stove mirror allows the individual to see what is on the stove and burners from a seated position and is easy to install. Options A and D are options for an individual with tetraplegia or hemiparesis.

Sherman AL, Dalal KL, Taylor J. Activities of daily living and upper limb orthotics. In: Kirshblum S, Lin VS, editors. Spinal cord medicine. 3rd ed. New York City: Springer Publishing Company; 2019. p. 709–27.

12. A 52-year-old woman with C6 AIS A tetraplegia secondary to a fall 2 weeks ago expresses her motivation to work hard towards recovery and maximizing her independence. She practices a tenodesis grip in her occupational therapy sessions, however, notes difficulty maintaining a grasp on objects due to weakness in her fingers. Which orthosis can augment her tenodesis grip and help increase her function?

    A. Universal cuff
    B. Tenodesis splint
    C. Wrist extension splint
    D. Resting hand ball splint

Answer: B.

Tenodesis techniques are commonly utilized in individuals with a C6 level of injury due to preserved ≥3/5 strength of the wrist extensors. With tenodesis grip, active wrist extension results in passive closing of the fingers, which allows for a gross grasp or pinch. This occurs because the tendons of the finger flexors and thumb flexors cross the wrist, and active wrist extension creates passive tension of the flexors. There are several strategies to maximize the benefits of tenodesis.

Tenodesis splints are custom splints that can be utilized to further augment pinch/gross grasp abilities in individuals with active wrist extension and weak finger flexion. It stabilizes the thumb and holds digits 2–3 in a slightly flexed position while stabilizing the wrist in 20–30° of wrist extension allowing for functional use of the fingers.

A universal cuff is worn proximal to the metacarpophalangeal joints and allows for the insertion of functional objects into a narrow opening on the cuff. This utilizes wrist extension to increase function, however it does not take advantage of a tenodesis grip as it does not involve the use of the fingers. A wrist extension orthosis supports the wrist in an extended position for individuals with impaired or absent wrist strength (C5 level of injury and above), and commonly has a universal cuff component attached. At the C6 level of injury, a wrist extension splint is not needed as a person would have ≥3/5 strength of the wrist extensors. A resting hand ball splint is utilized to stretch the finger flexors and to prevent contractures. For this patient, it is important to allow the development of some finger flexor tone ("selective tightening") to promote a tenodesis grip. Of note, a long opponens splint stabilizes the wrist in a neutral position while allowing full wrist extension for a pinch grasp. It may be useful in individuals with a C5–C7 level of injury.

Assistive devices are helpful in the compensatory training process (as compared to restorative training) for people living with spinal cord injury. In considering assistive devices, it must be the correct device based upon individual needs and capabilities and increase function significantly in order to justify the costs. The costs of assistive devices include the financial cost and the time spent in repetitive training in order to benefit from its use.

Bell P, Hinojosa J. Perception of the impact of assistive devices on daily life of three individuals with quadriplegia. Assist Technol. 1995;7(2):87–94.

Curtin M. Development of a tetraplegic hand assessment and splinting protocol. Paraplegia. 1994;32(3):159–69.

Garber SL, Gregorio TL. Upper extremity assistive devices: assessment of use by spinal cord-injured patients with quadriplegia. Am J Occup Ther. 1990;44(2):126–31.

Jung HY, Lee J, Shin HI. The natural course of passive tenodesis grip in individuals with spinal cord injury with preserved wrist extension power but paralyzed fingers and thumbs. Spinal Cord. 2018;56(9):900–6.

Sherman AL, Dalal KL, Taylor J. Activities of daily living and upper limb orthotics. In: Kirshblum S, Lin VS, editors. Spinal cord medicine. 3rd ed. New York City: Springer Publishing Company; 2019. p. 709–27.

13. You are in the process of discharge planning for a patient with C6 complete tetraplegia. The family asks how the patient is performing his transfers and if equipment is needed. What is the most likely expected functional outcome for transfers for an individual with C6 complete tetraplegia?

    A. Total assistance for transfers with mechanical lift
    B. Contact guard for level surfaces with transfer board
    C. Independent with or without transfer board for level surfaces
    D. Independent without assistive equipment

    Answer: B.

Although C7 complete tetraplegia is the most common key level for independence, some individuals with C6 complete tetraplegia are able to achieve independence with most activities at the manual wheelchair level. Most commonly, individuals with C6 complete tetraplegia require contact guard assistance for transfers on level surfaces with a transfer board due to a lack of triceps strength for stability. For uneven transfers, some assistance with a transfer board, or total assistance with a mechanical lift, is utilized.

Answer A: C5 or higher complete tetraplegia. Answer C: C7 complete tetraplegia. Answer D: T1 or lower complete tetraplegia.

Consortium for Spinal Cord Medicine. Outcomes following traumatic spinal cord injury: clinical practice guidelines for health-care professionals. J Spinal Cord Med. 2000;23(4):289–316. https://doi.org/10.1080/10790268.2000.11753539.

14. A 34-year-old woman with C5 AIS A tetraplegia completed her inpatient acute rehabilitation course and is looking forward to making more gains in outpatient therapy. She is being discharged with a loaner power wheelchair with tilt and recline features, air floatation cushion, a full electric hospital bed with Trendelenburg feature, specialty mattress, and a mechanical lift. Which is an expected functional mobility outcome at 1-year post-injury?

A. Shifting in bed with total assistance
B. Rolling side to side in bed with some assistance
C. Sitting unsupported
D. Transferring from bed to wheelchair with a transfer board and some assistance

Answer: B.

Individuals with a C1–C4 motor level will require total assistance for bed mobility. Individuals with C5–C6 motor level are expected to require some assistance for bed mobility. Individuals with C7 motor level may require some assistance or be independent. Individuals with C8–T1 motor level are expected to be independent in bed mobility. An individual's motivation, body habitus, comorbidities, and medical complications (for example, spasticity, skin, and other traumatic injuries) will influence the expected outcome.

Functional mobility is a goal of both physical and occupational therapy utilizing both restorative and compensatory techniques. The first stage consists of independence in bed mobility (shifting, rolling, sitting up). This is helpful in the prevention of pressure injuries and for respiratory function. Once the patient is sitting up, the patient can learn weight shifting, truncal stability, and balance. The second stage consists of independence in transfers. There are multiple transfer techniques: transfer board-assisted transfers, lateral transfers, squat-pivot transfers, stand-pivot transfers, and sit-to-stand transfers with varying degrees of assistance. "Functional transfers" include bed to wheelchair, wheelchair to bed/toilet/shower chair/car, and floor to chair. Transfer training includes optimizing upper extremity strength, truncal stability, balance, endurance, and vasomotor stability. The next stage of mobility is standing and walking. Spastic muscle tone can be helpful for standing.

Consortium for Spinal Cord Medicine. Outcomes following traumatic spinal cord injury: clinical practice guidelines for health-care professionals. J Spinal Cord Med. 2000;23(4):289–316. https://doi.org/10.1080/10790268.2000.11753539.
Sherman AL, Dalal KL, Taylor J. Activities of daily living and upper limb orthotics. In: Kirshblum S, Lin VS, editors. Spinal cord medicine. 3rd ed. New York City: Springer Publishing Company; 2019. p. 709–27.

15. A 53-year-old right-handed woman with tetraplegia is preparing for discharge home. For neurogenic bladder, she is on an intermittent catheterization program every 6 h. For neurogenic bowel, she is on docusate sodium 100 mg three times per day (TID) with meals, senna 17.2 mg at lunch, and a bisacodyl suppository followed by digital stimulation in the evening. For spasticity, she is on baclofen 10 mg TID and has bilateral multi podus boots. She has spasticity of bilateral adductors, hip flexors, knee flexors and plantar flexors graded as MAS 2. She has an ultra-lightweight manual wheelchair. This is her examination on discharge from acute inpatient rehabilitation.

Myotome	Right	Left
C5	5	5
C6	5	5
C7	5	3
C8	4	2
T1	3	2
L2	1	0
L3	0	0
L4	0	0
L5	0	0
S1	0	0
VAC	Present	

Which of the following adaptive equipment would you expect to prescribe on discharge?

A. Mechanical lift
B. Universal cuff
C. Zipper loops
D. Knee spreader with mirror

Answer: D.

This patient has C7 AIS C paraplegia and is expected to be modified independent at the wheelchair level. She has the functional strength and hand dexterity to perform IC independently, however spasticity and visualization of her anatomy will make it more challenging. She would benefit from a knee spreader with a mirror for her intermittent catheterization program. The knee spreader helps keep her lower extremities apart, especially in the presence of adductor spasticity. The mirror assists in locating the urethra. This adaptive equipment can help her achieve independence in bladder management and decrease caregiver burden.

She is expected to transfer independently with a transfer board. She would not benefit from a universal cuff as she has the finger strength and dexterity to hold the necessary items (feeding utensils, writing utensils, toothbrush, etc.). She also has the dexterity to manipulate zippers, thus zipper loops would not be indicated. Other adaptive equipment that may be useful to the patient include a button hook, shoehorn, reacher, dressing stick, sock aid, suppository inserter, digital stimulator device, razor adaptor, and long handled mirror. Bathroom equipment would include padded shower/commode chair, handheld showerhead, grab bars, safety floor treads, and waterproof timers.

Seth JH, Haslam C, Panicker JN. Ensuring patient adherence to clean intermittent self-catheterization. Patient Prefer Adherence. 2014;8:191–8.
Sherman AL, Dalal KL, Taylor J. Activities of daily living and upper limb orthotics. In: Kirshblum S, Lin VS, editors. Spinal cord medicine. 3rd ed. New York City: Springer Publishing Company; 2019. p. 709–27.

16. Which of the following weighs between 30 and 35 lb?

    A. Depot wheelchair
    B. Lightweight manual wheelchair
    C. Ultra-lightweight manual wheelchair, crafted with aluminum
    D. Ultra-lightweight manual wheelchair, crafted with titanium

Answer: B.

Depot wheelchairs are typically 40–60 lb and constructed with steel. They are indicated for institutional use (for example, hospitals, nursing facilities, and airports). They are designed to accommodate people of varying body habitus and to be propelled by another person. Lightweight and ultra-lightweight manual wheelchairs are indicated for individuals who use wheelchairs as their primary means of mobility. A lightweight wheelchair is 30–35 lb and is typically crafted with steel or aluminum. An ultra-lightweight wheelchair is <30 lb and is typically crafted with aircraft quality aluminum. A titanium ultra-lightweight manual wheelchair is <20 lb.

Cooper RA, Cooper R, Boninger ML, Teodorski E, Thorman T, Pelleschi T, Sundaram A, Daveler B, Kamaraj DC, Schein R. Wheelchairs and seating for people with spinal cord injury. In: Kirshblum S, Lin VS, editors. Spinal cord medicine. 3rd ed. New York City: Springer Publishing Company; 2019. p. 754–8.
Ragnarsson KT. Prescription considerations and a comparison of conventional and lightweight wheelchairs. J Rehabil Res Dev Clin Suppl. 1990;(2):8–16.

17. A 62-year-old man with chronic C8 AIS B tetraplegia presents to your clinic for a new wheelchair. He currently has an ultra-lightweight manual wheelchair that is 6 years old. He reports bilateral shoulder pain, worse with wheelchair propulsion and transfers. What type of wheelchair do you prescribe?

A. An ultra-lightweight aluminum manual wheelchair
B. An ultra-lightweight titanium manual wheelchair
C. An ultra-lightweight manual wheelchair with pushrim-activated power-assisted features
D. A power wheelchair

Answer: C.

At this time, he would benefit most from a pushrim-activated power-assisted wheelchair (PAPAW). This offers him the accessibility and maneuverability of a manual wheelchair, with the benefits of decreased stress on his upper extremities. A PAPAW is a hybrid wheelchair that utilizes in-wheel motors to augment the power applied by the wheelchair user to the pushrim. It decreases stress on the upper extremities by decreasing stroke force, stroke frequency, and energy demands. It is a consideration when an individual is aging or in a transition period between a manual and a power wheelchair.

The ultra-lightweight manual wheelchair weighs <30 lb. A wheelchair made of titanium parts is lighter and more durable than aluminum parts, however it is more expensive. A power wheelchair is not recommended at this time as his environment and mode of transportation may not be accessible.

Algood SD, Cooper RA, Fitzgerald SG, Cooper R, Boninger ML. Impact of a pushrim-activated power-assisted wheelchair on the metabolic demands, stroke frequency, and range of motion among subjects with tetraplegia. Arch Phys Med Rehabil. 2004;85(11):1865–71.

18. A 50-year-old woman with C4 AIS C tetraplegia is being prescribed a power mobility device on discharge from acute rehabilitation, and she is concerned about the accessibility of her home. A home evaluation reveals ramp entry, elevator access, and adequate doorway widths. Which type of powered mobility device offers the smallest turning radius?

A. Front-wheel drive power wheelchair
B. Mid-wheel drive power wheelchair
C. Rear-wheel drive power wheelchair
D. Powered scooter

Answer: B.

Power bases have three different drive wheel configurations: front-wheel drive, mid-wheel drive, rear-wheel drive. A front-wheel drive base has two drive wheels in the front, and two casters in the rear. It is advantageous for propelling over rough terrain or over large obstacles as the larger driving wheels contact the obstacle first. A mid-wheel drive base has two driving wheels in the middle, two casters in the front, and two casters in the rear. It offers the most maneuverability, because the base can turn 360° within its wheelbase. A rear-wheel drive base has two drive wheels in the rear, and two casters in the front. It is the most stable at higher speeds, however it has the least amount of maneuverability. A powered scooter generally has three or four equally sized wheels and are operated by a tiller and handlebars as opposed to a joystick. They also have a larger turning radius.

Cooper RA, Cooper R, Boninger ML, Teodorski E, Thorman T, Pelleschi T, Sundaram A, Daveler B, Kamaraj DC, Schein R. Wheelchairs and seating for people with spinal cord injury. In: Kirshblum S, Lin VS, editors. Spinal cord medicine. 3rd ed. New York City: Springer Publishing Company; 2019. p. 763–8.
Koontz AM, Brindle ED, Kankipati P, Feathers D, Cooper RA. Design features that affect the maneuverability of wheelchairs and scooters. Arch Phys Med Rehabil. 2010;91(5):759–64.

19. A 48-year-old man with T4 AIS B paraplegia and a pressure injury on his ischial tuberosity undergoes a pressure mapping evaluation. It is determined that a specific type of cushion would best redistribute his pressure, however he reports feeling unstable on this cushion. Which specific type of cushion was most likely initially recommended based on the pressure mapping?

    A. Foam cushion
    B. Honeycomb cushion
    C. Viscoelastic fluid cushion
    D. Air floatation cushion

Answer: D.

The material of the seating cushion affects skin integrity, body positioning, and pelvic stability. Air floatation cushions (commonly ROHO™ brand) provide great pressure redistribution. When an individual sits on the cushion and a localized force is applied on the cushion, the air in the loaded cells is redistributed to the neighboring cells. This allows the cushion to contour to the user and adapt to changes in position. However, the air causes a "floating" effect, which can result in loss of pelvic stability. Disadvantages include less postural stability, cost, and frequent maintenance to ensure that the air cells are properly inflated.

    Foam cushions are the most cost-effective and low maintenance, however, may need frequent replacement. Foam cushions come in different densities and contours. Honeycomb cushions behave like a collection of springs and can also be contoured. They have greater air flow and moisture wicking properties. Viscoelastic fluid cushions equalize pressures over the entire seating surface for an even pressure distribution. It offers a more stable seating surface than an air cushion. It is heavier than other cushions, which can affect a wheelchair user's ability to independently perform car transfers.

Ferguson-Pell MW. Seat cushion selection. J Rehabil Res Dev Clin Suppl. 1990;(2):49–73.

20. Which of the following occurs with increased camber of a wheelchair?

    A. Increased forward stability
    B. Increased lateral stability
    C. Slower turns
    D. Less ergonomic propulsion

Answer: B.

Camber is the angle of the wheels towards the wheelchair seat in the vertical plane. For wheelchairs used as a primary means of mobility, the camber is normally 0–4°. For sports wheelchairs, the average camber can be up to 15–20°. Advantages of increased camber include greater side-to-side stability, quicker turns, hand protection, and ergonomic propulsion. Disadvantages include a larger footprint, decreased accessibility, and increased wear on tires.

Veeger D, van der Woude LH, Rozendal RH. The effect of rear wheel camber in manual wheelchair propulsion. J Rehabil Res Dev. 1989;26(2):37–46.

21. What type of power wheelchair access device would you prescribe to an individual with C4 AIS A tetraplegia with bilateral 3/5 elbow flexion strength and no shoulder pain?

    A. Head array
    B. Sip and puff access device
    C. Chin proportional joystick
    D. Goal post U-shaped joystick

Answer: D.

In this case, the individual has a C4 neurologic level of injury, however, functionally has a motor level of C5. An individual with a C5 motor level will be able to operate an upper extremity access device. The goal post U-shaped joystick provides driving control with gross movements of the shoulder and elbow, without fine motor control of the fingers. An individual with motor levels C3 or C4 should be independent in operating a power wheelchair with a head array, mouth/lip/chin joystick, or sip-and-puff control.

Cooper RA, Cooper R, Boninger ML, Teodorski E, Thorman T, Pelleschi T, Sundaram A, Daveler B, Kamaraj DC, Schein R. Wheelchairs and seating for people with spinal cord injury. In: Kirshblum S, Lin VS, editors. Spinal cord medicine. 3rd ed. New York City: Springer Publishing Company; 2019. p. 767–8.
Dicianno BE, Cooper RA, Coltellaro J. Joystick control for powered mobility: current state of technology and future directions. Phys Med Rehabil Clin N Am. 2010;21(1):79–86.

22. What is the most important modifiable factor associated with increased post-injury employment?

    A. Pre-injury employment
    B. Post-injury education
    C. Financial disincentives
    D. Use of assistive technology

Answer: B.

There are modifiable and non-modifiable factors associated with return to work. Non-modifiable factors include age, sex, race, SCI etiology, duration of injury, pre-existing comorbidities, pre-injury education, and pre-injury employment. Modifiable factors include functional independence, medical complications, vocational rehabilitation, social support, financial disincentives, and post-injury education. By targeting modifiable factors, the SCI interdisciplinary team can maximize employment outcomes.

Education is an important predictor of employment post-injury. Literature demonstrates that each additional educational level completed post-injury significantly increases the odds of obtaining employment post-injury. Encouraging individuals to return to education is important. This can inform further interventions to support return to education and return to work.

Pre-injury employment is a non-modifiable risk factor. There have been mixed findings regarding the relationship between financial disincentives and assistive technology and employment.

Yasuda S, Wehman P, Targett P, Cifu DX, West M. Return to work after spinal cord injury: a review of recent research. NeuroRehabilitation. 2002;17(3):177–86.
Trenaman L, Miller WC, Querée M, Escorpizo R, SCIRE Research Team. Modifiable and non-modifiable factors associated with employment outcomes following spinal cord injury: a systematic review. J Spinal Cord Med. 2015;38(4):422–31.
Krause JS, Reed KS. Obtaining employment after spinal cord injury: relationship with pre- and postinjury education. Rehabil Couns Bull. 2009;53(1):27–33.

23. A 36-year-old male construction foreman sustained a C7 AIS C spinal cord injury after a work accident. He expresses interest in returning to work during his acute inpatient rehabilitation course. You refer him for vocational rehabilitation services. What factor is associated with a decreased time to first job after injury?

    A. Age at injury
    B. Gender
    C. Returning to pre-injury employer
    D. Working in management pre-injury

Answer: C.

Factors associated with a shorter time to first job (part-time or full-time) include returning to pre-injury employer, higher levels of education, less severe injury and being Caucasian. In addition to the above factors, gender was associated with a shorter time to return to a first *full-time* job, with men returning earlier than women. Age at injury and working in management pre-injury was not associated with a shorter time to return to first job.

Krause JS, Terza JV, Saunders LL, Dismuke CE. Delayed entry into employment after spinal cord injury: factors related to time to first job. Spinal Cord. 2010;48(6):487–91.

24. Which Minnesota Theory of Work Adjustment (MTWA) value describes a situation in which employment provides financial, health, and security to a person with SCI, which may be perceived as more important benefits than salary itself?

    A. Comfort
    B. Safety
    C. Autonomy
    D. Achievement

Answer: A.

The Minnesota Theory of Work Adjustment (MTWA) describes six values that can be utilized to understand the benefits of employment in the SCI population: comfort, safety, autonomy, achievement, altruism, and status. Comfort describes the benefits of employment including a salary and fringe benefits (for example, health insurance, medical leave, and a retirement plan). Salary itself is typically not perceived as the main benefit of working, however salary enables a person to pursue avocational interests and employment includes fringe benefits.

Safety describes a stable and fair work environment. Autonomy describes a personal sense of responsibility and initiative and feeling that the work is meaningful and contributing to self-identity. Achievement encourages progress and accomplishment. Altruism describes the moral obligation to be a contributing member of society; through this, individuals also have the opportunity to develop relationships with coworkers. Status describes the recognition one would receive through employment, and how it would positively impact self-esteem. Employment is often seen as necessary to a person's social identity.

Dawis RV, Lofquist LH. A psychological theory of work adjustment: an individual-differences model and its applications. Minneapolis: University of Minnesota Press; 1984.

Meade MA, Reed KS, Saunders LL, Krause JS. It's all of the above: benefits of working for individuals with spinal cord injury. Top Spinal Cord Inj Rehabil. 2015;21(1):1–9.
O'Neill JO, Ottomanelli L. Vocational rehabilitation for individuals with spinal cord injury. In: Kirshblum S, Lin VS, editors. Spinal cord medicine. 3rd ed. New York City: Springer Publishing Company; 2019. p. 776–88.

25. You are discussing home modifications with your patient with paraplegia. His family member states that the entrance doorway is 30 in. in width. What is the minimum width of entrance doorways to ensure accessibility to a manual wheelchair user?

    A. 28 in.
    B. 30 in.
    C. 32 in.
    D. 34 in.

    Answer: C.

    The entrance doorway should be at least 32 in. in width from the face of the door (opened to 90°) to the opposite door jamb for a manual wheelchair. It should be at least 34 in. for a power wheelchair. Swing clear offset hinges can be utilized to maximize the width of the doorway when the door is open. There should be clearance on both sides of the door to allow the wheelchair user to open the door, enter the room and close the door. Lever door handles are easier to operate than round door knobs.

    Sebring-Cale NJ. Accessibility issues with long-term disabilities. Neurol Res. 2008;30(5):437–40.

26. Your patient's home evaluation reveals that there are five steps to enter the first floor. The family member is prepared to build a ramp and asks you about ramp requirements. Per American with Disabilities Act (ADA) standards, what is the maximum ramp running slope (rise-to-run ratio)?

    A. 1:8
    B. 1:12
    C. 1:16
    D. 1:20

    Answer: B.

    The ramp rise-to-run ratio describes the number of inches in rise compared to the number of inches in length of the ramp (run). The maximum slope is 1:12 as recommended by the ADA. This means that for every inch of rise, you need one foot of ramp. The ideal slope is a 1:20 rise to run ratio. For private homes, a steeper ramp (for example, 2:12) may be acceptable. Other characteristics to consider when building a ramp include width, type of surface and handrails.

    2010 ADA standards for accessible design. 2010. https://www.ada.gov/regs2010/2010ADAStandards/2010ADAStandards_prt.pdf. Accessed 1 Jan 2021.

27. Your patient is concerned about using his manual wheelchair in his current home, which he describes as a small apartment. What is the minimum circular turning space of a manual wheelchair?

A. 4 × 4 ft
B. 5 × 5 ft
C. 6 × 6 ft
D. 7 × 7 ft

Answer: B.

The circular turning space requires less space as compared to a T-shaped turning space. For a manual wheelchair, at least a 5 ft × 5 ft (60-in. diameter) space is necessary to accommodate a 360°. The turning space for a power wheelchair or bariatric wheelchair may require at least 6 ft × 6 ft. The ideal dimensions will vary based upon the individual and their mobility device, and more clear space is always preferable when building home modifications.

2010 ADA standards for accessible design. 2010. https://www.ada.gov/regs2010/2010ADAS tandards/2010ADAStandards_prt.pdf. Accessed 1 Jan 2021.

28. Which statement is true regarding optimal heights above the floor?

A. Bed; 15 in.
B. Toilet seat; 15 in.
C. Sink; 30 in.
D. Light switch; 34 in.

Answer: D.

The optimal height of light switches and electrical outlets is no higher than 36 in. from the floor level, and no lower than 15 in. above the floor. The optimal height of a bed should be around 20–22 in., or the approximate height of an individual's wheelchair seat. The standard toilet height is 14–15 in. from the floor. The optimal height of a toilet seat for a wheelchair user is 17–19 in. above the floor, as it allows easier wheelchair-toilet transfers. The optimal height of a bathroom or kitchen sink should ideally be 32–34 in. with an open area below the sink, allowing for 27 in. of knee clearance, width of 30 in. and a depth of 19 in.

2010 ADA standards for accessible design. 2010. https://www.ada.gov/regs2010/2010ADAS tandards/2010ADAStandards_prt.pdf. Accessed 1 Jan 2021.
Lee JJ. Home modifications and architectural changes for spinal cord injury patients. In: Kirshblum S, Lin VS, editors. Spinal cord medicine. 3rd ed. New York City: Springer Publishing Company; 2019. p. 849–56.

29. At 1-year postinjury, what is the highest motor level an individual with complete tetraplegia would be expected to perform both upper and lower body dressing at a modified independent level?

A. C4
B. C5
C. C6
D. C7

Answer: D.

Persons with a C7 motor level are usually able to perform upper body dressing independently and are capable of completing lower body dressing at a modified independent level. Clothing modifications such as loops on zippers and velcro shoe closures allow for increased independence. Persons with a C4 injury (and above) will be dependent for upper and lower body dressing. Individuals with a C5 motor level will require assistance, often moderate for upper body dressing and will be dependent for lower body dressing. Those with a C6 motor level typically can complete upper body dressing independently with adaptive equipment. Although it is possible for persons with a C6 motor level to be modified independent with lower body dressing, they usually require some level of assistance for this task.

Donovan J, Kirshblum S, Didesch M, McNiece M. Spinal cord rehabilitation. In: Kirshblum S, Lin VS, editors. Spinal cord medicine. 3rd ed. New York City: Springer Publishing Company; 2019. p. 690–708.

30. A person with a diagnosis of C5 AIS A SCI expresses concern about his family assisting with his bowel program. He asks what level of assistance he will need in completing his bowel program when returning home. You explain:

A. He will likely require total assistance.
B. He will require some assistance with clean up but otherwise independent.
C. He will be independent with adaptive equipment.
D. He will be independent without adaptive equipment.

Answer: A.

Persons with a complete C5 (and above) SCI will usually require total assistance to complete their bowel program. Those with a C6 motor level typically require some to total assistance with their bowel program. Modified independence can be achieved at the C7 motor level with the use of adaptive equipment to aid in digital stimulation and suppository insertion. Individuals with thoracic level injuries should be independent in their bowel programs.

Donovan J, Kirshblum S, Didesch M, McNiece M. Spinal cord rehabilitation. In: Kirshblum S, Lin VS, editors. Spinal cord medicine. 3rd ed. New York City: Springer Publishing Company; 2019. p. 690–708.

31. Walking is a desired goal for most persons following acute SCI. Which of the following is the minimum walking speed necessary for persons with SCI to utilize walking as the primary means of outdoor mobility with or without assistive devices?

    A. 0.09 ± 0.01 m/s
    B. 0.15 ± 0.08 m/s
    C. 0.44 ± 0.14 m/s
    D. Walking speed is not an indicator for community ambulation

Answer: C.

Community ambulators have the ability to transfer from sit-to-stand and walk >150 ft independently, with or without an assistive device. SCI literature suggests a walking speed of at least 0.44 m/s is necessary for an individual to use walking as a primary means of mobility outside of the home. A minimal walking speed of 0.70 m/s separates community ambulates who need mobility aids from those who do not. A walking speed of 0.09 m/s corresponds to an individual or would perform walking in a controlled, supervised setting such as therapy. A walking speed of 0.15 m/s is indicative of a person who ambulates within the home and utilizes a wheelchair for outdoor/community mobility.

van Hedel HJA, EM-SCI Study Group. Gait speed in relation to categories of functional ambulation after spinal cord injury. Neurorehabil Neural Repair. 2008;23(4):343–50. https://doi.org/10.1177/1545968308324224.

Oleson CV, Flanders AE. Predicting outcomes following spinal cord injury. In: Spinal cord medicine. 3rd ed. New York, NY: Springer; 2019. p. 149–63.

Field-Fote EC, Nieves L, Hartigan C. Advanced mobility and strategies to promote walking function after spinal cord injury. In: Kirshblum S, Lin VS, editors. Spinal cord medicine. 3rd ed. New York City: Springer Publishing Company; 2019. p. 728–43.

32. A 58-year-old male presents to clinic for follow-up 1 year after his acute inpatient rehabilitation. He reports significant progress with therapy including ambulation with assistive devices while in the gym. He questions his prognosis and ability to become a community ambulator. Repeat examination today reveals a C7 AIS C SCI consistent with central cord syndrome. Which of the following is a positive predictor for this patient to return to community ambulation?

    A. Ability to complete a 10-m walk test in 50 s
    B. Total lower extremity motor score of 34
    C. Bilateral hip flexor strength of 2/5 and left knee extensor strength of 2/5
    D. Exam findings consistent with central cord syndrome

Answer: B.

Ambulation is dependent on many factors aside from neurologic level alone. Waters et al. (1994) found that a lower extremity motor score (LEMS) ≥30 is conducive to community ambulation. The 10-m walk test is a tool used to calculate walking speed. Traversing 10 m in 45 s equates to a walking speed of 0.20 m/s. A minimum walking speed of 0.44 ± 0.14 m/s is indicative of returning to community ambulation. A reciprocal gait pattern that may lead to community ambulation requires ≥3/5 strength in the bilateral hip flexors and at least one knee extensor. Although 57–86% of patients with central cord syndrome will ambulate independently, the patient's age >50 years and more importantly, AIS C classification, makes it less likely he will walk at the community level. Of the incomplete spinal cord injury syndromes, Brown-Séquard syndrome carries the best prognosis for functional ambulation.

Waters RL, Adkins R, Yakura J, Vigil D. Prediction of ambulatory performance based on motor scores derived from standards of the American Spinal Injury Association. Arch Phys Med Rehabil. 1994;75:756–60.

van Hedel HJA, EM-SCI Study Group. Gait speed in relation to categories of functional ambulation after spinal cord injury. Neurorehabil Neural Repair. 2008;23(4):343–50. https://doi.org/10.1177/1545968308324224.

Crozier KS, Cheng LL, Graziani V, Zorn G, Herbison G, Ditunno JF. Spinal cord injury: prognosis for ambulation based on quadriceps recovery. Paraplegia. 1992;30:762–7. https://doi.org/10.1038/sc.1992.147.

Oleson CV, Flanders AE. Predicting outcomes following spinal cord injury. In: Kirshblum S, Lin VS, editors. Spinal cord medicine. 3rd ed. New York City: Springer Publishing Company; 2019. p. 49–163.

33. Which of the following is true in regards to performing standing activities in the SCI population?

    A. It increases bone mineral density.
    B. It improves psychological well-being.
    C. It has no impact on lower limb spasticity.
    D. It has no impact on bowel function.

Answer: B.

In the spinal cord injury population, standing has a positive psychological impact and can improve well-being. A standing program alone has not been shown to increase bone mineral density. Literature exists to suggest the benefit of standing on spasticity. Additionally, there is evidence standing can improve bowel function.

Kunkel CF, Scremin AM, Eisenberg B, Garcia JF, Roberts S, Martinez S. Effect of "standing" on spasticity, contracture, and osteoporosis in paralyzed males. Arch Phys Med Rehabil. 1993;74:73–8. https://doi.org/10.5555/uri:pii:000399939390387P.

Janice JE, Levins SM, Townson AF, Mahjones D, Bremner J, Huston G. Use of prolonged standing for individuals with spinal cord injuries. Phys Ther. 2001;81(8):1392–9. https://doi.org/10.1090/ptj/81.8.1392.

Biering-Sorensen F, Hansen B, Lee BS. Non-pharmacological treatment and prevention of bone loss after spinal cord injury: a systematic review. Spinal Cord. 2009;47(7):508–18. https://doi.org/10.1038/sc.2008.177.

Kwok S, Harvey L, Glinsky J, Bowden JL, Coggrave M, Tussler D. Does regular standing improve bowel function in people with spinal cord injury? A randomized crossover trial. Spinal Cord. 2015;53:36–41. https://doi.org/10.1038/sc.2014.189.

Bohannon RW. Tilt table standing for reducing spasticity after spinal cord injury. Arch Phys Med Rehabil. 1993;74(10):1121–2. https://doi.org/10.1016/0003-9993(93)90073-J.

Donovan J, Kirshblum S, Didesch M, McNiece M. Spinal cord rehabilitation. In: Kirshblum S, Lin VS, editors. Spinal cord medicine. 3rd ed. New York City: Springer Publishing Company; 2019. p. 690–708.

34. During a new outpatient evaluation of an individual with a C7 AIS B SCI sustained 10 years ago, the patient questions his risk of fracture as he has known osteoporosis. You advise him he carries an increased risk of lower limb fracture due to the chronicity of his injury. Specifically, the most common site of fracture in chronic spinal cord injury is the:

A. Proximal tibia
B. Distal fibula
C. Supracondylar femur
D. Femoral neck

Answer: C.

Individuals with chronic spinal cord injury have a bone mineral density of the proximal femur that reaches fracture threshold at 1–5 years after injury. Supracondylar femur fractures are the most common site of fracture in chronic SCI followed by the proximal tibia, distal tibia, femoral shaft and neck, and humerus.

Szollar SM, Martin EM, Sartoris DJ, Parthemore JG, Deftos LJ. Bone mineral density and indexes of bone metabolism in spinal cord injury. Am J Phys Med Rehabil. 1998;77(1):28–35. https://doi.org/10.1097/00002060-199801000-00005.

Scelza WM, Dyson-Hudson TA. Neuromusculoskeletal complications of spinal cord injury. In: Kirshblum S, Campagnolo DI, editors. Spinal cord medicine. 2nd ed. Philadelphia: Lippincott Williams & Wilkins; 2011. p. 282–308.

Kiratli BJ, Smith AE, Nauenberg T, Kallfelz CF, Perkash I. Bone mineral and geometric changes through the femur with immobilization due to spinal cord injury. J Rehabil Res Dev. 2000;37(2):225–33.

Garland DE, Adkins RH, Scott M, Singh H, Massih M, Stewart C. Bone loss at the os calcis compared with bone loss at the knee in individuals with spinal cord injury. J Spinal Cord Med. 2004;27(3):207–11. https://doi.org/10.1080/10790268.2004.11753749.

35. For individuals with SCI, walking is often a primary concern. Which of the following is FALSE in regards to the potential impact of walking in the SCI population?

    A. Walking may lead to decreased medical costs.
    B. Walking minimizes fracture risk in chronic SCI.
    C. Walking may result in lower rates of hospitalization.
    D. Walking can lead to improved levels of spasticity.

    Answer: B.

    Ambulatory patients with SCI have a greater risk of falling compared to full-time wheelchair users. Due to the associated loss of bone density in chronic SCI, a fall after SCI increases the risk of fracture. Despite this risk, there are many proven benefits to ambulation in the SCI population. Walking may lead to improved mobility, as those who ambulate may often be able to access parts of their environments that are inaccessible by wheelchair. Individuals with SCI who have the ability to ambulate have lower associated medical costs over the 5-year period following injury. Literature also suggests the ability to ambulate is associated with a lower annual probability of hospitalization. Other potential benefits of walking include decreased spasticity, improved bowel/bladder function, cardiovascular benefits, and improved psychological wellbeing.

    Saunders LL, Dipiro ND, Krause JS, Brotherton S, Kraft S. Risk of fall-related injuries among ambulatory participants with spinal cord injury. Top Spinal Cord Inj Rehabil. 2013;19(4):259–66. https://doi.org/10.1310/sci1904-259.
    Jørgensen V, Butler Forslund E, Franzén E, Opheim A, Seiger Å, Ståhle A, Hultling C, Stanghelle JK, Wahman K, Skavberg Roaldsen K. Factors associated with recurrent falls in individuals with traumatic spinal cord injury: a multicenter study. Arch Phys Med Rehabil. 2016;97(11):1908–16. https://doi.org/10.1016/j.apmr.2016.04.024.
    Miller LE, Anderson LH. Association of ambulatory ability on complications and medical costs in patients with traumatic spinal cord injury: a decision-analytic model. Cureus. 2019;11(8):e5337. https://doi.org/10.7759/cureus.5337.
    Le Fort M, Espagnacq M, Perrouin-Verbe B, Ravaud JF. Risk analyses of pressure ulcer in tetraplegic spinal cord-injured persons: a French long-term survey. Arch Phys Med Rehabil. 2017;98(9):1782–91. https://doi.org/10.1016/j.apmr.2016.12.017.
    Karimi MT. Evidence-based evaluation of physiological effects of standing and walking in individuals with spinal cord injury. Iran J Med Sci. 2011;36(4):242–53.
    Donovan J, Snider B, Miller A, Kirshblum S. Walking after spinal cord injury: current clinical approaches and future directions. Curr Phys Med Rehabil. 2020;8:149–58. https://doi.org/10.1007/s40141-020-00277-1.

36. Compared to wheelchair use, all of the following are potential disadvantages to ambulation with assistive devices in the SCI population EXCEPT:

    A. Increased energy expenditure
    B. Increased incidence of joint pain

C. Greater risk of falling

D. Worsened bladder/bowel function

Answer: D.

Despite numerous physical and psychological benefits to walking in the SCI population, not all aspects of ambulation may be advantageous. There may be pronounced increases in energy expenditure. Excessive upper body weight-bearing coupled with pathological lower limb movement patterns (due to weakness) can be detrimental to joint health. Those who ambulate with the use of assistive devices have a greater risk of falling compared to full-time wheelchair users. Ambulation may lead to improved bladder/bowel function.

Donovan J, Snider B, Miller A, Kirshblum S. Walking after spinal cord injury: current clinical approaches and future directions. Curr Phys Med Rehabil. 2020;8:149–58. https://doi.org/10.1007/s40141-020-00277-1.

Field-Fote EC, Nieves L, Hartigan C. Advanced mobility and strategies to promote walking function after spinal cord injury. In: Kirshblum S, Lin VS, editors. Spinal cord medicine. 3rd ed. New York City: Springer Publishing Company; 2019. p. 728–43.

37. Which of the following is most accurate in regards to locomotor gait training in the SCI population?

    A. Locomotor training has consistently been shown to improve ambulation in those with motor complete SCI.
    B. The use of appropriate lower limb bracing is a necessary component of locomotor training.
    C. Locomotor training relies on specific, therapist driven feedback and compensatory strategies to overcome motor impairments.
    D. Locomotor training utilizes use-dependent neuroplasticity through repetitive practice intended to activate neural locomotor centers.

Answer: D.

Locomotor training is distinguished from gait training by its emphasis on neuroplasticity through repetitive practice while gait training places emphasis on functional ambulation with the use of lower extremity orthotics and therapist feedback. Both locomotor and gait training are typically combined in rehabilitation.

Individuals with chronic, motor incomplete SCI who complete locomotor training may have improvements with balance, strength, limb coordination, and energy expenditure in addition to the known health benefits of walking. In people with chronic, motor incomplete SCI, walking speed can improve with both overground training and treadmill-based training. Aside from a limited number of case reports, locomotor training has not led to functional ambulation in persons with motor complete injuries.

Field-Fote EC, Roach KE. Influence of a locomotor training approach on walking speed and distance in people with chronic spinal cord injury: a randomized clinical trial. Phys Ther. 2011;91(1):48–60. https://doi.org/10.2522/ptj.20090359.

Donovan J, Snider B, Miller A, Kirshblum S. Walking after spinal cord injury: current clinical approaches and future directions. Curr Phys Med Rehabil. 2020;8:149–58. https://doi.org/10.1007/s40141-020-00277-1.

Field-Fote EC, Nieves L, Hartigan C. Advanced mobility and strategies to promote walking function after spinal cord injury. In: Kirshblum S, Lin VS, editors. Spinal cord medicine. 3rd ed. New York City: Springer Publishing Company; 2019. p. 728–43.

38. Your patient with an SCI asks about lower limb bracing that will allow him to return to community ambulation. You perform an updated ISNCSCI examination and determine his classification to be T10 AIS C. His lower extremity motor scores are as follows:

Left: L2: 2/5, L3: 1/5, L4: 1/5, L5: 1/5, S1: 1/5.
Right: L2: 4/5, L3: 3/5, L4: 1/5, L5: 2/5, S1: 3/5.

Which of the following lower limb orthotics is most appropriate and provides the best chance of returning to community ambulation?

A. Hip-knee-ankle-foot orthosis
B. Bilateral knee-ankle-foot orthosis
C. Left knee-ankle-foot orthosis, right solid ankle-foot orthosis
D. Bilateral solid ankle ankle-foot orthoses

Answer: C.

The most appropriate lower extremity bracing option for this patient is a left KAFO and a right AFO. KAFOs provide multipoint stability and are typically indicated for those with manual muscle grades of less than 2/5 in hip extensors, knee extensors, and ankle dorsi- and plantar flexors. An AFO is indicated on his right lower extremity as he has knee extensor strength of 3/5. For patients who require a unilateral KAFO, community ambulation may be achieved in combination with a walker or forearm crutches. A HKAFO provides maximum lower extremity stability. Appropriate individuals for an HKAFO are those with complete paraplegia as well as trunk/pelvis paralysis. A reciprocal gait orthosis (RGO) includes thoracic support and can facilitate reciprocal leg movement through the use of a duplicable system. Although HKAFOs in conjunction with a walker can allow for locomotion, it requires significant energy expenditure and is likely reserved for exercise only as opposed to community ambulation. Bilateral solid ankle AFOs are not indicated in this individual as his left knee extensors are only 2/5. A solid ankle AFO is indicated when muscle test grades of the knee extensors are at least 3/5 while hip extensors are at least 2/5.

Field-Fote EC, Nieves L, Hartigan C. Advanced mobility and strategies to promote walking function after spinal cord injury. In: Kirshblum S, Lin VS, editors. Spinal cord medicine. 3rd ed. New York City: Springer Publishing Company; 2019. p. 728–43.

39. Which of the following assistive devices requires the greatest energy expenditure in an experienced individual with motor complete T11 paraplegia?

    A. Manual wheelchair propulsion
    B. Functional electrical stimulation-assisted walking
    C. Reciprocating gait orthosis
    D. Bilateral KAFOs using crutches with swing to gait

Answer: B.

The energy cost of overground walking can be measured in terms of oxygen consumption (mL O_2/kg/min). Of the above choices, functional electrical stimulation (FES) assisted walking requires the greatest energy expenditure at 23 mL/kg/min. Bilateral KAFOs with crutches utilizing swing to gait requires 16.5 mL/kg/min. Use of reciprocating gait orthosis requires 14 mL/kg/min. Wheeling a manual wheelchair is relatively energy-efficient. The metabolic demand of wheeling inside on tile and outside on even pavement is 7–8 and 8–11 mL/kg/min respectively.

Field-Fote EC, Nieves L, Hartigan C. Advanced mobility and strategies to promote walking function after spinal cord injury. In: Kirshblum S, Lin VS, editors. Spinal cord medicine. 3rd ed. New York City: Springer Publishing Company; 2019. p. 728–43.

40. Compared to those who do not participate in adaptive sports, individuals with SCI who participate in adaptive recreation activities:

    A. Have decreased rates of employment
    B. Describe higher daily pain levels
    C. Are more likely to be tetraplegic
    D. Report improved quality of life

Answer: D.

Participation in adaptive physical activity has been shown to have a positive impact on quality of life. This is particularly true within the psychological and physical domains of quality of life. Those involved in adaptive sports have higher rates of employment than inactive individuals with SCI. Participating in adaptive exercise can result in overall decreased daily pain levels in the SCI population. Those with paraplegia are more frequently involved in adaptive sports than those with tetraplegia.

Anneken V, Hanssen-Doose A, Hirschfeld S, Scheuer t, Thietje R. Influence of physical exercise on quality of life in individuals with spinal cord injury. Spinal Cord. 2010;48(5):393–99. https://doi.org/10.1038/sc.2009.137.

Hicks AL, Martin KA, Ditor DS, Latimer AE, Craven C, Bugaresti J, McCartney N. Long-term exercise training in persons with spinal cord injury: effects on strength, arm ergometry performance and psychological well-being. Spinal Cord. 2003;41:34–43. https://doi.org/10.1038/sj.sc.3101389.

41. During routine follow up with an otherwise healthy 22-year-old male with a T6
    AIS B SCI, he asks about participating in wheelchair rugby. Once he purchases
    an adaptive rugby wheelchair, he plans to transfer his air flotation cushion he
    obtained after completing pressure mapping. The league he intends to join
    requires medical clearance from a physician. He inquires about the associated
    risks with adaptive sports in the SCI population particularly as it pertains to his
    injury. During your discussion you explain:

    A. He is at high risk of developing autonomic dysreflexia and should consider
       other means of exercise.
    B. He should purchase a low-cost foam cushion to prevent damage to his pri-
       mary cushion.
    C. He is unable to participate in wheelchair rugby until an echocardiogram is
       completed.
    D. He is at risk for hyperthermia due to altered thermoregulation.

    Answer: D.

    Individuals with SCI are susceptible to hyperthermia due to impaired ability to
    regulate body temperature particularly in high heat and during sport. Because
    of this, it is important to have adequate hydration. The neurologic level of injury
    that predisposes individuals with SCI to hyperthermia is debated as some litera-
    ture reports T6 while others use T8. To combat hyperthermia due to impaired
    thermoregulation, individuals can complete precooling prior to activity. This
    can be accomplished by applying ice towels to the body, cold water immer-
    sion, and air circulation with fans. Precooling can minimize risk of heat illness
    and may improve athletic performance. For outdoor activities, it is also impor-
    tant to protect from sunburns as patients with SCI are at increased risk due to
    decreased sensation. Numerous skin injury risk factors exist while participating
    in sport including pressure, shear, moisture, and friction. For this reason, close
    monitoring of skin and injury prevention should be a high priority as skin injury
    is one of the most common issues requiring medical assistance in wheelchair
    sport athletes. There is no indication for this otherwise healthy individual to
    undergo echocardiogram prior to sports clearance.

Rosenbluth J, Lee V, Campbell C, Piatt J, Sandwick S, Kari T. Sports and recreation. In:
    Kirshblum S, Lin VS, editors. Spinal cord medicine. 3rd ed. New York City: Springer
    Publishing Company; 2019. p. 789–98.
Krassioukov A. Autonomic dysfunction and management. In: Kirshblum S, Lin VS, edi-
    tors. Spinal cord medicine. 3rd ed. New York City: Springer Publishing Company; 2019.
    p. 230–45.
Helkowski WM, Ditunno JF Jr, Boninger M. Autonomic dysreflexia: incidence in persons with
    neurologically complete and incomplete tetraplegia. J Spinal Cord Med. 2003;26:244–47.
    https://doi.org/10.1080/10790268.2003.11753691.
Lee V, Rudolph T, Campbell R, et al. Presentation abstracts 1–37 injury epidemiology of
    spinal cord injured participants in the National Veterans Wheelchair Games. J Spinal Cord
    Med. 2017;40(5):579–604.

42. What was the primary reason the practice known as 'boosting' was outlawed by the International Paralympic Committee (IPC)?

    A. Boosting puts those with SCI at an unfair competitive advantage compared to other competitors.
    B. Paralympic records were being broken at an accelerated rate.
    C. Boosting leads to injuries of athletes not participating in this practice.
    D. There are serious health risks related to this practice.

Answer: D.

Boosting is the practice of intentionally causing dysreflexia in those with SCI at or above the level of T6. This is often accomplished by purposefully inducing pain or kinking a Foley catheter. Athletes who partake in 'boosting' experience increased physical performance and a decrease in perceived exertion. Serious health risks exist in those who experience autonomic dysreflexia due to boosting including but not limited to severe hypertension, stroke, seizure, and death. Although boosting may provide an advantage over non-SCI athletes, this is not the primary reason for the IPC's decision to make this practice illegal.

Mazzeo F, Santamaria S, Iavarone A. "Boosting" in paralympic athletes with spinal cord injury: doping without drugs. Funct Neurol. 2015;30(2):91–8.
Rosenbluth J, Lee V, Campbell C, Piatt J, Sandwick S, Kari T. Sports and recreation. In: Kirshblum S, Lin VS, editors. Spinal cord medicine. 3rd ed. New York City: Springer Publishing Company; 2019. p. 789–98.

43. A patient with C6 AIS A SCI who was injured 3 years ago presents for her yearly SCI evaluation. Since you last saw her, she has been doing well overall with no significant medical changes. She continues to participate in outpatient physical and occupational therapy. Her blood pressure today is 92/78, without lightheadedness or dizziness. She monitors her BP at home and does not have reported episodes of autonomic dysreflexia. On examination, you note severe upper limb spasticity with involuntary spasms of the upper and lower limbs. The remainder of her exam is otherwise unremarkable and consistent with her known injury. She requests referral to a Driver Rehabilitation Specialist (DRS) to return to driving. You advise she is not a candidate to drive with an adapted vehicle at this time. What is your reasoning?

    A. Those with complete SCI cannot return to driving.
    B. Severe, uncontrolled upper limb spasticity with involuntary spasms make it dangerous to return to driving.
    C. Patients with a C6 level of injury do not have the necessary hand dexterity to return to driving.
    D. Her low blood pressure puts her at risk for orthostasis and prevents her from being able to drive.

Answer: B.

Severe upper extremity spasticity can prevent an individual with tetraplegia from returning to driving due to their potential inability to manage the adaptive equipment. Increased tone secondary to spasticity can impact the amount of force applied to adaptive controls as well as an individual's reaction time. Involuntary spasms of the upper or lower limbs can unintentionally engage controls. The neurologic level of injury and ASIA impairment scale guide what type of adaptive equipment is needed for an individual to drive an adapted vehicle. The patient's relative hypotension does not preclude her from driving as she does not have any symptoms. Once her upper limb spasticity is under better control, it would be reasonable for her to trial return to driving so long as the medications used to treat spasticity do not affect her reaction time and alertness.

Patopea M, Asanza JL. Driver training after spinal cord injury. In: Kirshblum S, Lin VS, editors. Spinal cord medicine. 3rd ed. New York City: Springer Publishing Company; 2019. p. 799–805.

44. Which acceleration and braking terminal device is most appropriate for an individual with C6 incomplete tetraplegia to utilize in their adapted vehicle?

   A. Tri-pin attached to push–pull angle hand control
   B. Spinner knob attached to push–right angle hand control
   C. Push–rock grip
   D. Classic gas/brake pedal system

Answer: A.

Drivers who have impaired lower extremity strength may benefit from adaptive hand controls. Various styles of hand controls exist to allow for acceleration and braking with the upper extremities. The push-pull hand control is a common hand control for braking and accelerating. To accelerate, the hand control is pulled while it is pushed to brake. Those with tetraplegia often have difficulty operating the mechanical hand controls due to impaired gripping, twisting, or pushing motions. Thus, a terminal device can be fitted to accommodate people with limited hand function. A tri-pin is commonly used in those with proximal arm strength who lack hand functioning. The wrist is placed in a neutral position with three vertical posts located at the medial and lateral sides of the wrist and at the thumb's web space. This allows for the driver to perform the necessary push-pull motions. This is for individuals lacking the necessary wrist and hand function required to grip a spinner knob. A push–rock grip is similar to the function of a motorcycle control. The handle is rotated to accelerate and pushed toward the floor to brake. This would likely not be appropriate in an individual with a C6 level injury.

Patopea M, Asanza JL. Driver training after spinal cord injury. In: Kirshblum S, Lin VS, editors. Spinal cord medicine. 3rd ed. New York City: Springer Publishing Company; 2019. p. 799–805.

45. In which of the following spinal cord injury classifications would it be appropriate to utilize functional electrical stimulation in combination with body-weight supported treadmill training (BWSTT)?

A. L3 AIS A with concomitant lumbosacral plexopathy
B. T4 AIS B with significant lower extremity spasticity
C. T10 AIS C with acute left popliteal DVT
D. C3 AIS B with a phrenic nerve stimulator implanted

Answer: B.

Functional electrical stimulation (FES) is generally categorized into one of three methods of action: direct neuromuscular activation, sensory afferent stimulation, or electrical conduction block. FES, particularly direct neuromuscular activation, can be paired with various types of locomotor training to provide stepping assistance to advance the lower limbs. A patient with a T4 AIS B SCI is an appropriate candidate to utilize FES in combination with BWSTT as several publications have demonstrated improvements in walking speed and distance when FES was combined with BWSTT. Additionally, FES has been shown to have a positive impact on spasticity in persons with SCI.

Those with lower motor neuron (LMN) injuries are not optimal candidates for FES use. When LMN injuries exist, the muscle will not be excitable and will not achieve the necessary contractile forces. Additionally, LMN injuries prevent the benefit of muscle atrophy prevention seen with FES.

Multiple contraindications exist to using FES including but not limited to acute venous thrombosis, an implanted electrical device, malignancy, infection, and epilepsy.

Donovan J, Snider B, Miller A, Kirshblum S. Walking after spinal cord injury: current clinical approaches and future directions. Curr Phys Med Rehabil. 2020;8:149–58. https://doi.org/10.1007/s40141-020-00277-1.

Mills PB, Dossa F. Transcutaneous electrical nerve stimulation for management of limb spasticity. Am J Phys Med Rehabil. 2016;95(4):309–18. https://doi.org/10.1097/PHM.0000000000000437.

Brose SW, Kilgore KL, Triolo R, DiMarco AF, Bourbeau DJ, Nemunaitis G. Functional electric stimulation for patients with spinal cord injury. In: Kirshblum S, Lin VS, editors. Spinal cord medicine. 3rd ed. New York City: Springer Publishing Company; 2019. p. 806–30.

46. In regards to improving functional independence in cervical level SCI patients with surgical reconstruction, which of the following motor levels and treatment options is correctly paired?

A. C5; brachioradialis to extensor carpi radialis brevis for wrist extension
B. C6; extensor carpi radialis brevis to flexor digitorum pollicis to restore palmar grasp

C. C7; posterior deltoid to triceps to restore elbow extension

D. C8; brachioradialis to extensor pollicis longus for lateral pinch

Answer: A.

The brachioradialis (BR) is the most readily available and versatile muscle for reconstructive transfers in tetraplegia. Since C5 SCI patients have a strong biceps brachii and brachialis, the BR is commonly sacrificed without impact on the patient's elbow flexion. A variety of tendon transfers using the BR have been described: BR to extensor carpi radialis brevis (ECRB) for wrist extension, BR to flexor digitorum profundus (FDP) for palmar grasp, BR to flexor pollicis longus (FPL) for lateral pinch.

Because wrist extension is critical to the tenodesis grasp function, extreme care is needed before sacrificing in surgical hand restoration. A wrist extensor is only a suitable donor when there are at least two muscles under voluntary control. The ECRB, has a central insertion on the base of the long finger metacarpal which produces wrist extension with minimal radial/ulnar deviation. When transferring one of the voluntary wrist extensors, the extensor carpi radialis (ECRL) is chosen to restore lateral pinch or palmar grasp depending on functional needs.

A patient with a C7 motor level will have $\geq 4/5$ strength with elbow extension and will not require surgical reconstruction to improve triceps strength. A posterior deltoid to triceps to restore elbow extension would be more appropriate in a patient with a C5 or C6 motor level.

Lateral pinch involves four phases: object acquisition, pinch/grasp, hold/manipulation, and object release. The BR can be transferred around the radius before inserting onto the FPL to allow for lateral pinch of the thumb against the index finger. Option D is incorrect as transfer should be to the FPL, not EPL.

Mills PB, Dossa F. Transcutaneous electrical nerve stimulation for management of limb spasticity. Am J Phys Med Rehabil. 2016;95(4):309–18. https://doi.org/10.1097/PHM.0000000000000437.

Brose SW, Kilgore KL, Triolo R, DiMarco AF, Bourbeau DJ, Nemunaitis G. Functional electric stimulation for patients with spinal cord injury. In: Kirshblum S, Lin VS, editors. Spinal cord medicine. 3rd ed. New York City: Springer Publishing Company; 2019. p. 806–30.

47. Which of the following is true regarding ankle dorsiflexion-assist surface stimulators?

    A. They are associated with decreased metabolic cost of walking compared to an ankle-foot orthosis.
    B. Use leads to slower gait speeds compared to ankle-foot orthoses.
    C. Users often prefer standard ankle-foot orthoses over dorsiflexion-assist stimulators.
    D. They are most appropriate for those with $\leq 2/5$ knee extension strength.

Answer: A.

Ankle dorsiflexion-assist surface stimulators, also called foot drop stimulators, are a form of functional electrical stimulation that utilizes surface electrical stimulation to activate the user's neuromuscular system to assist with gait. Stimulation of the common peroneal nerve results in assisted dorsiflexion. Compared to an ankle-foot orthosis (AFO), dorsiflexion-assist stimulators have been found to have a decreased metabolic cost of walking. Review of ambulation speed did not differ between standard AFO and dorsiflexion-assist stimulators. Literature suggests users prefer dorsiflexion-assist stimulators as they provide active assistance through muscle stimulation and can be worn with a wide variety of shoe types. Dorsiflexion-assist stimulators are most useful for those with good hip and knee control and who simply require some assistance for toe clearance during the swing phase of gait.

Stein RB, Everaert DG, Thompson AK, Chong Sl, Whittaker M, Robertson J, Kuether Get. Long-term therapeutic and orthotic effects of a foot drop stimulator on walking performance in progressive and nonprogressive neurological disorders. Neurorehabil Neural Repair. 2010;24(2):152–167. https://doi.org/10.1177/1545968309347681.

Everaert DG, Stein RB, Abrams GM, Dromerick AW, Francisco GE, Hafner BJ, Huskey TN, Munin MC, Nolan KJ, Kufta VK. Effect of a foot-drop stimulator and ankle–foot orthosis on walking performance after stroke: a multicenter randomized controlled trial. Neurorehabil Neural Repair. 2013;27(7):579–91. https://doi.org/10.1177/1545968313481278.

Burridge JH, Taylor PN, Hagan SA, Wood DE, Swain ID. The effects of common peroneal stimulation on the effort and speed of walking: a randomized controlled trial with chronic hemiplegic patients. Clin Rehabil. 1997;11(3):201–10. https://doi.org/10.1177/026921559701100303.

Field-Fote EC, Nieves L, Hartigan C. Advanced mobility and strategies to promote walking function after spinal cord injury. In: Kirshblum S, Lin VS, editors. Spinal cord medicine. 3rd ed. New York City: Springer Publishing Company; 2019. p. 728–43.

48. Which of the following is true of an intramuscular (IM) diaphragm pacing system compared to conventional phrenic nerve stimulators?

A. There are no advantages of IM diaphragm pacing over conventional phrenic nerve stimulators.
B. IM diaphragm pacing electrode wires are tunneled subcutaneously without wires exiting the body.
C. IM diaphragm pacing reduces the risk of potential surgical injuries as manipulation of the phrenic nerve is avoided.
D. Surgical implantation of IM diaphragm pacing electrodes requires an open surgical approach which leads to significantly increased costs.

Answer: C.

There are two basic diaphragm pacing configurations including conventional systems that are fully implanted with activation via radio frequency transmission which stimulate the phrenic nerve and the more recently designed IM diaphragm pacing. The latter involves a percutaneous system from which electrode wires exit the skin. With IM diaphragm pacing, stimulators are placed on the phrenic nerve motor points within the diaphragm so signal transduction through the diaphragm is uniform and contraction is coordinated. Thus, both configurations require an intact phrenic nerve for maximal efficacy.

Literature suggests IM diaphragm pacing and conventional pacing devices are able to maintain ventilatory support in patients with ventilator-dependent tetraplegia at similar success rates. IM diaphragm pacing does have some advantages due to implantation via a laparoscopic procedure resulting in avoidance of phrenic nerve manipulation, decreased costs, and overall reduced surgical risk. One limitation of the IM system is the percutaneous nature of the system resulting in electrode wires exiting the skin.

Brose SW, Kilgore KL, Triolo R, DiMarco AF, Bourbeau DJ, Nemunaitis G. Functional electric stimulation for patients with spinal cord injury. In: Kirshblum S, Lin VS, editors. Spinal cord medicine. 3rd ed. New York City: Springer Publishing Company; 2019. p. 806–30.

DiMarco AF, Onders RP, Ignagni A, Kowalski KA, Mortimer JT. Phrenic nerve pacing via intramuscular diaphragm electrodes in tetraplegic subjects. Chest. 2005;127(2):671–8. https://doi.org/10.1378/chest.127.2.671.

DiMarco AF, Onders RP, Kowalski KE, Miller ME, Ferek S, Mortimer JT. Phrenic nerve pacing in a tetraplegic patient via intramuscular diaphragm electrodes. Am J Respir Crit Care Med. 2002;166:1604–6. https://doi.org/10.1164/rccm.200203-175CR.

Elefteriades JA, Quin JA, Hogan JF, Holcomb WG, Lets GV, Chlosta WF, Glenn W. Long-term follow-up of pacing of the conditioned diaphragm in quadriplegia. Pacing Clin Electrophysiol. 2002;25(6):897–906. https://doi.org/10.1046/j.1460-9592.2002.00897.

49. A 33-year-old male with a diagnosis of T8 AIS B SCI sustained 5 years ago after falling off a ladder is seen in clinic for routine, yearly evaluation. He has been doing very well and for the past few months has been completing an exercise program with a personal trainer. Now that he has established a routine, he requests an exercise prescription to improve his body composition and decrease his cardiovascular risk. He has otherwise been healthy with no notable contraindications to exercise. Your prescription includes:

A. 3–5 sessions per week of moderate to vigorous intensity upper-body aerobic exercise for 30–44 min
B. 5–7 sessions per week of vigorous intensity upper-body aerobic exercise for 45–60 min
C. 2–3 sessions per week of moderate to vigorous intensity upper-body aerobic exercise for 50–60 min combined with upper-body strength exercise of 3 sets of 12 repetitions, at 75–90% 1 rep max for all large muscle groups
D. 2–3 sessions per week of moderate to vigorous intensity upper-body aerobic exercise for 20–30 min combined with upper-body strength exercise of 3 sets of 10 repetitions, at 50–80% 1 rep max for all large muscle groups

Answer: A.

Ginis et al. (2017) completed a systematic review to develop exercise guidelines for cardiometabolic health benefits in the SCI population. Guidelines were published regarding two types of exercises: combined upper-body aerobic plus strength exercise (options C and D); and upper-body aerobic exercise only (options A and B). For cardiometabolic health benefits including body composition and reducing cardiovascular risk, adults with a SCI are suggested to engage in 3–5 sessions per week of moderate to vigorous intensity upper-body aerobic exercise for 30–44 min. Performing the same regimen for 20–44 min resulted in improved cardiorespiratory fitness without evidence of improved body composition or cardiovascular risk.

Regarding combined upper-body aerobic plus strength training, 2–3 sessions per week of moderate to vigorous intensity upper-body aerobic exercise for 20–30 min combined with upper-body strength exercise [3 sets of 10 repetitions, at 50–80% of 1 rep max for all large muscle groups] resulted in improved cardiorespiratory fitness, power output, and muscle strength.

Option B provides an exercise prescription where the aerobic training is too frequent, too intense, and for too long. Option C provides a prescription where the aerobic training is too long, with a strengthening program that is too intense.

Ginis KAM, van der Scheer JW, Latimer-Cheung AE, et al. Evidence-based scientific exercise guidelines for adults with spinal cord injury: an update and a new guideline. Spinal Cord. 2017;56(4):308–21. https://doi.org/10.1038/s41393-017-0017-3.

Nash MS, Bilzon JLJ. Therapeutic exercise after spinal cord injury. In: Kirshblum S, Lin VS, editors. Spinal cord medicine. 3rd ed. New York City: Springer Publishing Company; 2019. p. 806–30.

50. Which of the following is a benefit of voluntary arm exercising training with moderate-intensity arm crank ergometry in the SCI population?

    A. Improved high-density lipoprotein (HDL) levels
    B. Decreased peripheral insulin sensitivity
    C. Increased shoulder abduction and adduction strength
    D. Increased VO$_2$peak

Answer: A.

SCI literature suggests the presence of selective dyslipidemia involving low HDL levels (<40 mg/dL) in up to 47% of persons with SCI. Evidence shows moderate intensity voluntary arm ergometry performed three times per week has a favorable impact on HDL levels. Additionally, low-density lipoprotein (LDL) has been shown to decrease with similar exercise regimens. Although Nightingale et al. (2017) showed moderate-intensity arm exercise improved hepatic insulin sensitivity, there is limited evidence to suggest peripheral insulin sensitivity improvement in chronic paraplegia with arm exercise. Moderate to high-intensity arm ergometry has been shown to increase strength of the elbow flexors and shoulder extensors. The same training regimen has not been shown to increase shoulder abduction or adduction strength nor has arm ergometry been shown to strengthen scapulothoracic motion.

Hooker SP, Wells CL. Effects of low- and moderate-intensity training in spinal cord-injured persons. Med Sci Sports Exerc. 1989;21(1):18–22. https://doi.org/10.1249/000057 68-198902000-00004.

Jacobs PL, Nash MS, Rusinowski JW. Circuit resistance training enhances cardiorespiratory endurance and muscular strength in persons with paraplegia. Med Sci Sports Exerc. 2001;33(5):711–7.

Nash MS, Jacobs PL, Mendez AJ, Goldberg RB. Circuit resistance training improves the atherogenic lipid profile in persons with chronic paraplegia. J Spinal Cord Med. 2001;24(1):2–9. https://doi.org/10.1080/10790268.2001.11753548.

de Groot PC, Hjeltnes N, Heijboer AC, Stal W, Birkeland K. Effect of training intensity on physical capacity, lipid profile and insulin sensitivity in early rehabilitation of spinal cord injured individuals. Spinal Cord. 2003;41(12):673–9. https://doi.org/10.1038/ sj.sc.3101534.

Nightingale TE, Walhin J-P, Thompson D, Bilzon JLJ. Impact of exercise on cardiometabolic component risks in spinal cord-injured humans. Med Sci Sport Exerc. 2017;49(12):2469. https://doi.org/10.1249/MSS.0000000000001390.

Nash MS, Bilzon JLJ. Therapeutic exercise after spinal cord injury. In: Kirshblum S, Lin VS, editors. Spinal cord medicine. 3rd ed. New York City: Springer Publishing Company; 2019. p. 806–30.

51. In a person with a C7 AIS A SCI, which of the following is true regarding physiologic response to exercise?

    A. Energy expenditure during upper body exercise is equivalent to able-bodied individuals.
    B. Oxygen uptake is higher with lower limb exercise at equivalent power output when compared to upper limb exercise.
    C. At equivalent power output, arm cranking leads to decreased heart rate and decreased peripheral resistance compared to lower extremity exercise.
    D. Heart rate during maximal exercise will rarely exceed 110–130 beats/min.

Answer: D.

Individuals with complete lesions above the T1 level rely on circulating catecholamines and parasympathetic withdrawal to increase their heart rate due to lack of central control sympathetic innervation to the heart. Because of this, heart rate during maximal exercise rarely exceeds 110–130 beats/min.

Energy expenditure during exercise in persons with SCI is reduced when compared to equivalent able-bodied individuals, often with expenditure values 30–75% that of able-bodied counterparts. The capacity to expend energy during exercise is reduced in persons with SCI. At any given equivalent power output, oxygen uptake is higher for arm than leg work due to lower mechanical efficiency of arm exercise. This discrepancy in oxygen uptake may be due to a greater reliance on less efficient muscle fibers and varying cardiovascular responses elicited by arm cycling. Arm exercise results in lower mechanical and metabolic efficiency which increases susceptibility to fatigue and reduces exercise tolerance time.

Although cardiac output is similar in both upper and lower limb exercise at equivalent power output, arm cranking results in a higher HR and increased total peripheral resistance.

Price M. Energy expenditure and metabolism during exercise in persons with a spinal cord injury. Sports Mede. 2010;40(8):681–96. https://doi.org/10.2165/115319 60-000000000-00000.

Pendergast DR. Cardiovascular, respiratory, and metabolic responses to upper body exercise. Med Sci Sport Exerc. 1989;21(5 Suppl):S121–5. https://doi.org/10.1249/000057 68-198910001-00002.

Nash MS, Bilzon JLJ. Therapeutic exercise after spinal cord injury. In: Kirshblum S, Lin VS, editors. Spinal cord medicine. 3rd ed. New York City: Springer Publishing Company; 2019. p. 806–30.

52. Regarding high intensity interval training (HIIT) in the SCI population, which of the following is true?

A. HIIT can improve VO_2peak.
B. Body composition is improved at greater rates with HIIT compared to moderate intensity training.
C. HIIT is not appropriate for those with motor complete lesions.
D. Arm ergometry exercise cannot be used for HIIT.

Answer: A.

High intensity interval training (HIIT) involves exercise performed in intervals at vigorous intensities above the steady state of lactate production. This results in accumulation of intramuscular and systemic metabolites that cause fatigue. For this reason, vigorous intervals are separated by low intensity or resting recovery. HIIT in SCI patients has demonstrated substantial improvements in VO2peak compared to moderate intensity continuous training. This improvement may be secondary to peripheral muscle adaptations, particularly increases in absolute mitochondrial capacity allowing for greater muscle oxygen utilization. Body composition changes appear to be similar with HIIT and moderate intensity continuous training protocols. Motor complete injuries have been studied in HIIT protocols without reported adverse outcomes when age and comorbidity are matched to motor incomplete injuries. Multiple studies have conducted HIIT protocols with the use of an arm ergometry.

de Groot PC, Hjeltnes N, Heijboer AC, Stal W, Birkeland K. Effect of training intensity on physical capacity, lipid profile and insulin sensitivity in early rehabilitation of spinal cord injured individuals. Spinal Cord. 2003;41(12):673–9. https://doi.org/10.1038/sj.sc.3101534.

Harnish CR, Daniels JA, Caruso D. Training response to high-intensity interval training in a 42-year-old man with chronic spinal cord injury. J Spinal Cord Med. 2017;40(2):246–9. https://doi.org/10.1080/10790268.2015.1136783.

Tjønna AE, Lee SJ, Rognmo Ø, et al. Aerobic interval training versus continuous moderate exercise as a treatment for the metabolic syndrome: a pilot study. Circulation. 2008;118(4):346–54. https://doi.org/10.1161/CIRCULATIONAHA.108.772822.

Nash MS, Bilzon JLJ. Therapeutic exercise after spinal cord injury. In: Kirshblum S, Lin VS, editors. Spinal cord medicine. 3rd ed. New York City: Springer Publishing Company; 2019. p. 806–30.

53. You are seeing a 40-year-old female who is 8 years post-injury who has a classification of C6 AIS C. She has recently initiated an exercise program with hopes of improving upper extremity function. She has been performing moderate intensity arm ergometry three times per week for three months but notes no change in upper extremity strength or improved performance with ADLs. She asks for advice to change her regimen to improve her daily tasks, particularly feeding and household cleaning. You advise:

    A. Increase frequency of arm ergometry exercises.
    B. Increase intensity of arm ergometry exercises.
    C. Incorporate resistance training of the upper extremities.
    D. There is little that can be done to improve function given the chronicity of her injury.

    Answer: C.

    Literature suggests that resistance exercise of the upper limbs is more effective than arm ergometry exercises for arm strengthening. Arm ergometry exercises fail to target strength improvement of the scapular stabilizers which are involved in the performance of ADLs. Strength training of the scapular muscles utilizing rowing and standard scapular retraction exercises resulted in improvement of scapular retractor strength.

    Cooney MM, Walker JB. Hydraulic resistance exercise benefits cardiovascular fitness of spinal cord injured. Med Sci Sports Exerc. 1986;18(5):522–5. https://doi.org/10.1249/00005768-198610000-00005.

    Olenik LM, Laskin JJ, Burnham R, Wheeler GD, Steadward RD. Efficacy of rowing, backward wheeling and isolated scapular retractor exercise as remedial strength activities for wheelchair users: application of electromyography. Paraplegia. 1995;33(3):148–52. https://doi.org/10.1038/sc.1995.32.

    Nash MS, Bilzon JLJ. Therapeutic exercise after spinal cord injury. In: Kirshblum S, Lin VS, editors. Spinal cord medicine. 3rd ed. New York City: Springer Publishing Company; 2019. p. 806–30.

54. While completing rounds on your acute inpatient SCI rehabilitation unit, the speech therapist stops you to discuss one of your patients. The 23-year-old patient was diagnosed with a C4 AIS C spinal cord injury 4 weeks ago after diving into shallow water. He recently initiated ventilator weaning and is now tolerating being off the ventilator for 6 h/day. He has a plastic, cuffed, 8 mm tracheostomy tube in place with the cuff inflated. The speech therapist reports

the patient's frustration about inability to produce audible speech at this time which is making communication with staff difficult. To improve the patient's voice quality, you would recommend:

A. Application of a speaking valve to the end of the tracheostomy tube with the cuff inflated.
B. Tracheostomy cuff deflation to allow air to the vocal cords for speech improved production.
C. Removing the patient's abdominal binder while upright to allow for more air movement.
D. Referral for phrenic nerve stimulator implantation to improve speech.

Answer: B.

Aiding patients with tetraplegia in speech production is extremely important, as it allows for effective communication with the family and hospital staff. Deflating the tracheostomy cuff is the first step as it allows for air flow across the vocal cords resulting in improved speech production. While on the ventilator, after deflating the tracheostomy cuff, tidal volume can be maintained by increasing the tidal volume setting on the ventilator to compensate for air loss across the larynx. Cuff deflation also reduces pressure on the esophagus posteriorly which may facilitate swallowing.

Some studies have also shown that cuff deflation reduces the time to decannulation and the incidence of respiratory tract infections. A speaking valve is a one-way valve designed to open when the patient takes a breath and close when they exhale. With the valve closed, air is forced into the airway across the vocal cords. If a speaking valve is going to be used, the tracheostomy cuff must be deflated. Failure to deflate the cuff will result in the patient being unable to exhale.

Use of abdominal binders has been shown to increase vital capacity allowing for more air movement.

Given the acuity of this patient's injury and his ability to tolerate early ventilator weaning trials, phrenic nerve stimulation would not be an appropriate consideration at this time.

Brown R, DiMarco AF, Hoit JD, et al. Respiratory Dysfunction and Management in Spinal Cord Injury. Respir Care. 2006;51(8):853–70.

MacBean N, Ward E, Murdoch B, Cahill L, Solley M, Geraghty T, Hukins C. Optimizing speech production in the ventilator-assisted individual following cervical spinal cord injury: a preliminary investigation. Int Lang Commun Disord. 2009;44:382–93. https://doi.org/10.1080/13682820802190339.

Goldman JM, Rose LS, Williams SJ, Silver JR, Denison DM. Effect of abdominal binders on breathing in tetraplegic patients. Thorax. 1986;41:940–5. https://doi.org/10.1136/thx.41.12.940.

DiMarco AF. Respiratory and sleep disorders in spinal cord dysfunction. In: Kirshblum S, Lin VS, editors. Spinal cord medicine. 3rd ed. New York City: Springer Publishing Company; 2019. p. 246–68.

55. You are caring for a 32-year-old male with a C4 AIS B SCI in acute inpatient rehabilitation who is currently ventilator dependent. His wife feels he is ready to start ventilator weaning trials. Which of the following is true regarding when it is appropriate to begin weaning trials?

   A. Initial weaning should occur while the patient is asleep to prevent anxiety.
   B. When vital capacity exceeds 10–15 mL/kg.
   C. When maximum inspiratory pressure is greater than 40 cmH$_2$O.
   D. When oxygen saturation can be maintained with 70% FiO$_2$.

Answer: B.

Prior to weaning attempts in the SCI population, pulmonary function must be assessed. Certain parameters should be met before ventilator weaning takes place. Vital capacity (VC) is a measure of overall pulmonary function. Those with severely reduced VC may require assisted ventilation. VC should be evaluated and weaning attempts should be withheld until VC measurements exceed 10–15 mL/kg of ideal body weight.

   Additionally, patients should be awake, have alert mental status, and be able to manage airway secretions. Maximum inspiratory pressure (MIP) can be used to assess inspiratory muscle strength. MIP values should be −20 cmH$_2$O or more negative. Adequate oxygenation should be maintained with use of <50% FiO$_2$ and PEEP <5 cmH$_2$O.

Vázquez RG, Sedes PR, Fariña MM, Marqués AM, Velasco MEF. Respiratory management in the patient with spinal cord injury. BioMed Res Int. 2013;2013:1–12. https://doi.org/10.1155/2013/168757.

DiMarco AF. Respiratory and sleep disorders in spinal cord dysfunction. In: Kirshblum S, Lin VS, editors. Spinal cord medicine. 3rd ed. New York City: Springer Publishing Company; 2019. p. 246–68.

Non-Traumatic Spinal Cord Injury

18

Samir R. Belagaje

Questions

1. A 52-year-old male presents with slowly progressive spasticity and paresthesias in their lower extremities. Neurological examination shows increased deep tendon reflexes with positive Babinski's sign bilaterally and a stocking-glove distribution pattern of sensory loss in their lower extremities. Which of the following pieces of information would NOT support the diagnosis of nitrous oxide toxicity?

   A. The patient is a dentist.
   B. Vitamin B12 deficiency seen on lab evaluations.
   C. Patient admits to using "Whippets" (whip cream canisters) recreationally.
   D. Patient works as a residential and commercial lead inspector.

   Answer: D.

   Nitrous oxide toxicity can cause a myelopathy in the spinal cord. The pathophysiology is thought to involve interference with vitamin B12 metabolism leading to a B12 deficiency. This is seen serologically with a decreased vitamin B12 level as well as clinically through a syndrome of subacute combined degeneration similar to traditional vitamin B12 deficiency. The risk factors for developing nitrous oxide toxicity include being a dentist because of its use as an anesthetic and recreational drug abuse in the form of nitrous oxide chargers traditionally used in whip cream canisters (hence the name "whippets").

S. R. Belagaje (✉)
Department of Neurology, Emory University, Atlanta, GA, USA

Department of Rehabilitation Medicine, Emory University, Atlanta, GA, USA
e-mail: sbelaga@emory.edu

Thompson AG, Leite MI, Lunn MP, Bennett DL. Whippits, nitrous oxide and the dangers of legal highs. Pract Neurol. 2015;15(3):207–9. https://doi.org/10.1136/practneurol-2014-001071.

Layzer RB. Myeloneuropathy after prolonged exposure to nitrous oxide. Lancet. 1978;2(8102):1227–30. https://doi.org/10.1016/s0140-6736(78)92101-3.

2. Which of the following is true of hereditary spastic paraplegia?

   A. It is transmitted through generations solely through an autosomal dominant pattern.
   B. Treatment involves riluzole.
   C. It is a slowly progressive spastic paraparesis due to degeneration of cortico-spinal and spinocerebellar tracts.
   D. Baclofen should be avoided in the management of spasticity.

   Answer: C.

   Hereditary spastic paraplegia is a group of inherited neurological diseases characterized by slowly progressive spastic paraparesis. There is a wide variety of genetic causes. While 2/3 of the causes are autosomal dominant variants, there are also autosomal recessive and X-linked forms. The mutations cause degeneration of corticospinal tracts as well spinocerebellar tracts. It should be suspected if there is a positive familial history, association with other signs, such as cerebellar ataxia, early cognitive impairment, or peripheral neuropathy.

   Riluzole does not have a role in the treatment of these diseases as it is a treatment in amyotrophic lateral sclerosis (ALS). There is no cure for these diseases so management primarily aimed at symptomatic treatments, with one example being baclofen for spasticity.

Lallemant-Dudek P, Durr A. Clinical and genetic update of hereditary spastic paraparesis. Rev Neurol (Paris). 2021;177(5):550–6. https://doi.org/10.1016/j.neurol.2020.07.001. Epub 2020 Aug 15.

3. A 48-year-old male presents with a 10-year history of a slowly progressive motor neuron disease. Based on evaluation and testing, patient is given the diagnosis of Kennedy's disease. Assuming the diagnosis is correct, which of the following is NOT true?

   A. The condition is associated with testicular atrophy
   B. This is an X-linked recessive genetic disorder due to a CAG trinucleotide repeat in the androgen receptor gene
   C. It can mimic ALS
   D. Females get more fatal versions of this disease

   Answer: D.

Kennedy's Disease also known as Spinal and Bulbar Muscular Atrophy (SBMA) is caused by a polyglutamine (polyQ) expansion in the androgen receptor (AR). This is due to a CAG trinucleotide repeat in the androgen receptor gene on the X-chromosome. The majority of SBMA patients have a clinical presentation which initially begins with proximal lower limb weakness, with symptom onset typically occurring in men between 30 and 50 years of age. Additional symptoms appear over time and include tremor, muscle cramps, fasciculations, dysarthria, and dysphagia. The predominance of neuromuscular symptoms in SBMA corresponds with disease pathology, which is characterized by a loss of lower motor neurons in the anterior horn of the spinal cord and in the brainstem. This is similar to ALS. Females display a markedly less severe phenotype, but it is notable that they can develop weight loss and motor function deficits later in life.

Arnold FJ, Merry DE. Molecular mechanisms and therapeutics for SBMA/Kennedy's disease. Neurotherapeutics. 2019;16(4):928–47. https://doi.org/10.1007/s13311-019-00790-9.

4. A 29-year-old female presents with gradual onset of parasthesias in the hands and feet and fatigue, followed by slow progression of spastic paraparesis. Assuming the patient has vitamin B12 deficiency, which of the following is false?

   A. Patient's vegetarian diet may be contributing.
   B. Labs can show microcytosis, and decreased serum level of methylmalonic acid.
   C. Subacute combined degeneration tends to affect the corticospinal tracts and dorsal columns of the spinal cords.
   D. The underlying cause is due to defective methionine production.

Answer: B.

Vitamin B12 is an important cofactor for enzyme methionine synthase which catalyzes synthesis of methionine from homocysteine. The deficit in methionine production is thought to be responsible for the neurologic symptoms. Vitamin B12 deficiency causes several neurologic conditions including optic atrophy (leading to visual loss), and spinal cord injury. In the spinal cord, it preferentially affects the dorsal columns and corticospinal tracts leading to the syndrome of subacute combined degeneration where patients experience insidious onset of parasthesias in hands and feet, gait problems due to sensory ataxia, and subsequent paraparesis.

The diagnosis is made with clinical suspicions and laboratory work-up which show macrocytic (megaloblastic) anemia, decreased serum B12, increased serum homocysteine and methylmalonic acid.

Risk factors include those on vegetarian diet, malnutrition, alcoholism, elderly age and those with gastrointestinal disease.

Langan RC, Goodbred AJ. Vitamin B12 deficiency: recognition and management. Am Fam Physician. 2017;96(6):384–89.

Rizzo G, Laganà AS, Rapisarda AM, La Ferrera GM, Buscema M, Rossetti P, Nigro A, Muscia V, Valenti G, Sapia F, Sarpietro G, Zigarelli M, Vitale SG. Vitamin B12 among vegetarians: status, assessment and supplementation. Nutrients. 2016;8(12):767. https://doi.org/10.3390/nu8120767.

5. What is the most common cause of extradural spinal tumors in elderly?

   A. Metastases
   B. Osteoid sarcomas
   C. Lymphoma
   D. Primary intramedullary tumors

Answer: A.

There are a wide variety of neoplasms in an adult. In elderly individuals, the most common type of tumor is of metastatic origin. Health care providers should attempt to identify the primary cancer through a systemic evaluation. The most frequent spinal metastases (60%) are from breast, lung, or prostate cancer. The chance that an elderly patient (60–79 years old) is affected by bony metastases is four times higher in men and three times higher in women than a middle-aged patient (40–59 years old).

Aebi M. Spinal metastasis in the elderly. Eur Spine J. 2003;12(Suppl 2):S202–13. https://doi.org/10.1007/s00586-003-0609-9. Epub 2003 Sept 23.

6. The pathology of ALS:

   A. Is due to neuronal loss of anterior horn cells
   B. Occurs in the majority of patients
   C. Responds to immunosuppressive treatments such as intravenous immunoglobulins
   D. Can be associated with a history of prior heavy metal exposure

Answer: A.

Amyotrophic lateral sclerosis (ALS) is a progressive neurodegenerative disorder of motor systems. Gross pathology of the spinal cord reveals neuronal loss of anterior horn cells and rarefaction of ventral horns.

The majority of cases are sporadic with only 10% of cases having a familial and hereditary causes with SOD1 gene mutations.

van den Bos MAJ, Geevasinga N, Higashihara M, Menon P, Vucic S. Pathophysiology and diagnosis of ALS: insights from advances in neurophysiological techniques. Int J Mol Sci. 2019;20(11):2818. https://doi.org/10.3390/ijms20112818.

7. Which of the following vignettes is most consistent with the diagnosis of surfer's myelopathy?

   A. 23-year-old female with history of multiple sclerosis who presents with myalgias and numbness in her right arm after getting stung by a jellyfish while surfing in the Pacific Ocean
   B. 54-year-old male who is an experienced surfer who presents with bilateral lower extremity weakness, a T11 sensory level and bladder and bowel incontinence after suffering a fall while surfing. Imaging shows thoracic spine fractures.
   C. 27-year-old male novice surfer who felt progressive and rapid lower extremity weakness while surfing. Magnetic resonance imaging (MRI) of the spine shows T2 longitudinal hyperintensities from the mid-thoracic level to the conus
   D. 35-year-old male who is a professional surfer presents with quadriplegia. Imaging shows cervical spine hyperintensities as well as lesions in the brain.

Answer: C.

Surfer's myelopathy is a rare, nontraumatic spinal cord injury. Spinal MRI appears similar to ischemic lesions and may demonstrate longitudinally extensive, central T2 hyperintense signal abnormality in the spinal cord and is associated with spinal cord swelling. It is seen in beginner surfers and the etiology is suspected to be due to ischemia of the thoracic region due to compression of vasculature (particularly the artery of Adamkiewicz) due to prolonged prone hyperextension.

Choi JH, Ha JK, Kim CH, Park JH. Surfer's myelopathy: case series and literature review. J Korean Neurosurg Soc. 2018;61(6):767–73. https://doi.org/10.3340/jkns.2017.0262. Epub 2018 Oct 30.

8. Which of the following is a typical feature of early myelopathy due to radiation?

   A. It is usually transient with a good prognosis.
   B. The onset occurs within days of radiation treatment.
   C. The symptoms involve diaphragmatic paralysis and weakness of the arms.
   D. The amount of radiation is not related to the risk.

Answer: A.

Acute myelopathy is a transient syndrome with a good prognosis. It usually occurs 3–6 months after completion of radiation therapy. The symptoms are limited to Lhermitte's sign and parasthesias in the extremities and has a good prognosis. Patients receiving radiation of 4000 cGy to the spinal cord appear to be at the highest risk.

Rampling R, Symonds P. Radiation myelopathy. Curr Opin Neurol. 1998;11(6):627–32. https://doi.org/10.1097/00019052-199812000-00003.

9. Which of the following is FALSE regarding adrenomyeloneuropathy?

   A. This disease is due to mutation in the gene producing very long chain fatty acids (VLCFA).
   B. Unlike adrenoleukodystrophy, this condition presents later in life (i.e. adulthood) and has a milder phenotype.
   C. Females are affected more severely than males.
   D. Treatment involves steroid replacement for adrenal insufficiency, physical therapy and treatment of symptomatic spasticity.

Answer: C.

Adrenomyeloneuropathy is a variant of adrenoleukodystrophy and tends to affect young adults. Adrenoleukodystrophy is a genetic disease which is inherited as X-linked recessive pattern. Therefore, females tend to be asymptomatic or develop myelopathy later in life. A gene mutation in the ABCD gene affects metabolism of very long fatty acid chains (VLFAC). It mostly affects boys between 5 and 8 years old. It may cause behavioral changes, muscle cramps, difficulty walking, swallowing problems, hearing loss, seizures and other symptoms.

By contrast, those with adrenomyeloneuropathy generally begin to develop features in their late 20s. Signs and symptoms may include progressive stiffness and weakness of the legs, ataxia, speech difficulties, adrenal insufficiency, sexual dysfunction, and bladder control issues. Treatment of adrenomyeloneuropathy varies based on the signs and symptoms in each affected person. For instance, steroid replacement therapy may be prescribed in people with adrenal insufficiency. Physical therapy is also be recommended to help build and maintain muscle strength.

Azar C, Shor N, Nadjar Y. Adrenomyeloneuropathy masquerading as chronic myelitis. JAMA Neurol. 2020;77(4):522–3. https://doi.org/10.1001/jamaneurol.2020.0019.

10. Which of the following is true regarding bilevel positive airway pressure (BiPAP) ventilation in the management of ALS?

   A. It should be avoided to minimize chances of life-long dependence.
   B. It can be used in prevention of ALS.
   C. It can significantly prolong survival and slow the decline of FVC.
   D. It should only be used concomitantly with riluzole to see any benefit.

Answer: C.

Amyotrophic lateral sclerosis (ALS) is a progressive, neurodegenerative disease affecting motor tracts in the brain and spinal cord. There is no definitive cure. Non-invasive BiPAP-ventilation has proven to be helpful to manage the increasing hypoventilation due to weakness in ventilatory muscles in ALS.

Moreover, studies have shown that it can significantly prolong survival and maintain pulmonary function. Therefore, patients with ALS should have periodic pulmonary function testing and start BIPAP ventilation as early as possible in the course of the disease.

Kleopa KA, Sherman M, Neal B, Romano GJ, Heiman-Patterson T. Bipap improves survival and rate of pulmonary function decline in patients with ALS. J Neurol Sci. 1999;164(1):82–8. https://doi.org/10.1016/s0022-510x(99)00045-3.

11. Lhermitte's sign is specifically indicative of:

    A. Lesions involving dorsal columns of cervical/thoracic spinal cord
    B. Human T-lymphotropic virus type 1 (HTLV-1)
    C. Neuromyelitis optica
    D. Multiple sclerosis

Answer: A.

Lhermitte's sign describes a transient sensation of an electric shock extending down the spine and/or extremities upon flexion of the neck, often a sequela of neurologic disease. It was first described by Marie and Chatelin in 1917. Lhermitte described it in multiple sclerosis (MS) with which it is most commonly associated. Although most associated with MS, any myelopathic process affecting the dorsal columns can lead to this sign, including demyelinating infections, radiation treatment, and neuromyelitis optica.

Gemici C. Lhermitte's sign: Review with special emphasis in oncology practice. Crit Rev Oncol Hematol. 2010;74(2):79–86. https://doi.org/10.1016/j.critrevonc.2009.04.009. Epub 2009 Jun 2.

12. A 45-year-old male choreographer presented with progressive left leg paresis and decreased sensation on the right side of his body from his abdomen to his thigh. Physical examination revealed trace weakness of the left leg and decreased sensation to pinprick in the right leg without a clear sensory level. MRI revealed a fluid filled cavity in the middle of the c-spine between C5 and C8.

    His findings are most consistent with:

    A. Subacute combined degeneration
    B. Syringohydromyelia
    C. Cervical stenosis
    D. Radiation exposure

Answer: B.

The MRI findings and imaging are most consistent with syringohydromyelia. Syringohydromyelia is characterized by a fluid-filled cavity within the spinal cord. While terminology is often used interchangeably, hydromyelia refers to distention of the central canal which is lined by ependyma, syringomyelia refers to a cavitary lesion within the cord parenchyma which is not lined by ependyma, syringohydromeylia, hydrosyringomyelia, and syrinx refer to both of these conditions (which is often difficult to discriminate on imaging).

While the pathogenesis of syringomhydromyelia is currently debated, the relationship of with other conditions, such as Chiari I malformation and cord/column trauma, is well established. While it can be seen in trauma, nontraumatic (idiopathic) mechanisms are also possible. Clinical suspicion is associated with the cape-like sensory loss distribution across the back. Diagnosis is confirmed with spinal imaging, usually MRI. Treatment may involve surgery along with rehabilitation.

Milhorat TH, Johnson WD, Miller JI, Bergland RM, Hollenberg-Sher J. Surgical treatment of syringomyelia based on magnetic resonance imaging criteria. Neurosurgery. 1992;31(2):231–44; discussion 244–5. https://doi.org/10.1227/00006123-199208000-00008.

Porensky P, Muro K, Ganju A. Nontraumatic cervicothoracic syrinx as a cause of progressive neurologic dysfunction. J Spinal Cord Med. 2007;30(3):276–81. https://doi.org/10.1080/10790268.2007.11753937.

13. Mutations on the superoxide dismutase-1 (SOD1) gene cause which of the following spinal cord disorders?

   A. Familial variants of amyotrophic lateral sclerosis (ALS)
   B. Adrenomyeloneuropathy
   C. Brown-Sequard syndrome
   D. Spinocerebellar ataxia, type 2

Answer: A.

Approximately 10% of ALS are inherited and the most common genetic abnormality is mutations in the superoxide dismutase-1 (SOD1) gene. It is believed these mutations cause a toxic gain of function which increase free radical formation which in turn injures neuronal cells.

Adrenomyeloneuropathy is caused by mutations on the gene, ABCD1. Spinocerebellar Ataxia, type 2 is caused by caused by an expansion of polyglutamine in the ataxin-2 protein. Brown-Sequard syndrome is a clinical syndrome of hemicord injuries and is caused by a variety of different pathologies and not directly associated with a particular hereditary link.

Mackenzie IR, Bigio EH, Ince PG, Geser F, Neumann M, Cairns NJ, Kwong LK, Forman MS, Ravits J, Stewart H, Eisen A, McClusky L, Kretzschmar HA, Monoranu CM, Highley JR, Kirby J, Siddique T, Shaw PJ, Lee VM, Trojanowski JQ. Pathological TDP-43 distinguishes sporadic amyotrophic lateral sclerosis from amyotrophic lateral sclerosis with SOD1 mutations. Ann Neurol. 2007;61(5):427–34. https://doi.org/10.1002/ana.21147.

Wang C, Liu H, Han B, Zhu H, Liu J. A novel ABCD1 gene mutation causes adrenomyeloneuropathy in a Chinese family. Brain Behav. 2019;9(10):e01416. https://doi.org/10.1002/brb3.1416. Epub 2019 Sept 26.

Egorova PA, Bezprozvanny IB. Molecular mechanisms and therapeutics for spinocerebellar ataxia type 2. Neurotherapeutics 2019;16:1050–73. https://doi.org/10.1007/s13311-019-00777-6

14. A 52-year-old male is found to have a metastasis in the spinal cord after presenting with bilateral lower extremity weakness and sensory deficits. He is subsequently found to have prostate cancer. The tumor is treated with radiation with good results. Subsequent imaging does not show any residual tumor and patient's deficits have improved with therapy.

Approximately, 18 months later, the patient is found to have progressive weakness to the point of developing paraplegia over 6 weeks. MRI shows thoracic spinal cord enlargement and edema with T2 hyperintensity and no clear evidence of a tumor.

What is the most likely diagnosis?

A. Early radiation myelopathy
B. Delayed radiation myelopathy
C. Tumor recurrence
D. Multiple sclerosis

Answer: B.

Delayed myelopathy begins with gradual onset of symptoms with average onset 14 months (range 4 months-19 years) after completing radiation. The MRI findings are highly suggestive especially in the absence of any neoplasia recurrence. Over time, the MRI can also show atrophy. The symptoms generally begin with paresthesias. Higher risk is correlated with increased radiation dosage. Injury is usually noted in the previous radiation field.

Rampling R, Symonds P. Radiation myelopathy. Curr Opin Neurol. 1998;11(6):627–32. https://doi.org/10.1097/00019052-199812000-00003.

15. A 35-year-old woman presented with lower extremity weakness, bladder/bowel dysfunction and a sensory deficit in her legs. Five years ago, the patient had new onset diplopia and visual disturbance which was treated with steroids. Current MRI of her spine showed lesions in the lower cervical and upper thoracic cord consisting of swelling and contiguous hyperintensity which spanned more than five vertebral segments.

The cerebrospinal fluid (CSF) was negative for oligoclonal bands and showed a normal myelin basic protein level of 40.4 pg/mL (normal range, <102 pg/mL). Antibodies to which protein would confirm the diagnosis in this case?

A. Gliadin
B. Amphysin
C. SLE
D. Aquaporin 4

Answer: D.

The vignette most describes neuromyelitis optica (NMO) AKA Devic's disease. This is a demyelinating disorder characterized by a myelopathy and optic neuritis. The pathology is related to antibodies against aquaporin 4, a water channel protein.

Isobe N, Yonekawa T, Matsushita T, Masaki K, Yoshimura S, Fichna J, Chen S, Furmaniak J, Smith BR, Kira J. Clinical relevance of serum aquaporin-4 antibody levels in neuromyelitis optica. Neurochem Res. 2013;38(5):997–1001. https://doi.org/10.1007/s11064-013-1009-0. Epub 2013 Mar 2.

Scott TF, Kassab SL, Pittock SJ. Neuromyelitis optica IgG status in acute partial transverse myelitis. Arch Neurol. 2006;63(10):1398–400. https://doi.org/10.1001/archneur.63.10.1398.

16. Which of the following is true regarding treatment of spinomuscular atrophy (SMA)?

A. Immunosuppression works well as a first-line agent.
B. Antispasticity treatments are important to consider.
C. Nusinersen makes significant changes in survival and function.
D. Polio survivors need to take extra caution.

Answer: C.

Spinomuscular atrophy (SMA) is a rare neuromuscular disorder that results in the loss of motor neurons and progressive muscle wasting. SMA is due to an abnormality (mutation) in the *SMN1* gene. SMA types and 2 used to be considered highly fatal childhood diseases.

However, more recently, medical advancements in gene therapy have improved the course. In an open-label study of nusinersen in type-1 SMA, there was a higher rate of survival and an incremental improvement in achievement of motor milestones. Furthermore, a placebo-controlled trial in type-2 SMA patients revealed that nusinersen-treated patients had a significantly higher increase in motor function than patients who received placebo. Because this is a genetic disease and not an autoimmune issue, immunosuppression has no role here. Also, patients with SMA tend to be hypotonic (traditionally referred to as "floppy babies"), so there is no indication for antispastic agents. There is no relation or known indication for polio survivors.

Finkel RS, Chiriboga CA, Vajsar J, Day JW, Montes J, De Vivo DC, Yamashita M, Rigo F, Hung G, Schneider E, Norris DA, Xia S, Bennett CF, Bishop KM. Treatment of infantile-onset spinal muscular atrophy with nusinersen: a phase 2, open-label, dose-escalation study. Lancet. 2016;388(10063):3017–26. https://doi.org/10.1016/S0140-6736(16)31408-8. Epub 2016 Dec 7.

17. Which of the following is NOT a risk factor for cervical spondylotic myelopathy?

    A. Having an age >50 years
    B. Osteophytes and herniated discs
    C. Ligamentous flava hypertrophy
    D. Female gender

Answer: D.

Cervical spondylotic myelopathy (also known as degenerative myelopathy) encompasses a collection of pathologic conditions that result in progressive spinal cord dysfunction secondary to cord compression. Pathological conditions include a combination of spondylosis (including herniated discs and osteophytes), spondylolisthesis, congenital narrowing of spinal canal, and ligamentum flava hypertrophy. Patients are typically male with an average age of presentation of 64 years. Treatment depends on the presence and severity of symptoms. Surgery is recommended for patients with moderate to severe symptoms or rapidly progressive disease.

Kane SF, Abadie KV, Willson A. Degenerative cervical myelopathy: recognition and management. Am Fam Physician. 2020;102(12):740–50.

18. Which of the following is NOT a typical clinical presentation of lumbar spinal stenosis?

    A. 64-year-old female with intermittent leg discomfort and parasthesias produced by walking or standing straight for a long period of time.
    B. 73-year-old male with persistent progressive back and left leg pain for 7 months.
    C. 72-year-old male with persistent back and leg pain which is improved immediately after rest as well as by leaning backward.
    D. 66-year-old female without any clinical symptoms. Lumbar stenosis found incidentally on imaging.

Answer: C.

Lumbar spinal stenosis can present in a variety of different ways and therefore the clinician must have a low threshold and keep this in consideration for a variety of back and lower extremity complaints. The symptoms can range from being asymptomatic (answer D) to spinal/neurogenic claudication (answer A). Individuals can have chronic pain which can present in radicular distribution. Features of neurogenic claudication include slow relief with rest (as opposed to vascular claudication where immediate relief occurs with rest) and improvement by leaning forward (as opposed to leaning backward). This is often referred to as the "shopping cart sign" with patients leaning forward over the shopping cart when going to a store in order to relief their claudication.

Cook CJ, Cook CE, Reiman MP, Joshi AB, Richardson W, Garcia AN. Systematic review of diagnostic accuracy of patient history, clinical findings, and physical tests in the diagnosis of lumbar spinal stenosis. Eur Spine J. 2020;29(1):93–112. https://doi.org/10.1007/s00586-019-06048-4. Epub 2019 Jul 16.

19. Which of the following is NOT true about monomyelic atrophy (Hirayama's disease)?

    A. The sensory exam on such patients will be normal.
    B. Treatment addresses genetic causes.
    C. The initial differential diagnosis includes amyotrophic lateral sclerosis (ALS).
    D. Cervical spine surgery may be a treatment.

Answer: B.

Monomelic amyotrophy (MMA) or Hirayama's disease is a rare motor neuron disease. Its symptoms usually present between 15 and 25 years of age and males are more typically affected. Characteristics include insidious onset of muscle atrophy of an upper limb, which plateaus after 2–5 years from after which it generally neither improves nor worsens. There is no pain or sensory loss associated with MMA. MMA is not believed to be hereditary but rather the etiology is suspected to be due to compression of the spinal cord during cervical flexion leading to ischemia of anterior horn cells.

Symptoms are similar to ALS but unlike ALS, the symptoms do not progress after a few years and usually only involves one limb. Given that this is a motor neuron disease, the symptoms involve weakness, muscle atrophy, fasiculations, and tremors; the sensory exam should be normal. There is no clear treatment although usage of cervical collars and anterior cervical discectomy and fusion may lead to clinical and imaging improvement.

Zhang H, Wang S, Li Z, Shen R, Lin R, Wu W, Lin J. Anterior cervical surgery for the treatment of hirayama disease. World Neurosurg. 2019;127:e910–8. https://doi.org/10.1016/j.wneu.2019.03.295. Epub 2019 Apr 6.

20. Which of the following is FALSE in regards to spinal epidural abscesses in adults?

    A. The most frequent organism is *Staphylococcus aureus*.
    B. Treatment involves IV antibiotics and possible surgery.
    C. Risk factors include IV drug abuse and spinal surgery.
    D. It is most commonly found in the cervical region.

Answer: D.

Spinal epidural abscess is a severe infection of the epidural space that leads to devastating neurological deficits and may be fatal. It is considered an emergency. The diagnosis is difficult due to clinical symptoms not being specific and it can mimic many benign conditions. The classical triad of symptoms includes back pain, fever and neurological deterioration. Epidural abscesses are usually located in the thoracic and lumbar regions of the vertebral column and injures the spine by direct compression or local ischemia. Spinal cord injury may be prevented if surgical and medical interventions are implemented early.

Vakili M, Crum-Cianflone NF. Spinal epidural abscess: a series of 101 cases. Am J Med. 2017;130(12):1458–63. https://doi.org/10.1016/j.amjmed.2017.07.017. Epub 2017 Aug 7.

21. Which of the following viruses is not commonly associated with leading to myelopathy?

    A. Human T-lymphotropic virus type 1 (HTLV-1)
    B. Human immunodeficiency virus (HIV)
    C. Rotavirus
    D. West-Nile virus

Answer: C.

Infectious causes of myelopathy are a common cause of non-traumatic myelopathies. In addition to bacterial and fungal causes, several viruses can cause myelopathies. Specific viruses include HTLV, HIV, West-Nile virus, polio virus, influenza and herpesviruses. While there have been case reports of rotavirus leading to Guillain Barre syndrome, there is no evidence for this virus causing myelopathy. Specific diagnosis is based on careful review of history, determination of risk factors, spinal cord imaging and CSF serology.

Grill MF. Infectious myelopathies. Continuum (Minneap Minn). 2018;24(2, Spinal Cord Disorders):441–73. https://doi.org/10.1212/CON.0000000000000597.
Ho EL. Infectious etiologies of myelopathy. Semin Neurol. 2012;32(2):154–60. https://doi.org/10.1055/s-0032-1322588. Epub 2012 Sept 8.

Nowak DA, Griebl G, Bock A. Acute myelopathy associated with H1N1 virus infection. J Neurol. 2011;258:34–6. https://doi.org/10.1007/s00415-010-5676-3

Smeets CC, Brussel W, Leyten QH, Brus F. First report of Guillain-Barré syndrome after rotavirus-induced gastroenteritis in a very young infant. Eur J Pediatr. 2000;159(3):224. https://doi.org/10.1007/s004310050057.

22. Lathyrism is caused by ingestion of which of the following:

    A. Grass peas
    B. Fluoride
    C. Cassava root
    D. Organophosphates

Answer: A.

While all of the above answers are known toxins which can cause myelopathies, lathyrism is caused by consumption of the grass pea, *Lathyrus sativus*. The disease manifests as an acute or insidiously evolving spastic paraparesis following consumption. While extremely rare in the western hemisphere, it continues to occur sporadically throughout Africa and Asia. Cassava root ingestion leads to a condition known as Konzo.

Bick AS, Meiner Z, Gotkine M, Levin N. Using advanced imaging methods to study neuro-lathyrism. Isr Med Assoc J. 2016;18(6):341–5.

23. All of the following are true of tabes dorsalis EXCEPT:

    A. It involves primarily the dorsal columns of the spinal cords.
    B. It may be associated with pupillary findings.
    C. It is caused by *Mycobacterium tuberculosis*.
    D. It is slowly progressive.

Answer: D.

Tabes dorsalis is a late consequence of neurosyphilis and is characterized by the slowly progressive demyelination of the dorsal columns and dorsal root ganglia of the spinal cord. Symptoms may not appear for decades after the initial infection. In addition to symptoms such as weakness, pain, sensory, coordination loss, infected individuals will have signs unrelated to their spinal cord. This includes an Argyll-Robertson pupil (near-light dissociation). Once diagnosis is made, intravenous (IV) penicillin is the primary treatment.

   Mycobacterium tuberculosis infections of the spine can lead to Pott's disease (not tabes dorsalis).

Osman C, Clark TW. Tabes dorsalis and Argyll Robertson pupils. N Engl J Med. 2016;375(20):e40. https://doi.org/10.1056/NEJMicm1507564.

Reinoso J, Arias J, Santana G. Case of Pott's disease in a 17-year-old patient in the dominican republic. Cureus. 2019;11(6):e4922. https://doi.org/10.7759/cureus.4922.

The following vignette should be used to answer questions 24–25.

A 70-year-old male developed painful vesicular rash around his right hemithoracic area. Fifteen days later, the patient developed lower extremity weakness and urinary incontinence which continued to progress over the next few weeks. Exam showed lower extremity paraplegia, superficial sensory loss up to the T4 level and loss of vibratory sensation. MRI of spine showed increased T2 signal extending from T4 to T7 with spinal cord swelling and contrast enhancement. CSF studies showed 6 WBC/mm^3, elevated protein level: 0.65 g/L and positive anti-varicella-zoster virus antibodies.

24. What is the treatment for this suspected diagnosis?

    A. High dose radiation and initiation of chemotherapeutic
    B. Surgical placement of lumbar drain
    C. IV Acyclovir (10 mg/kg/8H) × 21 days
    D. IV Vancomycin × 21 days

25. In which part of the spine does the pathological process tend to remain latently during remission?

    A. Dorsal columns
    B. Dorsal root ganglion
    C. Anterior horn cells
    D. Lumbar bodies

Answer for question 24: C.
Answer for question 25: B.

The vignette most likely describes myelopathy secondary to varicella-zoster virus (VZV). This virus causes chicken pox as well as shingles. After initial infection, VZV becomes latent in the neurons of the dorsal root ganglia. If immunity declines, VZV is reactivated and can spread to the dermatome associated with the dorsal root ganglion leading to the rash (known as zoster) and in some cases to the spinal cord. Myelopathy is rare and may develop in the absence of skin rash making the diagnosis challenging.

Farhat N, Daoud S, Hdiji O, Sakka S, Damak M, Mhiri C. Myelopathy after zoster virus infection in immunocompetent patients: a case series. J Spinal Cord Med. 2021;44(2):334–8. https://doi.org/10.1080/10790268.2019.1607053. Epub 2019 Apr 23.

26. Which of the following spinal disorders preferentially affects anterior columns of the spinal cord?

    A. Neurosyphyllis
    B. Vitamin B12 deficiency
    C. Freidrich's ataxia
    D. Ischemia due to cross-clamping of the aorta

Answer: D.

The posterior cord syndrome is one of the incomplete spinal cord syndromes and results from pathology affecting the dorsal columns and potentially (in larger lesions) the lateral corticospinal tracts of the spinal cord. The syndrome is clinically characterized by isolated loss of proprioception and vibratory sensation. There are a variety of pathologies which can cause the syndrome. These include: inflammatory (e.g. multiple sclerosis), infectious (e.g. tabes dorsalis secondary to neurosyphyllis, HIV-related vacuolar myelopathy), ischemia (e.g. posterior spinal artery syndrome), metabolic (e.g. subacute combined degeneration of the cord secondary to vitamin B12 deficiency), and hereditary (e.g. Friedreich ataxia).

Ischemia due to cross-clamping of the aorta or disruption of blood flow through the artery of Adamkiewicz typically leads to an anterior spinal cord injury or a complete spinal cord injury.

Kunam VK, Velayudhan V, Chaudhry ZA, Bobinski M, Smoker WRK, Reede DL. Incomplete cord syndromes: clinical and imaging review. Radiographics. 2018;38(4):1201–22. https://doi.org/10.1148/rg.2018170178.

27. Spinomuscular atrophy (SMA) occurs due to:

    A. Organophosphate toxicity
    B. Genetic mutations of the ABCD1 gene
    C. Degeneration of anterior horn cells in the spinal cord
    D. Maternal inhalation of nitrous oxide

Answer: D.

Spinal muscular atrophy (SMA) is a rare neuromuscular disorder that results in the loss of motor neurons and progressive muscle wasting. Depending on the type, it can lead to premature death or have a mild disease course which does not change life expectancy. Common features in more severe types include progressive weakness of voluntary muscles, with arm, leg and respiratory muscles being affected first. Associated problems may include poor head control, difficulties swallowing, scoliosis, and joint contractures.

Spinal muscular atrophy types 1 and 2 are genetic diseases due to a mutation in the *SMN1* gene which encodes SMN (survival motor neuron), a protein necessary for survival of motor neurons. Loss of these neurons in the anterior horn of the spinal cord prevents signaling between the brain and skeletal muscles. Another gene, *SMN2*, is considered a disease modifying gene; more *SMN2* copies is generally associated with milder disease course. The diagnosis of SMA is based on symptoms and confirmed by genetic testing.

Genetic mutations of the ABCD1 gene lead to adrenomyeloneuropathy.

Inhalation of nitrous oxide can lead to spinal cord injury through nitrous oxide's inactivation of B12 by oxidation.

Farrar MA, Kiernan MC. The genetics of spinal muscular atrophy: progress and challenges. Neurotherapeutics. 2015;12(2):290–302. https://doi.org/10.1007/s13311-014-0314-x.

28. Acute poliomyelitis is due to infection by the virus to which part of the spinal cord?

    A. Anterior horn cell
    B. Dorsal column
    C. Lateral corticospinal tract
    D. Anterior commissure

Answer: A.

Certain infectious agents have a predilection towards certain parts of the spinal cord. In the case of the poliovirus, it has an affinity to the anterior horn cells of the spinal cord. Therefore, it follows that the symptoms include an asymmetric paralytic illness leading to hypotonia, areflexia, and muscle atrophy. Acute infection is not seen in the developed world due to the previous development and dissemination of the polio vaccine.

Rao DG, Bateman DE. Hyperintensities of the anterior horn cells on MRI due to poliomyelitis. J Neurol Neurosurg Psychiatry. 1997;63(6):720. https://doi.org/10.1136/jnnp.63.6.720.

29. A 70-year-old man presents with complaints of progressive left lower limb weakness for past 2 years. He has a previous history of an infectious disease as a child (unknown to him) affecting his right lower limb but that has been stable for 40 years. Exam shows weakness and atrophy in large muscles of both lower extremities, muscle fasiculations, and areflexia. MRI of his spine is normal. Electromyograph of the left lower extremity shows low amplitude compound muscle action potentials and fibrillation potentials suggestive of denervation. Of the possible differential diagnosis, which of the following is the most likely diagnosis?

    A. Transverse myelitis
    B. Monomyelic amyotrophy
    C. Post-polio syndrome
    D. Chronic spinal cord ischemia

Answer: C.

The vignette is most consistent with post-polio syndrome. The exam and findings are suggestive of a lower motor neuron disorder. Therefore, multiple sclerosis and stroke (a central nervous system diseases which would cause upper motor neuron findings) are unlikely. Monomyelic atrophy (also known as Haryama's disease) would occur at a younger age and not progress.

Post-polio syndrome is a rare sequela of acute poliomyelitis. It is usually seen 30–40 years after an acute episode. It is characterized by new muscle weakness seen in survivors of acute polio infection. It is characterized by muscular atrophy, weakness, pain, and fatigue in limbs and can be seen in limbs that were originally affected or in limbs that did not seem to have been affected at the time of the initial polio illness. The etiology is unknown.

Abrar A, Ahmad A. Post poliomyelitis syndrome: a rare sequel of acute poliomyelitis (author reply). J Pak Med Assoc. 2015;65(5):577.

30. Myelopathy secondary to copper deficiency may be caused by:

   A. Increased zinc in the diet
   B. Vitamin B12 deficiency
   C. A mutation in the cobalmin gene
   D. By HTLV-2 infection

Answer: A.

Myelopathy secondary to copper deficiency represents a treatable cause of myelopathy which closely mimics subacute combined degeneration due to vitamin B12 deficiency. Based on data, risk factors include previous upper gastrointestinal surgery, zinc overload and malabsorption syndromes, all of which impair copper absorption in the upper gastrointestinal tract and subsequently copper deficiency.

Jaiser SR, Winston GP. Copper deficiency myelopathy. J Neurol. 2010;257(6):869–81. https://doi.org/10.1007/s00415-010-5511-x. Epub 2010 Mar 16.

Questions 31–34 pertain to following vignette.

A 22-year-old female presented with sudden onset tetraplegia that improved upon arrival to the hospital. The neurological exam demonstrated residual weakness on the left upper and lower extremities. Brain MRI was normal, however, a spinal MRI revealed cord edema at multiple spinal cord levels (C2–T4).

Assuming this myelitis is secondary to an autoimmune process, match the hypothetical additional exam finding which could help identify the underlying cause of the myelitis.

31. Malar rash

32. Oral and genital ulcers

33. Bilateral hilar lymphadenopathy

34. Dry mouth

    A. Sjogren's
    B. Sarcoidosis
    C. Behcet's disease
    D. Systemic lupus erythematous (SLE)

Answer for question 31: D.
Answer for question 32: C.
Answer for question 33: B.
Answer for question 34: A.

There are multiple autoimmune causes of transverse myelitis/myelopathy. Clinically and radiologically, they can appear similar to each other. If the underlying autoimmune condition is known, the diagnosis becomes easier. However, the neurological abnormality can be the initial presenting sign which can make the diagnosis more difficult and therefore, it is important to use ancillary clues such as exam findings and history.

A malar rash is an erythematous rash in the shape of a butterfly (hence, also called butterfly rash) and is a medical sign often associated with systemic lupus erythematosus. A malar rash is present in approximately 46–65% of people with lupus.

Nearly all people with Behçet's disease present with some form of painful ulcerations inside the mouth. They are a form of aphthous ulcers or non-scarring oral lesions. Painful genital ulcerations usually develop around the anus, vulva, or scrotum and are another feature of Behçet's disease.

Bilateral hilar lymphadenopathy consists of bilateral enlargement of the lymph nodes of the pulmonary hila. It is a radiographic term for the enlargement of mediastinal lymph nodes. This is associated with sarcoidosis.

Sjögren's syndrome is a long-term autoimmune disease that affects the body's moisture-producing (lacrimal and salivary) glands. Consequently, patients' primary complaints include dryness, including dry mouth and dry eyes.

Mehmood T, Munir I, Abduraimova M, Ramirez MA, Paghdal S, McFarlane IM. Longitudinally extensive transverse myelitis associated with systemic lupus erythematosus: a case report and literature review. Am J Med Case Rep. 2019;7(10):244–9. https://doi.org/10.12691/ajmcr-7-10-6. Epub 2019 Jul 31.

Lee HS, Kim do Y, Shin HY, Choi YC, Kim SM. Spinal cord involvement in Behçet's disease. Mult Scler. 2016;22(7):960–3. https://doi.org/10.1177/1352458515613642. Epub 2015 Oct 19.

Pascuzzi RM, Shapiro SA, Rau AN, Schultz CE, Bowman RM, Caldemeyer KS, Wilkes DS. Sarcoid myelopathy. J Neuroimaging. 1996;6(1):61–2. https://doi.org/10.1111/jon19966161.

Ishikawa Y, Hattori K, Ishikawa J, Fujiwara M, Kita Y. Refractory Sjögren's syndrome myelopathy successfully treated with subcutaneous tocilizumab: a case report. Medicine (Baltimore). 2019;98(27):e16285. https://doi.org/10.1097/MD.0000000000016285.

35. Which of the following is true regarding postvaccination transverse myelitis?

    A. It is common
    B. Vaccines for Hepatitis B, Measles-Mumps-Rubella, Diphtheria-Pertussis-Tetanus, and Influenza have all been associated with it
    C. The most frequently involved spinal cord segment is the lumbar segment
    D. Intravenous steroid administration is the definitive treatment

Answer: B.

A variety of different causes of transverse myelitis exist. This includes following vaccination. There are several vaccines that have been associated as noted in answer B. However, it is quite rare with only case reports noted in the literature. Usually, the thoracic cord is involved. While steroids are often used in the treatment, there is not any strong evidence that they have clear benefit.

Agmon-Levin N, Kivity S, Szyper-Kravitz M, Shoenfeld Y. Transverse myelitis and vaccines: a multi-analysis. Lupus. 2009;18(13):1198–204. https://doi.org/10.1177/0961203309345730.

36. Which of the following scenarios is most likely to cause an artery of Adamkiewicz stroke?

    A. 62-year-old wakes-up after an abdominal aorta aneurysm repair surgery and is found to have paraparesis, urinary incontinence and a T10 sensory level
    B. 71-year-old develops new onset of atrial fibrillation
    C. 50-year-old with history of HTN, DM, and smoking history stops his medications due to loss of insurance and inability to afford his medications
    D. 54-year-old with Stage IV lung cancer with spinal metastasis.

Answer: A.

The great radicular artery of Adamkiewicz is a major supplier of blood to the lower spinal cord. When damaged or obstructed, it can result in a syndrome of spinal cord ischemia, often similar to anterior spinal artery syndrome with loss of urinary and fecal continence and impaired motor function of the legs. Sensory function may be preserved.

Taterra D, Skinningsrud B, Pękala PA, Hsieh WC, Cirocchi R, Walocha JA, Tubbs RS, Tomaszewski KA, Henry BM. Artery of Adamkiewicz: a meta-analysis of anatomical characteristics. Neuroradiology. 2019;61(8):869–80. https://doi.org/10.1007/s00234-019-02207-y. Epub 2019 Apr 27.

37. Which of the following clinical features is NOT seen in a stroke due to anterior spinal artery?

   A. Complete motor paralysis below the level of the lesion
   B. Loss of pain and temperature sensation at and below the level of the lesion due to interruption of the spinothalamic tract
   C. Loss of proprioception and vibratory sensation
   D. Autonomic dysfunction

Answer: C.

The anterior spinal artery the supplies anterior two-thirds of the spinal cord. The region affected includes the descending corticospinal tract, ascending spinothalamic tract, and autonomic fibers. It is characterized by a corresponding loss of motor function, loss of pain and temperature sensation, and autonomic dysfunction such as hypotension. It does not supply the dorsal columns which is supplied by two posterior spinal arteries. Therefore, proprioception and vibration are preserved.

Nakstad I, Randjelovic I, Bergan H, Evensen K. Fibrocartilaginous embolism as a cause of anterior spinal artery syndrome? Tidsskr Nor Laegeforen. 2020;140(5) (English, Norwegian). https://doi.org/10.4045/tidsskr.19.0261.

38. Primary progressive multiple sclerosis (MS)

   A. Is treated with steroids as a first line treatment
   B. Can have its progression halted with surgery
   C. Is treated with Riluzole
   D. Has a poor functional outcome despite treatment

Answer: D.

Primary progressive MS occurs in approximately 10–20% of individuals with MS. It is characterized by progression of disability from onset, with no, or only occasional and minor, remissions and improvements. The usual age of onset for the primary progressive subtype is later than of the relapsing-remitting subtype.

Bieniek M, Altmann DR, Davies GR, Ingle GT, Rashid W, Sastre-Garriga J, Thompson AJ, Miller DH. Cord atrophy separates early primary progressive and relapsing remitting multiple sclerosis. J Neurol Neurosurg Psychiatry. 2006;77(9):1036–9. https://doi.org/10.1136/jnnp.2006.094748. Epub 2006 Jun 22.

39. The difference in transverse myelitis between neuromyelitis optica (NMO) and multiple sclerosis (MS) is that:

    A. Greater than three vertebral segments are often affected in NMO.
    B. The myelitis in MS spares the highly myelinated tracts.
    C. The myelitis in NMO usually is confined to the dorsal columns.
    D. There is more hemorrhage seen in NMO.

Answer: A.

Unlike multiple sclerosis, the transverse myelitis in NMO usually affects longer cord segments (>3 segments) and multiple sclerosis usually affects <2 segments. Multiple sclerosis will usually have more numerous lesions. NMO usually affects greater than 50% of the spinal cord. MS has a predilection for the highly myelinated tracts (dorsal columns and corticospinal tracts).

Pekcevik Y, Mitchell CH, Mealy MA, Orman G, Lee IH, Newsome SD, Thompson CB, Pardo CA, Calabresi PA, Levy M, Izbudak I. Differentiating neuromyelitis optica from other causes of longitudinally extensive transverse myelitis on spinal magnetic resonance imaging. Mult Scler. 2016;22(3):302–11. https://doi.org/10.1177/1352458515591069. Epub 2015 Jul 24.

Presas-Rodríguez S, Grau-López L, Hervás-García JV, Massuet-Vilamajó A, Ramo-Tello C. Myelitis: differences between multiple sclerosis and other aetiologies. Neurologia. 2016;31(2):71–5 (English, Spanish). https://doi.org/10.1016/j.nrl.2015.07.006. Epub 2015 Sept 14.

Marrodan M, Gaitán MI, Correale J. Spinal cord involvement in MS and other demyelinating diseases. Biomedicines. 2020;8(5):130. https://doi.org/10.3390/biomedicines8050130.

40. Atlantoaxial subluxation of the cervical spine is associated with which of the following conditions?

    A. Multiple sclerosis
    B. Human immunodeficiency virus myelopathy
    C. Rheumatoid arthritis
    D. Neuromyelitis optica

Answer: C.

Cervical spine subluxations such as the anterior atlantoaxial subluxation are common disorders in patients with rheumatoid arthritis. At an early stage of the disease, rheumatoid inflammation of cervical spine structures may lead to subluxation. Sustained inflammation increases the prevalence of these subluxations. After a follow up period of 20 years, cervical spine subluxations were found in 42% of patients with destructive rheumatoid arthritis. It is believed that inflammatory mechanisms lead to ligament destruction which in turn causes subluxation. While patients may present with symptoms of myelopathy, there is a high percentage of asymptomatic cases as well. Risk factors for development include duration of disease, patient age, and severity of disease.

Neva MH, Häkkinen A, Mäkinen H, Hannonen P, Kauppi M, Sokka T. High prevalence of asymptomatic cervical spine subluxation in patients with rheumatoid arthritis waiting for orthopaedic surgery. Ann Rheum Dis. 2006;65(7):884–8. https://doi.org/10.1136/ard.2005.042135. Epub 2005 Nov 3.

41. Which of the following is the most common intramedullary spine tumor in children?

    A. Myxopapillary ependymoma
    B. Astrocytoma
    C. Paraganglioma
    D. Meningioma

Answer: B.

There are several types of tumors which can grow in the spine. Based on epidemiological data, astrocytomas are the most common intramedullary spine tumor in children. Most are low grade and slow growing. In contrast, ependymomas are the most common intramedullary spine tumor in adults.

Chatterjee S, Chatterjee U. Intramedullary tumors in children. J Pediatr Neurosci. 2011;6(Suppl 1):S86–90. https://doi.org/10.4103/1817-1745.85718.
Das JM, Hoang S, Mesfin FB. Intramedullary spinal cord tumors [Updated 2021 May 4]. In: StatPearls, editor. Treasure Island, FL: StatPearls Publishing; 2022. Available from: https://www.ncbi.nlm.nih.gov/books/NBK442031/

42. Which of the following best represents the evidence for riluzole in the treatment of amyotrophic lateral sclerosis (ALS)?

    A. Use of the medication prolongs independence in ALS by 8–10 years.
    B. Use of the medication prolongs survival in ALS by 2–3 months.
    C. It should only be used in extreme circumstances given the high rate of hypersensitivity reactions.
    D. It augments the effect of CPAP but not BIPAP ventilation in ALS.

Answer: B.

Riluzole was approved in the United States for the treatment of ALS by the U.S. Food and Drug Administration (FDA) in 1995. It can delay the onset of ventilator-dependence or tracheostomy and may increase survival by 2–3 months. CPAP does not have a clear role in the management of ALS whereas BIPAP does.

Miller RG, Mitchell JD, Lyon M, Moore DH. Riluzole for amyotrophic lateral sclerosis (ALS)/motor neuron disease (MND). Cochrane Database Syst Rev. 2002;(2):CD001447. https://doi.org/10.1002/14651858.CD001447. Update in: Cochrane Database Syst Rev. 2007;(1):CD001447.

43. A 40-year-old male with history of chronic asthma presents with back pain and lower extremity weakness. Exam was significant for a Cushingoid appearance and right lower extremity weakness. MRI revealed epidural lipomatosis. What is the next step in management?

A. Intravenous steroids
B. Urgent surgery referral
C. Reassurance
D. Cessation of any steroids that the patient is using to treat their asthma.

Answer: D.

Epidural lipomatosis refers to an excessive accumulation of fat within the spinal epidural space resulting in compression of the thecal sac. In severe cases, compression may be symptomatic. Symptoms are often non-specific and may be similar to other degenerative spinal conditions resulting in stenosis the lumbar region is most frequently affected.

Usually the etiology is due to glucocorticoid excess long term steroid administration (e.g. for asthma). The first steps in treatment is to decrease any exogenous glucocorticoids if possible and weight loss. Surgery is reserved for those who fail conservative therapy.

Sáez-Alegre M, Pérez López C, Giner García J, Junnior Palpán Flores A, García Feijoo P, Vivancos Sánchez C, Isla Guerrero A. Epidural lipomatosis and syringomyelia in adulthood: case report and literature review. World Neurosurg. 2019;129:341–4. https://doi.org/10.1016/j.wneu.2019.06.075. Epub 2019 Jun 20.

44. A 35-year-old previously healthy female presented with a 10-day history of high-grade fever, dry cough, and anosmia followed by acute onset of flaccid paralysis and numbness of both lower limbs with difficulty in voiding. One day later, she developed weakness and numbness of both upper limbs with retention of urine and fecal incontinence. Autonomic symptoms included fluctuations of heart rate with frequent attacks of palpitation, and dizziness and fainting upon sitting from recumbent position. She had received no vaccinations in previous months, and there was no history of a previous similar attack. On general examination, cardiac exam was normal with normal blood pressure and symmetry in both arms. On neurological examination, she had quadriplegia with greater involvement of the lower limbs, areflexia, and bilateral positive Babinski signs. Pain and temperature sensation was absent up to the C4 level with preserved touch, vibration, and joint position sense.

Visual and brain stem auditory evoked potentials were normal. Chest CT showed a bilateral ground glass appearance with no evidence of aortic dissection. Electrocardiography was normal.

MRI examination of the spine revealed an extensive hyperintense signal on T2-weighted imaging, extending from C5 to T7, and occupying the anterior two thirds of the cord with involvement of both gray and white matter.
What is the most likely diagnosis?

A. Multiple sclerosis
B. Guillain-Barré syndrome
C. COVID-19 myelopathy
D. HIV myelopathy

Answer: C.

The vignette supports the diagnosis of COVID myelopathy. The supporting features including the anosmia and the ground-glass appearance of lungs.
COVID-19 is caused by a SARS-CoV coronavirus and has been implicated as a
rare cause of myelitis/myelopathy. Guillian-Barré syndrome would not demonstrate Babinski signs and would not be associated with changes on MRI.

Khedr EM, Karim AA, Soliman RK. Case report: acute spinal cord myelopathy in patients with
    COVID-19. Front Neurol. 2020;11:610648. https://doi.org/10.3389/fneur.2020.610648.

45. A healthy individual admits to frequent recreational use of Whippets? What
    spinal cord pathology are they most at risk of?

    A. Epidural abscess
    B. Myelitis due to opportunistic infections secondary to immunosuppression
    C. Diabetic radiculopathy
    D. Nitrous oxide myelopathy

Answer: D.

Nitrous oxide (N_2O) is inhaled in anesthesia and as a recreational drug from
whipped cream dispensers (i.e. Whippets). Rates of use may reach up to 10% in
some age groups. By inactivating vitamin B12, N_2O can cause neurologic and
hematologic manifestations mimicking a B12 deficiency.

Diamond AL, Diamond R, Freedman SM, Thomas FP. "Whippets"-induced cobalamin defi-
    ciency manifesting as cervical myelopathy. J Neuroimaging. 2004;14(3):277–80. https://
    doi.org/10.1177/1051228404264956.

46. A 41-year-old woman presented with acute worsening of back pain, weakness
    in the left leg and urinary retention. Spinal angiography showed a spinal cord
    arteriovenous malformation (AVM). What is the best treatment?

    A. Intravenous steroids
    B. Embolization or surgical removal
    C. Blood thinners
    D. Chemotherapy

Answer: B.

Spinal arteriovenous malformations (AVMs) are a rare but treatable cause of myelopathy and spinal cord hemorrhage. The clinical presentation and ideal treatment of these lesions vary widely, primarily due to differences in anatomy and features of the AVM. They usually involve embolization or surgical treatment and will depend on clinical features. Immunosuppression does not have a role as this is not an autoimmune process. If possible, blood thinning medications should be avoided to reduce risk of hemorrhage into the spinal cord.

Drake B, Patro S, Quateen A, Cora EA, Finitsis S, Sinclair J, Lesiuk H, Iancu D. Metameric spinal AVM: long-term symptomatic relief achieved by embolization of the extradural component. Interv Neuroradiol. 2019;25(4):469–73. https://doi.org/10.1177/1591019919828135. Epub 2019 Mar 28.

47. Which of the following is true regarding acute flaccid myelitis?

    A. Adults are more likely than children to develop it.
    B. Possible viral etiologies include West Nile virus, enteroviruses, and the Epstein-Barr virus.
    C. Treatment involves vitamin B12 supplementation.
    D. Sensory findings are predominant.

Answer: B.

Acute flaccid myelitis (AFM) is a polio-like illness that affects the motor neurons in the gray matter of the spinal cord. It is thought to be due to a viral infection. Children with AFM have acute onset of flaccid paralysis, usually in an arm or leg. They may also have trouble moving their face or trouble swallowing. This weakness may progress to weakness of the muscles that control breathing. Cases of AFM have been attributable to oral trivalent attenuated polio vaccine and other viruses (including enterovirus, Epstein-Barr virus, and West Nile virus). As this affects motor neurons, sensation remains normal.

Hopkins SE. Acute flaccid myelitis: etiologic challenges, diagnostic and management considerations. Curr Treat Options Neurol. 2017;19(12):48. https://doi.org/10.1007/s11940-017-0480-3.

48. What is the pathophysiology of spinocerebellar ataxia (SCA) type 2?

    A. Mutations in SOD
    B. CAG repeat in the ataxin gene
    C. SMn1 homozygous deletions
    D. X-linked recessive

Answer: B.

Spinocerebellar ataxias (SCA) are a group of genetic disorders characterized by slowly progressive incoordination of gait and is often associated with poor coordination of hands, speech, and eye movements.

The polyglutamine tract in human ataxin-2 is unstable and can expand as it is transmitted across generations. Normal alleles usually have 22 or 23 repeats, but can contain up to 31 repeats. Longer expansions can cause spinocerebellar ataxia type 2 (SCA2), a fatal progressive genetic disorder in which neurons degenerate in the cerebellum, inferior olive, pons, and other areas.

Sun YM, Lu C, Wu ZY. Spinocerebellar ataxia: relationship between phenotype and geno-type—a review. Clin Genet. 2016;90(4):305–14. https://doi.org/10.1111/cge.12808. Epub 2016 Jun 30.

Karam A, Trottier Y. Molecular mechanisms and therapeutic strategies in spinocerebellar ataxia type 7. Adv Exp Med Biol. 2018;1049:197–218. https://doi.org/10.1007/978-3-319-71779-1_9.

49. Mutations in the gene for making frataxin are responsible for what disease?

    A. Neuromyelitis optica (NMO)
    B. Freidreich's ataxia
    C. Spinomuscular atrophy type III
    D. Spinocerebellar ataxia

Answer: B.

Friedreich's ataxia is an autosomal-recessive genetic disease that causes difficulty walking, a loss of sensation in the arms and legs, and impaired speech that worsens over time. Symptoms generally start between 5 and 20 years of age. Many develop hypertrophic cardiomyopathy and require a mobility aid such as a cane, walker, or wheelchair. As the disease progresses, people lose their sight and hearing. Other complications include scoliosis and diabetes mellitus. From a spinal pathology perspective, abnormal curvature of the spine can be seen. Degeneration of nerve tissue in the spinal cord causes the ataxia; particularly affected are the sensory neurons essential for directing muscle movement of the arms and legs through connections with the cerebellum. The spinal cord becomes thinner and atrophies during the course of the disease.

The condition is caused by mutations in the *FXN* gene on chromosome 9, which makes a protein called frataxin. In Freidreich's ataxia, cells produce less frataxin. In 96% of cases, the mutant *FXN* gene has 90–1300 GAA trinucleotide repeat expansions in Intron 1 of both alleles. In about 4% of cases, the disease is caused by a (missense, nonsense, or intronic) point mutation, with an expansion in one allele and a point mutation in the other.

Clark E, Strawser C, Schadt K, Lynch DR. Identification of a novel missense mutation in Friedreich's ataxia-FXN[W168R]. Ann Clin Transl Neurol. 2019;6(4):812–6. https://doi.org/10.1002/acn3.728.

Gottesfeld JM. Molecular mechanisms and therapeutics for the GAA·TTC expansion disease Friedreich ataxia. Neurotherapeutics. 2019;16(4):1032–49. https://doi.org/10.1007/s13311-019-00764-x.

50. A 42-year-old female who has a history of relapsing remitting multiple sclerosis (MS) develops transverse myelitis. All of the following would be considered a treatment of their acute MS flare EXCEPT:

    A. Intravenous methylprednisolone
    B. Plasma exchange
    C. Interferon therapy
    D. Immunoadsorption

Answer: C.

The management of multiple sclerosis involves acute exacerbation treatment and long-term treatment to prevent fewer exacerbations. Acute treatment includes steroids such as methylprednisolone as well as immune treatment such as plasma exchange or immunoadsorption. Often, larger lesion loads such as those seen in transverse myelitis need plasmapheresis and steroids combined. Long term management involves disease modifying treatment such as interferon therapy.

Hart FM, Bainbridge J. Current and emerging treatment of multiple sclerosis. Am J Manag Care. 2016;22(6 Suppl):s159–70.

Pediatric Spinal Cord Injury

19

Lauren Fetsko, Simra Javaid, and Glendaliz Bosques

Questions

1. ____ are the most common cause of traumatic spinal cord injury (tSCI) in children ≤5 years old.

   A. Motor vehicle collisions
   B. Falls
   C. Firearm injuries
   D. Sports-related injuries

   Answer: A.

   Motor vehicle collisions (MVCs) are still the most common cause of traumatic spinal cord injury (tSCI) in children ≤5 years old. They are most common in children 5 years and younger (50.9% of all tSCI) and less common in children aged 6–17 years (25.9–39.2%). In children aged 6–12, common causes of tSCI included road traffic accidents (30.2%), falls (29.5%), being struck by objects (13.9%), and sports injuries (8.2%). Children aged 13–17 are more likely to

L. Fetsko
Department of Pediatrics, University of Wisconsin School of Medicine and Public Health, American Family Children's Hospital, Madison, WI, USA
e-mail: lfetsko@wisc.edu

S. Javaid
Department of Physical Medicine and Rehabilitation, McGovern Medical School at UTHealth, Houston, TX, USA
e-mail: simra.javaid@uth.tmc.edu

G. Bosques (✉)
Department of Neurology, Dell Medical School at University of Texas, Austin, TX, USA
e-mail: Glendaliz.Bosques@austin.utexas.edu

© The Author(s), under exclusive license to Springer Nature Switzerland AG 2022
B. A. Abramoff et al. (eds.), *The Essential Spinal Cord Injury Medicine Question Bank*, https://doi.org/10.1007/978-3-031-07796-8_19

sustain tSCI from assaults and firearms (21.5% and 6.9%), both of which have been on the rise since the mid-1990s.

Selvarajah S, Schneider EB, Becker D, Sadowsky CL, Haider AH, Hammond ER. The epidemiology of childhood and adolescent traumatic spinal cord injury in the United States: 2007–2010. J Neurotrauma. 2014;31(18):1548–60. https://doi.org/10.1089/neu.2014.3332. Epub 2014 Aug 12.

2. Which of the following anatomic features do NOT make children susceptible to spinal cord injury without radiographic abnormality (SCIWORA)?

   A. Anterior wedging of ossifying vertebral bodies
   B. Large head-to-trunk radio
   C. Cervical ligamentous laxity
   D. Fully developed nuchal muscles

Answer: D.

In comparison to adult spine biomechanics, children have multiple anatomic features that make them more vulnerable to SCIWORA which include still developing nuchal muscles, large head-to-trunk ratio, anterior wedging of ossifying vertebral bodies, and cervical ligamentous laxity. These features allow for increased stretching of the vertebral column beyond the capabilities of the spinal cord.

Farrell CA, Hannon M, Lee LK. Pediatric spinal cord injury without radiographic abnormality in the era of advanced imaging. Curr Opin Pediatr. 2017;29(3):286–90. https://doi.org/10.1097/MOP.0000000000000481.

3. A 6-year-old male with achondroplasia, hip dysplasia, moderate sleep apnea, and recurrent ear infections is undergoing several procedures over the course of the next year. Upon reviewing his chart to clear him for surgery, you also note he has "spine-at-risk" findings which include cervical kyphosis and thoracic level stenosis. For which of the following procedures would you recommend neuromonitoring?

   A. Placement of bilateral ear tubes (30-min procedure, supine position, head rotated)
   B. Laryngoscopy for hypopharyngeal evaluation (15-min procedure, seated position)
   C. Hip osteotomy (2 h procedure, supine position)
   D. Extraction of left maxillary first molar (45-min procedure, supine position, mouth open)

Answer: C.

"Spine-at-risk" is a concept that describes certain features in patients with skeletal dysplasia that increases their risk of spinal cord injury with prolonged anesthesia (defined as duration exceeding 1 h). In the pre-operative period, features found on magnetic resonance imaging (MRI) can include foramen magnum stenosis, atlantoaxial instability, cervical stenosis, cervical kyphosis, cervicothoracic kyphosis, thoracic level stenosis, cord level thoracolumbar kyphosis, syrinx, and cord signal abnormalities. The upper thoracic level is the area of greatest risk. Spinal cord infarcts (in areas separate from the surgical area) have been reported in several cases after prolonged orthopedic or neurosurgical procedures. Neuromonitoring is not recommended for procedures lasting less than 1 h and these include, endoscopy, placement of ear tubes, etc.

White KK, Bober MB, Cho TJ, Goldberg MJ, Hoover-Fong J, Irving M, Kamps SE, Mackenzie WG, Raggio C, Spencer SA, Bompadre V, Savarirayan R, Skeletal Dysplasia Management Consortium. Best practice guidelines for management of spinal disorders in skeletal dysplasia. Orphanet J Rare Dis. 2020;15(1):161. https://doi.org/10.1186/s13023-020-01415-7.

4. At the age of ___ children with skeletal dysplasia should have _____ imaging done to assess for cervical spine stability.

   A. 2–3 years of age, AP-Lateral cervical spine radiographs
   B. 2–3 years of age, Flexion-extension cervical spine radiographs
   C. 5–6 years of age, AP-Lateral cervical spine radiographs
   D. 5–6 years of age, Flexion-extension cervical spine radiographs

   Answer: B.

   Children with short stature skeletal dysplasias have an increased risk of spinal cord injury due to hypoplasia of the odontoid, axis, or other cervical vertebrae. Flexion-extension cervical x-rays can help assess for instability of the occipital-cervical junction. Flexion-extension radiographs are recommended once a child can cooperate to perform the task, usually by the age of 2–3.

White KK, Bober MB, Cho TJ, Goldberg MJ, Hoover-Fong J, Irving M, Kamps SE, Mackenzie WG, Raggio C, Spencer SA, Bompadre V, Savarirayan R, Skeletal Dysplasia Management Consortium. Best practice guidelines for management of spinal disorders in skeletal dysplasia. Orphanet J Rare Dis. 2020;15(1):161. https://doi.org/10.1186/s13023-020-01415-7.

5. Which of the following is NOT recommended by the American Academy of Pediatrics (AAP) as part of routine screening for asymptomatic atlantoaxial instability in patients with trisomy 21 (Down Syndrome)?

   A. Focused history and neurological examination
   B. Discuss cervical spine-positioning precautions during procedures

C. Counsel regarding avoidance of trampoline use
D. Plain radiography (including neutral, lateral, flexion, and/or extension views)

Answer: D.

The AAP recommends that during biennial exams physicians discuss with parents the importance of cervical spine-positioning precautions during procedures as well as perform a careful history and physical exam with special attention to myelopathic-related signs and symptoms. Physicians should instruct parents to monitor for new onset of symptoms such as change in gait, change in bowel or bladder function, neck pain, stiff neck, head tilt, torticollis, change in general function or use of arms or hands, or weakness. Although children with trisomy 21 (Down Syndrome) are at an increased risk for atlantoaxial subluxation, routine radiographs in asymptomatic children are not recommended as they do not predict which children are at increased risk of developing spinal cord problems. However, in order to have accurate radiographic evaluation of the cervical spine, a child must be 3 years old for adequate vertebral mineralization and epiphyseal development. Children are at increased risk for spinal cord injury with participation in some sports (such as contact sports like football, soccer, and gymnastics) and parents should be advised of this risk. The AAP also recommends the avoidance of trampolines by all children younger than 6 (with or without Down Syndrome) and by older children unless under direct professional supervision.

Bull MJ, Committee on Genetics. Health supervision for children with Down syndrome. Pediatrics. 2011;128(2):393–406. https://doi.org/10.1542/peds.2011-1605. Epub 2011 Jul 25. Erratum in: Pediatrics. 2011;128(6):1212.

6. What is the most common finding in "seat belt syndrome" in a child who was involved in a MVC in which they were restrained with a 2-point restraint (lap belt)?

A. Burst fractures
B. Intra-abdominal injuries
C. Abdominal wall ecchymosis
D. Chance fracture

Answer: B.

"Seat belt syndrome" is the collection of clinical features seen after a MVC involving a 2-point restraint such as a lap belt. This includes: vertebral fractures with SCI, abdominal wall ecchymosis and intra-abdominal organ injuries. A 2007 review of pediatric seat belt syndrome and lap belt injuries found that the most common result of seat belt syndrome was intra-abdominal injuries. Lap belts are thought to cause injuries to the thoracolumbar spine via a flexion-distraction mechanism. Spinal injuries associated with seatbelt syndrome can include chance fractures, burst fractures, spinal cord injury without radiographic abnormality (SCIWORA) and compression fractures. Abdominal wall ecchymosis was associated with intra-abdominal injuries and vertebral fractures in this study.

Achildi O, Betz RR, Grewal H. Lapbelt injuries and the seatbelt syndrome in pediatric spinal cord injury. J Spinal Cord Med. 2007;30(Suppl 1):S21–4. https://doi.org/10.108 0/10790268.2007.11753964.

7. Spinal cord injuries associated with non-accidental trauma are most closely associated with which of the following characteristics:

A. Cervical spinal cord injuries
B. Children under the age of 2
C. Less severe spinal cord injuries
D. Similar length of stays as compared to injuries sustained from non-abusive trauma

Answer: B.

A study evaluating non-accidental and accidental spinal cord injuries found that spinal cord injuries associated with non-accidental trauma were more likely to occur in children under the age of 2 years-old, tend to have more severe spinal cord injuries, longer hospital stays and higher hospital costs. Studies on non-accidental pediatric spinal cord injury have been inconclusive, showing injury within cervical, thoracic and lumbar spinal regions within this population.

Jauregui JJ, Perfetti DC, Cautela FS, Frumberg DB, Naziri Q, Paulino CB. Spine injuries in child abuse. J Pediatr Orthop. 2019;39(2):85–9. https://doi.org/10.1097/ BPO.0000000000000877.

8. Within clinical studies the most common birth mechanism that has been found to be associated with birth-related spinal cord injury is:

A. Breech delivery
B. Vaginal delivery with shoulder dystocia
C. Emergency c-section
D. Vaginal delivery with forceps

Answer: D.

Previous reports of birth-related spinal cord injury have been associated with obstructed labor. Within these reports, vaginal delivery with forceps has been the most common etiology linked to birth-related spinal cord injury. Breech delivery, vaginal delivery with shoulder dystocia, uneventful vaginal deliveries and c-sections have also been associated. Diagnosis of a birth-related spinal cord injury can often be difficult to diagnose as the differential diagnosis includes neuromuscular disease, brachial plexus injury, and hypoxic ischemic encephalopathy.

Lee CC, Chou IJ, Chang YJ, Chiang MC. Unusual presentations of birth related cervical spinal cord injury. Front Pediatr. 2020;8:514. https://doi.org/10.3389/fped.2020.00514.

9. Which of the following statements regarding pediatric SCIWORA (spinal cord injury without radiographic abnormality) is true?

   A. The most common mechanism of injury across all age groups is sports-related.
   B. Initial neurologic impairment is a good prognostic indicator of recovery.
   C. Most require surgical management.
   D. It is uncommon for MRI imaging to be without neurologic findings in these patients.

Answer: B.

SCIWORA (spinal cord injury without radiographic abnormality) is defined as the clinical appearance of a spinal cord injury in the absence of spinal cord column injury visible on X-ray, computed tomography (CT) imaging or dynamic flexion/extension films. In a study examining 114 pediatric patients with SCIWORA, there was found to be a relatively even distribution in terms of American Spinal Injury Association impairment scale (AIS). The most common mechanism of injury was motor vehicle collisions, followed by sports-related injuries and falls. The vast majority were able to be treated conservatively. Initial neurologic impairment was a prognostic factor for later clinical recovery. Forty-three percent of patients were found to have no neurological findings on MRI.

Boese CK, Oppermann J, Siewe J, Eysel P, Scheyerer MJ, Lechler P. Spinal cord injury without radiologic abnormality in children: a systematic review and meta-analysis. J Trauma Acute Care Surg. 2015;78(4):874–82. https://doi.org/10.1097/TA.0000000000000579.

10. Higher rates of post laminectomy deformity in children have been associated with all of the following EXCEPT:

    A. Younger age
    B. The presence of a neoplasm
    C. 1–2 level laminectomies
    D. History of radiation treatments

Answer: C.

Iatrogenic deformities have been associated with the presence of neoplasms, radiation treatment, more expansive laminectomies involving multiple levels, and younger age. Laminoplasty may carry a decreased risk of iatrogenic deformities. If kyphotic deformities develop, standard management includes bracing and surgical correction.

Safain MG, Engelberg RB, Riesenburger R, Kryzanski J, Jea A, Hwang SW. Pediatric iatrogenic thoracic kyphosis and tension myelopathy treated with a thoracic pedicle subtraction osteotomy: a case report and review of the literature. Childs Nerv Syst. 2014;30(7):1293–9. https://doi.org/10.1007/s00381-014-2373-z. Epub 2014 Feb 7.

11. A 9-year-old male presents to your Emergency Department with symptoms of fever for 3 days, cough, difficulty swallowing, and right arm pain with flaccid weakness. Among his abnormal lab findings, you note that his CSF and respiratory cultures are positive for Enterovirus D68 (EV-D68). MRI of the brain and cervical spine without contrast revealed a brainstem T2-hyperintense lesion and right sided lesion spanning from C5 to C8. What is the most likely diagnosis?

A. Acute flaccid myelitis (AFM)
B. Multiple sclerosis
C. Acute disseminated encephalomyelitis (ADEM)
D. Neuromyelitis optica spectrum disorders

Answer: A.

Acute flaccid myelitis (AFM) typically affects children between 5 and 9 years of age. Similar to transverse myelitis (TM), AFM almost always follows a mild respiratory or other febrile illness. AFM presents with predominantly motor symptoms, though sensory changes can also be seen. Distinguishing features of AFM include (1) asymmetric onset of flaccid limb weakness, commonly starting in a single arm, and (2) positive complaints of pain or paresthesia in the affected limb without an apparent sensory deficit.

Flaccid tone and hyporeflexia/areflexia in the affected limb are hallmarks of AFM, but may also occur in the acute phase of TM. AFM leads to loss of the alpha-motor neuron and does not progress to upper motor neuron patterns of spasticity. Bowel and bladder dysfunction are less commonly seen in AFM compared to TM. Acutely though, they can look very similar, both in presentation and results of testing.

Cranial nerve involvement, bulbar weakness, or other deficits localizing to the brainstem are seen in AFM, but altered mental status is rare and should raise suspicion for an alternative diagnosis, such as ADEM. The presence of unique intrathecal oligoclonal bands are typically seen in patients who will ultimately meet criteria for a diagnosis of multiple sclerosis. Positive aquaphorin-4 antibodies are consistent with a diagnosis of neuromyelitis optica in the appropriate clinical context and should be tested in serum, as CSF testing is less sensitive.

Theroux LM, Brenton JN. Acute transverse and flaccid myelitis in children. Curr Treat Options Neurol. 2019;21(12):64. https://doi.org/10.1007/s11940-019-0603-0.

Cortese MM, Kambhampati AK, Schuster JE, Alhinai Z, Nelson GR, Guzman Perez-Carrillo GJ, Vossough A, Smit MA, McKinstry RC, Zinkus T, Moore KR, Rogg JM, Candee MS, Sejvar JJ, Hopkins SE. A ten-year retrospective evaluation of acute flaccid myelitis at 5 pediatric centers in the United States, 2005–2014. PLoS One. 2020;15(2):e0228671. https://doi.org/10.1371/journal.pone.0228671.

12. Which of the following features is NOT typical of transverse myelitis?

    A. Back pain followed by motor and sensory deficits
    B. Intrathecal oligoclonal bands
    C. Bowel and bladder dysfunction
    D. Bilateral weakness

Answer: B.

Neurologic symptoms of transverse myelitis (TM) often manifest with back pain that is followed by motor and sensory deficits. Bowel and bladder dysfunction are autonomic impairments that can also be seen in TM. These neurologic manifestations can evolve over the course of a few hours or over several days. Weakness in TM is typically bilateral, however, partial cord myelitis can result in asymmetric neurologic findings. While muscle tone and reflexes may be initially diminished, upper motor neuron signs, such as increased tone and hyperreflexia, become more apparent as the clinical course evolves. Sensory abnormalities include numbness, paresthesia, or hyperesthesias. A spinal level may be apparent in some cases, but deficits may be patchy depending on the distribution of the cord lesions. TM associated with persistent nausea, vomiting, or hiccups suggests involvement of the area postrema and is more suggestive of a neuromyelitis optica-associated myelitis. The presence of intrathecal oligoclonal bands are typically seen in patients who will ultimately meet criteria for a diagnosis of multiple sclerosis.

Theroux LM, Brenton JN. Acute transverse and flaccid myelitis in children. Curr Treat Options Neurol. 2019;21(12):64. https://doi.org/10.1007/s11940-019-0603-0.

13. ___ is the most common site of the spinal cord affected in pediatric transverse myelitis.

    A. Lumbar
    B. Lumbar and thoracolumbar
    C. Cervical
    D. Cervical and cervicothoracic

Answer: D.

Cervical and cervicothoracic lesions represent the majority of TM lesions (64–76%) and lesions spanning more than 3–5 segments are most commonly seen in children.

De Goede CG, Holmes EM, Pike MG. Acquired transverse myelopathy in children in the United Kingdom—a 2 year prospective study. Eur J Paediatr Neurol. 2010;14(6):479–87. https://doi.org/10.1016/j.ejpn.2009.12.002. Epub 2010 Jan 25.

Absoud M, Greenberg BM, Lim M, Lotze T, Thomas T, Deiva K. Pediatric transverse myelitis. Neurology. 2016;87(9 Suppl 2):S46–52. https://doi.org/10.1212/WNL.0000000000002820.

Pidcock FS, Krishnan C, Crawford TO, Salorio CF, Trovato M, Kerr DA. Acute transverse myelitis in childhood: center-based analysis of 47 cases. Neurology. 2007;68(18):1474–80. https://doi.org/10.1212/01.wnl.0000260609.11357.6f.

14. In pediatric patients diagnosed with acute transverse myelitis with abnormal brain MRI findings on initial presentation, which of the following demyelinating disorders are they subsequently at risk for developing?

A. Neuromyelitis optica
B. Acute flaccid myelitis
C. Multiple sclerosis (MS)
D. Acute disseminated encephalomyelitis (ADEM)

Answer: C.

Children with acute idiopathic transverse myelitis (TM) and brain MRI abnormalities at initial presentation were found to be at five times higher risk of subsequent MS diagnosis. Deiva et al. (2015) identified early predictors of relapse after acute idiopathic transverse myelitis including female sex, severe AIS at onset, gadolinium enhancement on spinal MRI, absence of pleocytosis, and absence of cervical or cervicothoracic lesion on spinal MRI. Within their study cohort, 16 (17%) relapsed. Of those, 13 (14%) subsequently received a diagnosis of MS in 13 (14%) and 3 (3%) a diagnosis of neuromyelitis optica.

Meyer P, Leboucq N, Molinari N, Roubertie A, Carneiro M, Walther-Louvier U, Cuntz-Shadfar D, Leydet J, Cheminal R, Cambonie G, Echenne B, Rondouin G, Deiva K, Mikaeloff Y, Rivier F. Partial acute transverse myelitis is a predictor of multiple sclerosis in children. Mult Scler. 2014;20(11):1485–93. https://doi.org/10.1177/1352458514526943. Epub 2014 Mar 11.

Deiva K, Absoud M, Hemingway C, Hernandez Y, Hussson B, Maurey H, Niotakis G, Wassmer E, Lim M, Tardieu M, United Kingdom Childhood Inflammatory Demyelination (UK-CID) Study and French Kidbiosep Study. Acute idiopathic transverse myelitis in children: early predictors of relapse and disability. Neurology. 2015;84(4):341–9. https://doi.org/10.1212/WNL.0000000000001179. Epub 2014 Dec 24.

15. Which of the following factors is NOT associated with a better functional outcome in pediatric transverse myelitis (TM)?

    A. Older age at diagnosis
    B. Shorter time to diagnosis
    C. Lower anatomic levels of spinal injury
    D. Presence of T1 hypointensities on spinal MRI during the acute period

Answer: D.

Absence, not presence, of T1 hypointensity on spinal MRI obtained during the acute period is associated with better functional outcome in pediatric TM. Other factors include older age at time of diagnosis, shorter time to diagnosis, lower sensory and anatomic levels of spinal injury, lack of white blood cells in the CSF, and fewer affected spinal cord segments. Rapid progression to maximum impairment in less than one day, any antecedent illness, immunization, or trauma were not associated with a worse outcome.

Pidcock FS, Krishnan C, Crawford TO, Salorio CF, Trovato M, Kerr DA. Acute transverse myelitis in childhood: center-based analysis of 47 cases. Neurology. 2007;68(18):1474–80. https://doi.org/10.1212/01.wnl.0000260609.11357.6f.

16. What is the most common location for pediatric spinal cord tumors?

    A. Intradural extramedullary
    B. Extradural
    C. Intradural intramedullary
    D. Conus medullaris

Answer: C.

Anatomically, spinal cord tumors can be described as extradural or intradural tumors. Intradural tumors can then be further classified as intramedullary or extramedullary. Extradural tumors exist between the dura and bones in the spine. Extramedullary tumors are within the dura, but are found outside the spinal cord. Intramedullary tumors are found within the spinal cord itself. Multiple studies have shown that the most common location for a pediatric spinal cord tumor is intramedullary. The most common intradural intramedullary tumor in children are astrocytomas.

Wilson PE, Oleszek JL, Clayton GH. Pediatric spinal cord tumors and masses. J Spinal Cord Med. 2007;30(Suppl 1):S15–20. https://doi.org/10.1080/10790268.2007.11753963.

17. Based on clinical reports, which is the most accurate statement when describing pediatric fibrocartilaginous emboli (FCE)?

    A. It is most common among the adolescent population
    B. Pain is an uncommon finding
    C. Neurogenic bowel and bladder is generally not seen in this population
    D. Weakness in the extremities is a later clinical finding in these cases

Answer: A.

Fibrocartilaginous emboli (FCE) appear to have a bimodal distribution, peaking in adolescence and late middle age. The etiology of this injury is thought to be due to ischemia, arising from the migration of the nucleus pulposus into the spinal artery. Presentation is rapid progression (in a matter of minutes to hours) of new onset of weakness (the most common presenting symptom), paresthesias, and pain (most commonly back pain). It can also be associated with bowel and bladder changes. Among a review of recent pediatric cases, half of those were associated with heavy exercise or tumbling.

Yamaguchi H, Nagase H, Nishiyama M, Tokumoto S, Toyoshima D, Akasaka Y, Maruyama A, Iijima K. Fibrocartilaginous embolism of the spinal cord in children: a case report and review of literature. Pediatr Neurol. 2019;99:3–6. https://doi.org/10.1016/j.pediatrneurol.2019.04.013. Epub 2019 Apr 26.

18. In children undergoing a tethered cord release, which of the following is NOT associated with higher complication rates?

    A. Male gender
    B. Use of operating microscope
    C. Increased operating time
    D. American Society of Anesthesiologists (ASA) class 3–4

Answer: A.

The American Society of Anesthesiologists (ASA) physical status classification system was developed in 1941 in order to categorize a patient's physiological status to help predict operative risk. ASA class 1 denotes a normal healthy patient while ASA class 2 is for patients with mild systemic disease. ASA class 3 is for patients with a severe systemic disease that is not life-threatening and class 4 is for patients with systemic disease that is a constant threat to life. Bhimani et al. (2019) paradoxically found that in children undergoing tethered cord releases, females were found to have a higher complication rate despite males having more comorbidities during presentation. Operative time, use of the surgical microscope, and [worse] ASA class were also associated with complications. Whether these associations represent higher complexity of cases or are direct risk factors is unclear.

Bhimani AD, Selner AN, Patel JB, Hobbs JG, Esfahani DR, Behbahani M, Zayyad Z, Nikas D, Mehta AI. Pediatric tethered cord release: an epidemiological and postoperative complication analysis. J Spine Surg. 2019;5(3):337–50. https://doi.org/10.21037/jss.2019.09.02.

19. In children with tethered cord syndrome-associated scoliosis, which of the following combination of factors leads to the greatest risk of scoliosis curve progression following untethering procedures?

    A. Cobb angle <40°, Risser Grades 3–5
    B. Cobb angle >40°, Risser Grades 0–2
    C. Cobb angle >40°, Risser Grades 3–5
    D. Cobb angle <40°, Risser Grades 0–2

    Answer: B.

    A baseline Cobb angle >40° was associated with a 5.9-fold increase in curve progression when compared with an angle <40° following tethered cord surgery. The Risser classification grades skeletal maturity based on how much ossification and fusion is present at the iliac crest apophyses, from stage 0 having no ossification to stage 5 with complete ossification and fusion. Patients with Risser Grades 0–2 were 3.4 times more likely to experience scoliosis progression compared to those with Risser Grades 3–5. In patients with curves <40°, particularly those with Risser Grades 3–5, a greater incidence of stabilization or improvement following cord untethering procedures was observed.

McGirt et al. Pediatric tethered cord syndrome: response of scoliosis to untethering procedures. J Neurosurg Pediatrics. 2009;4(3):270–4. https://doi.org/10.3171/2009.4. PEDS08463.

20. The absence of which of the following muscles is the most important predictor of the inability to ambulate in children with myelomeningocele?

    A. Iliopsoas muscles
    B. Hamstring muscles
    C. Anterior tibialis muscles
    D. Gastrocnemius muscles

    Answer: A.

    The relationship between patterns of strength and mobility was studied in 291 children with myelomeningocele, graded as community ambulators, partial (household) ambulators and nonambulators. All children with iliopsoas ≤3 relied on a wheelchair for some (11.5%) or all (88.5%) of their mobility. All of the children with iliopsoas strength of 0 or 1 were non-ambulatory. Grade 4–5 gluteal and anterior tibialis function was associated with community ambulation, without aids or braces.

McDonald CM, Jaffe KM, Mosca VS, Shurtleff DB. Ambulatory outcome of children with myelomeningocele: effect of lower-extremity muscle strength. Dev Med Child Neurol. 1991;33(6):482–90. https://doi.org/10.1111/j.1469-8749.1991.tb14913.x.

21. Formal AIS examination in pediatric patients should be delayed at least until the age of ___.

    A. 2 years
    B. 4–6 years
    C. 8 years
    D. 15 years

Answer: B.

Children under the age of 4 are unable to comprehend and follow standardized ISNSCI test instructions, regardless of the type or severity of the injury. Children older than 4 years are generally able to participate with high reliability in the total motor and sensory scores. Thus, according to Mulcahey et al. (2007), 4 years of age is the lower limit in which motor and sensory exams can generate reliable data and formal testing should be delayed until this age. Children injured at a young age and those with little or no prior experience with volitional bowel movements have difficulty with the anal motor exam and the anorectal examination is not reliable until after the age of 10. Also of note, despite being able to complete the sensory exam, children under 10 years of age have been noted to be anxious and stressed by the pinprick exam. Therefore, modifications of the exam for children under 10 years may be warranted.

Mulcahey MJ, Gaughan J, Betz RR, Johansen KJ. The International Standards for Neurological Classification of Spinal Cord Injury: reliability of data when applied to children and youths. Spinal Cord. 2007;45(6):452–9. https://doi.org/10.1038/sj.sc.3101987. Epub 2006 Oct 3.

22. Which shortened sensory exam for light touch and pin prick may be useful in evaluating children with SCI who cannot tolerate a full exam?

    A. 4-dermatome sensory exam
    B. 8-dermatome sensory exam
    C. 12-dermatome sensory exam
    D. 16-dermatome sensory exam

Answer: D.

Primary obstacles to International Standards for Neurological Classification of Spinal Cord Injury (ISNCSCI) examination administration in young children include test anxiety, especially concerning the pin prick (PP) test, as well as the inability to remain attentive and provide responses over the course of the exam. The 16-dermatome sensory exam has been shown to provide a good correlation to the usual 56-dermatome sensory exam on the ISNSCI. For both PP and light touch (LT), correlations between the full examination and the shortened 4-, 8-, 12-, or 16-dermatome tests, reveal the 16-dermatome test as the best fit to the 56-dermatome examination.

Krisa L, Mulcahey MJ, Gaughan JP, Smith B, Vogel LC. Using a limited number of derma-tomes as a predictor of the 56-dermatome test of the international standards for neuro-logical classification of spinal cord injury in the pediatric population. Top Spinal Cord Inj Rehabil. 2013;19(2):114–20. https://doi.org/10.1310/sci1902-114.

23. In adults with spinal cord injuries at T6 and above, a blood pressure of 20–40 mmHg above baseline may signify autonomic dysreflexia. In compari-son, a blood pressure of more than ___ above baseline in children and more than ___ above baseline in adolescents may signify autonomic dysreflexia.

    A. 10 mmHg, 15–20 mmHg
    B. 15 mmHg, 15–20 mmHg
    C. 15 mmHg, 20–40 mmHg
    D. 20 mmHg, 20–40 mmHg

Answer: B.

The Clinical Practice Guideline of the Consortium for Spinal Cord Medicine notes that an elevation of systolic blood pressure of 20–40 mmHg may be a sign of autonomic dysreflexia (AD) in adults with a spinal cord injury at or above T6. The Clinical Practice Guideline also notes that significant blood pressure elevations above baseline that may be a sign of AD are 15 mmHg in children and 15–20 mmHg for adolescents.

Consortium for Spinal Cord Medicine. Acute management of autonomic dysreflexia: indi-viduals with spinal cord injury presenting to health-care facilities. J Spinal Cord Med. 2002;25(Suppl 1):S67–88.

24. In children ≤13 years old, which of the following is NOT an appropriate inter-vention in the management of autonomic dysreflexia?

    A. Elevate patient's head
    B. Use 1 in. of topical nitroglycerine (Nitropaste) for systolic BP ≥10 mmHg above baseline
    C. Perform bladder management
    D. Loosen clothing and shoes

Answer: B.

The Shriners Hospitals for Children Task Force on Autonomic Dysreflexia in Children with Spinal Cord Injury has developed several algorithms specific to children in the treatment of autonomic dysreflexia (AD). In children who are 13 years old or younger, initial interventions include assessing the patient, including vital signs of blood pressure, pulse, and temperature. Subsequent steps involve elevating the patient's head or repositioning unless contraindicated, removing gradient elastic stockings/abdominal binders, loosening clothing and shoes, monitoring vital signs every 5 min, bladder management, bowel management if blood pressure continues to be >30 mmHg above baseline, and considering use of ½-in. of nitropaste for systolic pressures >30 mmHg above baseline.

McGinnis KB, Vogel LC, McDonald CM, Porth S, Hickey KJ, Davis M, Bush P, Jenkins D, Shriners Hospitals for Children Task Force on Autonomic Dysreflexia in Children with Spinal Cord Injury. Recognition and management of autonomic dysreflexia in pediatric spinal cord injury. J Spinal Cord Med. 2004;27(Suppl 1):S61–74. https://doi.org/10.108 0/10790268.2004.11753787.

25. Which newly diagnosed pediatric spinal cord injury patient below should receive anticoagulant thromboprophylaxis to prevent deep venous thrombosis (DVT)?

    A. 1-month-old with traumatic spinal cord injury due to injury during delivery
    B. 8-year-old male newly diagnosed with acute flaccid myelitis
    C. 10-year-old female diagnosed with SCIWORA
    D. 15-year-old male with a traumatic spinal cord injury (tSCI) and right tibial fracture

Answer: D.

Studies have shown that children are less likely than adults with SCI to develop a DVT or venous thromboembolisms (VTEs). The incidence of DVT/VTE development appears to increase during adolescence between the ages of 13–15 or at Tanner pubertal stage >2. The Consortium for Spinal Cord Medicine published guidelines in 2016 that recommended children with acute SCI are given mechanical prophylaxis with compression stockings and/or pneumatic compression devices. Given the lower risk of developing a DVT in this population, the consensus recommended that adolescents receive anticoagulants for thromboprophylaxis, particularly if a pelvic or lower extremity fracture is present and in the absence of contraindications such as active or increased bleeding risk.

Prevention of venous thromboembolism in individuals with spinal cord injury: clinical practice guidelines for health care providers, 3rd ed.: Consortium for Spinal Cord Medicine. Top Spinal Cord Inj Rehabil. 2016;22(3):209–40. https://doi.org/10.1310/sci2203-209.

Streif W. Perioperative thromboseprophylaxe bei kindern [Prevention of perioperative venous thromboembolism in children]. Wien Med Wochenschr. 2009;159(19–20):481–6 (German). https://doi.org/10.1007/s10354-009-0712-6.

26. Per Koff (1983), which of the following commonly used formulas most accurately estimates pediatric maximal bladder capacity in mL?

   A. Age + 2
   B. (Age + 3) × 20
   C. Age + 3
   D. (Age + 2) × 30

   Answer: D.

   Koff (1983) examined children of varying ages via cystogram. In this study they determined maximal bladder capacity existed when the pressure per unit of volume increased linearly within the study. They derived that bladder capacity was able to be estimated via the following equation: Age + 2. This original equation estimated maximal bladder capacity in ounces. To convert bladder capacity to mL the value must be multiplied by 30 making the formula (Age + 2) × 30.

   Koff SA. Estimating bladder capacity in children. Urology. 1983;21(3):248. https://doi.org/1
      0.1016/0090-4295(83)90079-1.

27. Self-catheterization by a child with spinal cord dysfunction can generally be accomplished if the patient's cognitive development is consistent with what age?

   A. 2–3 years old
   B. 6–7 years old
   C. 10–12 years old
   D. 15–16 years old

   Answer: B.

   A small cohort study conducted by Hannigan (1979) found that pre-school aged children who were cognitively appropriate for their age were able to learn self-catheterization techniques. This study first had them practice on dolls. A further study of a population of children with spina bifida found that 55% of their population greater than 3 years old were able to perform independent straight catheterization. This skill was acquired on average at 9.45 years of age. Lower rates of independent straight catheterization were associated with a higher level of lesion and female gender. 15% of those able to perform independent catheterization also had a diagnosis of intellectual disability.

   Hannigan KF. Teaching intermittent self-catheterization to young children with myelodysplasia. Dev Med Child Neurol. 1979;21(3):365–8. https://doi.org/10.1111/j.1469-8749.1979.
      tb01628.x.
   Castillo J, Ostermaier KK, Fremion E, Collier T, Zhu H, Huang GO, Tu D, Castillo H. Urologic self-management through intermittent self-catheterization among individuals with spina bifida: a journey to self-efficacy and autonomy. J Pediatr Rehabil Med. 2017;10(3–4):219–26. https://doi.org/10.3233/PRM-170447.

28. At what age range is it appropriate to start to work towards an independent bowel routine, with a goal of social continence, in a child with neurogenic bowel who is otherwise developmentally appropriate?

    A. Toddler
    B. Elementary school age
    C. Middle school age
    D. High school age

Answer: B.

Each child is different, so this milestone is assessed on a case-by-case basis. In general, transitioning towards a more independent bowel routine can be considered as the child approaches elementary school. It is important to understand how bowel patterns change as a child ages. In infants, prior to the initiation of solid foods, several stools are common throughout the day. As infants approach a year old, this decreases to 1–2 bowel movements per day and then becomes more formed by 18 months. Typically developing children become more aware of bowel movements by the age of 2 years, at which time toilet training usually commences. Neurotypical children complete toilet training by the age of 4. In children with neurogenic bowel, such as spina bifida, constipation can be seen and should be monitored for as solid foods are introduced to the child.

Children with spinal cord injury may have altered anal sensation and not know when they need to have a bowel movement. Starting as a toddler, a potty-chair can be utilized with diaper changes, suppository or enema administration, to allow for the child to make the association between the bathroom and defecation. As the child transitions into school, continence becomes of greater importance for social acceptance. At around the age of 6, if developmentally appropriate, families can start to work towards an independent bowel program with their child with incorporation of bowel routines typically recommended for the management of neurogenic bowel.

Leibold SR. Achieving continence with a neurogenic bowel. Pediatr Clin North Am. 2010;57(4):1013–25. https://doi.org/10.1016/j.pcl.2010.08.002.

29. Which of the following orthopedic problems is NOT prevalent in children with spinal cord injuries?

    A. Spine deformity
    B. Hip instability
    C. Pathologic vertebral fractures
    D. Soft tissue contractures

Answer: C.

The major orthopedic problems in a child with spinal cord injury (SCI) include spine deformity, hip instability, joint contractures, pathologic long bone fractures and spinal cord syrinx. Studies have shown a prevalence of spine deformity in 98%, hip instability in 43%, soft tissue contractures (almost universal), pathologic long bone fractures in 14% and spinal cord syrinx in 51%. Age at the time of SCI strongly influences the prevalence of spine deformity, with those injured prior to skeletal maturity being at highest risk.

The Symposium on Pediatric Spinal Cord Injury noted that age at the time of injury was also a very important factor in hip instability, and of those injured prior to age 5, 87% developed hip instability. Although children with SCI are initially contracture free, contractures can develop within weeks to months if prevention is not routinely done with positioning and range of motion. Children with SCI are at an increased risk for pathologic long bone fractures due to loss of bone mineral density. They often have 60% of normal age- and sex-matched bone density and can also have osteomalacia secondary to poor oral intake. Prevention is critical and weight bearing with braces as well as functional electrical stimulation (FES) is encouraged.

Vogel LC. Unique management needs of pediatric spinal cord injury patients: etiology and pathophysiology. J Spinal Cord Med. 1997;20(1):10–3.

30. Which of the following is the strongest predictor of neuromuscular scoliosis in children with spinal cord injury?

    A. Neurologic level
    B. Motor score
    C. Injury severity
    D. Age at injury

Answer: D.

Mulcahey et al. (2013) found that neurological level, motor score, and severity of injury were not predictors of neuromuscular scoliosis. Age at injury was found to be the only predictor of worsened curve and requirement for spinal fusion in children with SCI. Children who were injured at a younger age were more likely to have progressive neuromuscular scoliosis and need for a definitive spinal fusion. Injuries prior to the age of 12 were almost four times as likely to need spinal fusions.

Mulcahey MJ, Gaughan JP, Betz RR, Samdani AF, Barakat N, Hunter LN. Neuromuscular scoliosis in children with spinal cord injury. Top Spinal Cord Inj Rehabil. 2013;19(2):96–103. https://doi.org/10.1310/sci1902-96.

31. In adults with pediatric onset spinal cord injury, hip subluxation is associated with:

A. AIS motor score
B. Shorter duration of injury
C. Functional independence measure (FIM) scores
D. Age at injury

Answer: D.

Hip subluxation in adults with pediatric onset SCI is significantly associated with younger age at injury and longer duration of injury. Hip subluxation is not significantly associated with gender, neurological level, AIS motor score, or FIM scores. In contrast, hip contractures are more common in those with spinal cord injuries from violence and not associated with age at injury or duration of injury.

Vogel LC, Krajci KA, Anderson CJ. Adults with pediatric-onset spinal cord injury: part 2: musculoskeletal and neurological complications. J Spinal Cord Med. 2002;25(2):117–23. https://doi.org/10.1080/10790268.2002.11753611.

32. Emerging adults with spina bifida have been found to be similar to their peer counterparts in terms of which of the following:

A. Number of peer friendships
B. Number of romantic relationships
C. Attending college
D. Maintaining employment

Answer: A.

Young adults with spina bifida have been found in a study to be less likely than age matched peers to have romantic relationships, attend college, maintain employment and leave home. No difference was noted in regards to the number of peer friendships. Executive function and patient motivation is thought to be a positive predictor for the achievement of adult milestones.

Zukerman JM, Devine KA, Holmbeck GN. Adolescent predictors of emerging adulthood milestones in youth with spina bifida. J Pediatr Psychol. 2011;36(3):265–76. https://doi.org/10.1093/jpepsy/jsq075. Epub 2010 Sept 19.

33. When looking at education in children with acquired spinal cord injuries:

A. It is common for children to continue with part-time schooling years after their initial injury.
B. The intensity of school physical and occupational therapy support remains the same as a child progresses from elementary school towards high school.

C. Elementary students are more likely than their older counterparts to require curriculum modifications such as increased time to complete tasks and alternative assignments.
D. Student performance is generally at or above the level of their peers.

Answer: D.

A study that examined the educational performance of children with acquired spinal cord injuries found that children with spinal cord injury performed at or above the level of their peers. Most students were found to attend classes full time. Younger children tended to require more physical and occupational therapy support. This became less likely as the children progressed in school, likely related to age appropriate independence in mobility and activities of daily living. Therapy services may also be more common within elementary schools. As children aged, they were found to require more modifications such as increased time or alternative assignments which was thought to be related to increased academic rigor.

Massagli TL, Dudgeon BJ, Ross BW. Educational performance and vocational participation after spinal cord injury in childhood. Arch Phys Med Rehabil. 1996;77(10):995–9. https://doi.org/10.1016/s0003-9993(96)90058-1.

34. All of the following are true of individuals with pediatric-onset spinal cord injuries EXCEPT:

A. They have comparable or greater rates of college completion when compared to peers.
B. They have a higher employment rate than individuals who sustain a spinal cord injury as an adult.
C. They have about a 30% rate of independently driving in those with thoracolumbar injuries or AIS D impairments.
D. There is an equal or higher rates of completing college with AIS A–C C1–C4 level injuries compared to other spinal cord injury levels

Answer: C.

In a study evaluating long term outcome of pediatric onset spinal cord injury, across all impairment groups (AIS A–C C1–C4, AIS A–C C5–C8, AIS A–C T1–L4 and AIS D) college completion rates ranged from 28% to 39% of individuals compared to a national average of 26% to 29% of aged-matched peers. College completion rates were highest (39%) within the AIS A–C C1–C4 group. Employment rates ranged from 42% to 64%, averaging higher than those seen in adult-onset spinal cord injury (19% to 23%). Independent driving varied within this cohort with those with higher cervical levels of injury being less likely to drive independently. Among those with thoracolumbar injuries or AIS D impairments, independent driving ranged from 75% to 86%.

Vogel LC, Chlan KM, Zebracki K, Anderson CJ. Long-term outcomes of adults with pediatric-onset spinal cord injuries as a function of neurological impairment. J Spinal Cord Med. 2011;34(1):60–6. https://doi.org/10.1179/107902610X12883422813787.

35. Which of the following is true regarding ambulation after a pediatric onset spinal cord injury?

    A. A greater severity of neurologic impairment is associated with a greater likelihood of ambulation.
    B. Prolonged duration of ambulation years after initial spinal cord injury is longer in those who sustain their injury at an older age.
    C. An injury sustained at or before the age of 5 is a more positive predictive factor for ambulation.
    D. Individuals who sustain a spinal cord injury at an older age are more likely to be community ambulators.

Answer: C.

Children injured before or at the age of 5 were found in a study by Vogel et al. (2007) to be more likely to ambulate, ambulate at a household or community level, and maintain ambulation for a longer duration after their injury when compared to children injured at an older age. Neurological impairment scores as measured by the AIS were also predictive of ambulation, with more severe injuries associated with a decreased incidence of ambulation.

Vogel LC, Mendoza MM, Schottler JC, Chlan KM, Anderson CJ. Ambulation in children and youth with spinal cord injuries. J Spinal Cord Med. 2007;30(Suppl 1):S158–64. https://doi.org/10.1080/10790268.2007.11754595.

36. For women with spina bifida, which of the following is true:

    A. The risk of a woman with spina bifida having a child with spina bifida is equal to the general population.
    B. This population has a higher incidence of precocious puberty as compared to healthy counterparts.
    C. This population is noted to have decreased fertility as compared to peers.
    D. If pregnant, it is encouraged that a cesarean section be performed rather than vaginal delivery.

Answer: B.

Women with spina bifida have been found to be more likely to experience precocious puberty when compared to those without spina bifida. This is thought to be related to hydrocephalus and other central nervous system malformations and how this affects the release of growth hormone. If one parent is affected with spina bifida, that couple is at increased risk of having a child with spina bifida (or other neural tube defects), with the risk of recurrence increasing to 5%. If both parents have spina bifida, this risk increases to 15%. Women with spina bifida have an average fertility rate. During delivery of a pregnancy, it is currently recommended that women with spina bifida pursue a vaginal delivery, due to the prolonged recovery and increased surgical risks seen with cesarean sections in this population.

Visconti D, Noia G, Triarico S, Quattrocchi T, Pellegrino M, Carducci B, De Santis M, Caruso A. Sexuality, pre-conception counseling and urological management of pregnancy for young women with spina bifida. Eur J Obstet Gynecol Reprod Biol. 2012;163(2):129–33. https://doi.org/10.1016/j.ejogrb.2012.04.003. Epub 2012 Apr 28.

37. Which of the following birth control options for women with spina bifida most closely matches the associated contradiction to its use?

    A. Intrauterine device (IUD): hypertension
    B. Oral contraceptives containing estrogen: osteoporosis
    C. Oral contraceptives that are progesterone only: hypercoagulability
    D. Diaphragm use: latex allergy

Answer: D.

In women with spina bifida, latex allergy has been reported in up to 23% of individuals. Some birth control options such as diaphragms, condoms and cervical caps may contain latex and should be avoided. Progesterone only or oral contraceptives that contain primarily progesterone carry a risk of osteoporosis. Primarily estrogen contraceptives have the potential to induce a hypercoagulable state. IUD should be avoided in individuals with impaired pelvic sensation, a prolapsed uterus or a history of chronic urinary tract infections.

Jackson AB, Mott PK. Reproductive health care for women with spina bifida. ScientificWorldJournal. 2007;7:1875–83. https://doi.org/10.1100/tsw.2007.304.
Tong CMC, Tanaka ST. Let's talk about sex: special considerations in reproductive care and sexual education in young women with spina bifida. Urology. 2021;151:79–85. https://doi.org/10.1016/j.urology.2020.05.092. Epub 2020 Jul 18.

38. Regarding sexual health in men with spina bifida, which of the following is true?

    A. Men do not carry any increased risk of having a child with spina bifida.
    B. Infertility in men with spina bifida is infrequent.
    C. Sildenafil can be an effective treatment for individuals with ED and spina bifida.
    D. The level of neurologic lesion does not influence the presence or absence of erectile dysfunction.

Answer: C.

Sildenafil can be an effective treatment for men with spina bifida and ED. In men with spina bifida there are not usually any anatomical anomalies in the penile region, and sildenafil can be helpful to achieve an erection. Erectile dysfunction is dependent on the level of the lesion. Those who have intact continence and sacral reflexes are more likely to be potent. Compared to the general population, the risk of neural tube defects in offspring is greater regardless if the parent who has spina bifida is the mother or the father.

Bong GW, Rovner ES. Sexual health in adult men with spina bifida. ScientificWorldJournal. 2007;7:1466–9. https://doi.org/10.1100/tsw.2007.191.

39. Compared to individuals who sustain spinal cord injuries as an adult, individuals who experience a pediatric-onset spinal cord injury:

    A. Reported less physical activity participation when compared to those who sustained an injury as an adult.
    B. Reported similar levels of pain.
    C. Endorsed having more frequent physician visits over a period of 1 year.
    D. Were noted to have greater social participation.

Answer: D.

A study comparing self-reported health measures and participation between those who sustained an injury in childhood vs adulthood found that individuals who sustained an injury during childhood reported fewer physician visits within the last year and less pain. They were also noted to have greater social and occupational participation, more minutes per day of moderate/heavy physical activity and greater functional independence. Results were matched for lesion level, complete/incomplete nature of the injury, gender, education, age and ethnicity.

Ma JK, Post MW, Gorter JW, Martin Ginis KA. Differences in health, participation and life satisfaction outcomes in adults following paediatric-versus adult-sustained spinal cord injury. Spinal Cord. 2016;54(12):1197–202. https://doi.org/10.1038/sc.2016.45. Epub 2016 Sept 20. Erratum in: Spinal Cord. 2016;54(12):1220.

40. Common neurodevelopmental impairments seen in children with spina bifida include all of the following EXCEPT:

    A. Difficulties with executive functioning
    B. Deficits in visual spatial skill
    C. Impaired verbal learning skills
    D. Impaired working memory

Answer: B.

Throughout the years, several studies have characterized common patterns of intellectual functioning in children with spina bifida. Impairments in language functioning, visual-spatial skills, verbal learning, working memory and executive function have been noted. Difficulties in executive function and planning can be evident within daily activities and may have implications on future independence as the child becomes an adult.

Kelly NC, Ammerman RT, Rausch JR, Ris MD, Yeates KO, Oppenheimer SG, Enrile BG. Executive functioning and psychological adjustment in children and youth with spina bifida. Child Neuropsychol. 2012;18(5):417–31. https://doi.org/10.1080/09297049.201 1.613814. Epub 2011 Oct 3.

System Based Practice and Ethical Considerations Related to Spinal Cord Injuries

20

Elizabeth Twist, David Leong, and James Wilson

Questions

1. A 30-year-old male with a spinal cord injury (C8 AIS A) secondary to gunshot wound (GSW) has been under your care in acute inpatient rehab for 2 weeks. He goes to the garden with a friend and upon returning appears stuporous and slumped over in his wheelchair. While performing a thorough neurologic exam the patient becomes more awake and oriented. You talk with his friend who admits they injected heroin in the hospital courtyard. A small baggie of an unknown substance is incidentally found in the patient's sweatshirt pocket. Which of the following best encompasses your legal obligations as a physician?

    A. Notify police of drugs, give patient name as suspect, and discharge patient to authorities
    B. Notify police of drugs, give patient name as a suspect, and discharge patient from your rehabilitation facility to the community
    C. Immediately notify police of found drugs, but the physician is not obligated to provide additional information to the police about the patient
    D. Perform a citizen's arrest of the patient and his friend

    Answer: C.

    There are three things being addressed in this question: drug use, drug use on hospital grounds, and drug possession. Assuming the patient is not in life-threatening overdose, drug use alone would fall under the Health Insurance Portability and Accountability Act (HIPAA) and physician-patient confidentiality.

E. Twist · D. Leong · J. Wilson (✉)
Physical Medicine and Rehabilitation, MetroHealth Rehabilitation Institute,
Cleveland, OH, USA
e-mail: etwist@metrohealth.org; dleong@metrohealth.org; jwilson4@metrohealth.org

407

Of course, if the patient required additional medical attention, appropriate protected health information (PHI) handoff to other medical professionals would be acceptable. In general, physicians are permitted, but not obligated, to report this drug use to authorities under HIPAA "when responding to an off-site medical emergency, as necessary to alert law enforcement about criminal activity."

Since this occurred on hospital grounds, physicians would also be permitted, but not obligated, to report the patient to authorities under HIPPA which allows physicians "to report PHI that the covered entity in good faith believes to be evidence of a crime that occurred on the covered entity's premises."

The baggie of drugs is not protected under PHI and is evidence, which should be turned over to authorities immediately. While turning over the drugs is the only obligation you have as a physician, it is the physician's discretion what PHI to reveal when talking with police.

US Department of Health and Human Services. When does the privacy rule allow covered entities to disclose information to law enforcement. Available from: https://www.hhs.gov.

2. An 18-year-old previously healthy male presents to inpatient rehabilitation after sustaining a traumatic SCI (C4 AIS A) secondary to motor vehicle accident. His mood quickly becomes an issue with nursing staff and therapists. He refuses therapies, yells profanities at staff, and does not comply with medical management like intermittent catheterization or bowel regimen. He feels that he will be able to improve without anyone's help. He lives with his supportive parents, and his girlfriend comes to encourage him. Over his rehabilitation course the patient works with rehabilitation psychology and begins to adjust and cope with improved mood. Which quality was the strongest predictor of resilience in people with spinal cord injuries during a rehabilitation stay?

A. Self-efficacy
B. Positive mood
C. Social support
D. Lower level of comorbidities

Answer: A.

The work of Driver et al. (2016) determined that self-efficacy was the strongest predictor of resilience when inpatient, while at 3 months, an inverse relationship with depression was the strongest predictor. Other predictors like social support, lower level of comorbidities, and religious beliefs were also found to be important in long term coping and resilience in SCI patients.

Driver S, Warren AM, Reynolds M, Agtarap S, Hamilton R, Trost Z, Monden K. Identifying predictors of resilience at inpatient and 3-month post-spinal cord injury. J Spinal Cord Med. 2016;39(1):77–84. https://doi.org/10.1179/2045772314Y.0000000270. Epub 2014 Oct 9.

Guest R, Craig A, Tran Y, Middleton J. Factors predicting resilience in people with spinal cord injury during transition from inpatient rehabilitation to the community. Spinal Cord. 2015;53(9):682–6. https://doi.org/10.1038/sc.2015.32. Epub 2015 Feb 24.

Livneh H, Martz E. Coping strategies and resources as predictors of psychosocial adaptation among people with spinal cord injury. Rehabil Psychol. 2014;59(3):329–39. https://doi.org/10.1037/a0036733.

Jones K, Simpson GK, Briggs L, Dorsett P. Does spirituality facilitate adjustment and resilience among individuals and families after SCI? Disabil Rehabil. 2016;38(10):921–35. https://doi.org/10.3109/09638288.2015.1066884. Epub 2015 Jul 20.

3. Which of the following is NOT a strength of the National Spinal Cord Injury Database (NSCID) and Spinal Cord Injury Model Systems (SCIMS)?

A. Longitudinal data collection since 1970
B. Large sample size
C. Geographic and participant diversity
D. Direct reporting of regional incidence and prevalence

Answer: D.

The NSCID and SCIMS were started in 1970 which have collected data from 30 rehabilitation facilities throughout the US with ~44,000 subjects enrolled with SCI as of 2015. Data collection includes sociodemographics, information on acute care and rehabilitation experiences, and treatment outcomes. Current eligibility criteria (January 2005–present) include traumatic SCI with neurologic deficits, resident of SCIMS catchment area at time of injury, US citizen or non US citizen who is expected to stay in the catchment area, not having completed rehabilitation before SCIMS admission, admission to SCIMS within 1 year of injury, and discharge from SCIMS as either neurologically normal, having completed rehabilitation, or deceased.

As the answer choices imply, the NSCID has benefited from its long history of data collection. One constraint of the NSCID is that only persons with SCI that have been treated at SCIMS centers are included. The other drawback is that the data reflects a hospital based, rather than population based, study sample and therefore can only be presented as frequencies and percentages of the studied sample and not as community incidence or prevalence. A secondary analysis to assess the representativeness of the SCIMS National Database found that it was largely representative of the population of adults receiving inpatient rehabilitation for new onset traumatic SCI in the US.

Chen Y, DeVivo MJ, Richards JS, SanAgustin TB. Spinal cord injury model systems: review of program and national database from 1970 to 2015. Arch Phys Med Rehabil. 2016;97(10):1797–804. https://doi.org/10.1016/j.apmr.2016.02.027.

Ketchum JM, Cuthbert JP, Deutsch A, Chen Y, Charlifue S, Chen D, Dijkers MP, Graham JE, Heinemann AW, Lammertse DP, Whiteneck GG. Representativeness of the spinal cord injury model systems national database. Spinal Cord. 2018;56(2):126–32. https://doi.org/10.1038/s41393-017-0010-x. Epub 2017 Nov 6.

4. Which of the following is the most common health condition associated with re-hospitalization after inpatient rehabilitation?

   A. Pressure injury
   B. Pneumonia or non-infectious pulmonary issues
   C. Urinary tract infection
   D. Autonomic dysreflexia

Answer: C.

Multiple studies have found the most common cause of re-hospitalization after inpatient rehabilitation is UTI. Additionally, the proportion of SCI-related hospitalizations from any genitourinary complication has increased by 2.5% annually from 2006 to 2011 and 0.9% annually from 2011 to 2015. Acknowledgement of the increased risk of SCI patients for all of these possible complications make them a focus for rapid diagnosis, management, and prevention.

DeJong G, Tian W, Hsieh CH, Junn C, Karam C, Ballard PH, Smout RJ, Horn SD, Zanca JM, Heinemann AW, Hammond FM, Backus D. Rehospitalization in the first year of traumatic spinal cord injury after discharge from medical rehabilitation. Arch Phys Med Rehabil. 2013;94(4 Suppl):S87–97. https://doi.org/10.1016/j.apmr.2012.10.037.

Cardenas DD, Hoffman JM, Kirshblum S, McKinley W. Etiology and incidence of rehospitalization after traumatic spinal cord injury: a multicenter analysis. Arch Phys Med Rehabil. 2004;85(11):1757–63. https://doi.org/10.1016/j.apmr.2004.03.016.

Skelton F, Salemi JL, Akpati L, Silva S, Dongarwar D, Trautner BW, Salihu HM. Genitourinary complications are a leading and expensive cause of emergency department and inpatient encounters for persons with spinal cord injury. Arch Phys Med Rehabil. 2019;100(9):1614–21. https://doi.org/10.1016/j.apmr.2019.02.013. Epub 2019 Mar 30.

5. Which of the following is NOT a modifiable factor associated with employment outcomes following SCI?

   A. Level of injury
   B. Functional independence
   C. Social support
   D. Vocational rehabilitation

Answer: A.

Employment rates in individuals with SCI are about 35%. A systematic review by Treneman et al. found that education, vocational rehabilitation, functional independence, social support, and financial disincentives were modifiable factors that have been consistently and independently associated with employment outcomes. Non-modifiable risk factors include severity/level of injury, pre-injury chronic conditions, associated injuries, and pre-injury employment.

Trenaman L, Miller WC, Querée M, Escorpizo R, SCIRE Research Team. Modifiable and non-modifiable factors associated with employment outcomes following spinal cord injury: a systematic review. J Spinal Cord Med. 2015;38(4):422–31. https://doi.org/1 0.1179/2045772315Y.0000000031. Epub 2015 May 20.

6. Which of the following is true regarding falls in the first year after SCI?

A. 70% of SCI patients have a fall in the first year after injury
B. People with SCI are at disproportionately increased risk of falls compared to chronic neurologic conditions such as stroke and Parkinson's disease
C. Spasticity and contractures are the most common risk factors for falls
D. Fractures and loss of consciousness occur in more than half of all falls

Answer: B.

The work of Khan et al. (2019) showed that SCI patients are at a disproportionate risk of falls (30–41%) even compared to other individuals with diseases affecting motor function like stroke and Parkinson's. While the most commonly reported consequence was a minor injury, up 15% resulted in more serious injury like fracture or loss of consciousness. While there are many risk factors that contribute to falls in individuals with SCI the two most common biological factors of muscle weakness and impaired balance control are areas that could be improved with rehabilitation intervention.

Khan A, Pujol C, Laylor M, Unic N, Pakosh M, Dawe J, Musselman KE. Falls after spinal cord injury: a systematic review and meta-analysis of incidence proportion and contributing factors. Spinal Cord. 2019;57(7):526–39. https://doi.org/10.1038/s41393-019-0274-4. Epub 2019 Apr 9.

7. Racial disparities in SCI have been found in all the following areas EXCEPT?

A. Functional independence measure (FIM) scores at time of discharge from acute inpatient rehabilitation
B. Length of hospital admission
C. Rate of pressure injuries
D. Age at injury

Answer: D.

African American and Hispanic patients have been found to have significantly longer hospitalizations, lower FIM scores at time of discharge from acute inpatient rehabilitation, and all type complications. The work of Saunders et al. (2010) found that race was significantly associated with the presence of a pressure ulcer after SCI.

Fyffe DC, Deutsch A, Botticello AL, Kirshblum S, Ottenbacher KJ. Racial and ethnic disparities in functioning at discharge and follow-up among patients with motor complete spinal cord injury. Arch Phys Med Rehabil. 2014;95(11):2140–51. https://doi.org/10.1016/j.
apmr.2014.07.398. Epub 2014 Aug 2.

Saunders LL, Krause JS, Peters BA, Reed KS. The relationship of pressure ulcers, race, and
socioeconomic conditions after spinal cord injury. J Spinal Cord Med. 2010;33(4):387–95.
https://doi.org/10.1080/10790268.2010.11689717.

8. Spinal cord injury research trials that involve participants with the following
   patient characteristics require additional ethical, scientific, and regulatory considerations?

   A. Children
   B. Tetraplegia
   C. SCI resulting from drug abuse
   D. Ventilator dependence

   Answer: A.

   Children are considered a vulnerable population. A higher standard is applied
   that requires justification. Investigators should be prepared to answer why the
   intervention is likely to be particularly effective and beneficial in a younger
   population especially if it has not been previously tested in adults. Prisoners are
   similarly a vulnerable population but etiology of injury alone is not relevant.
   Vulnerable population broadly refers to a disadvantaged sub-segment of the
   community that may lack full ability to give free and informed consent. Other
   populations include but are not limited to pregnant women, fetuses, terminally
   ill, comatose, physically and intellectually challenged individuals, institutional-
   ized, elderly individuals and employees, military persons, and students in hier-
   archical organizations.

   Tuszynski MH, Steeves JD, Fawcett JW, Lammertse D, Kalichman M, Rask C, Curt A,
   Ditunno JF, Fehlings MG, Guest JD, Ellaway PH, Kleitman N, Bartlett PF, Blight AR,
   Dietz V, Dobkin BH, Grossman R, Privat A, International Campaign for Cures of Spinal
   Cord Injury Paralysis. Guidelines for the conduct of clinical trials for spinal cord injury as
   developed by the ICCP Panel: clinical trial inclusion/exclusion criteria and ethics. Spinal
   Cord. 2007;45(3):222–31. https://doi.org/10.1038/sj.sc.3102009. Epub 2006 Dec 19.

   Shivayogi P. Vulnerable population and methods for their safeguard. Perspect Clin Res.
   2013;4(1):53–7. https://doi.org/10.4103/2229-3485.106389.

9. Medical research of interventions may benefit from a sham control group; however, for central nervous system surgical therapies sham treatments often carry
   significant risks. Which of the following is FALSE regarding sham control
   groups in surgical trials?

   A. Similar standards apply to informed consent for projects with or without
      sham surgery
   B. Society may be injured when surgical procedures are adopted based on
      inadequate study of control groups

C. Sham treatments can have risk attenuated by careful procedure selection
D. There is often temporary, but unsustained postoperative improvement after any type of surgical manipulation of the spinal cord

Answer: A.

Sham surgery carries an increased risk to study participants. Informed consent in such cases demands higher standards. However, the benefit to future spinal cord injured persons may justify scientifically sound sham-controlled research. Historical and placebo controls are often inadequate due to the temporary effect of spinal manipulation due to decompression, lysis of adhesions (detethering), or other unknown factors. As such, researchers should include long term monitoring in such cases.

Tuszynski MH, Steeves JD, Fawcett JW, Lammertse D, Kalichman M, Rask C, Curt A, Ditunno JF, Fehlings MG, Guest JD, Ellaway PH, Kleitman N, Bartlett PF, Blight AR, Dietz V, Dobkin BH, Grossman R, Privat A, International Campaign for Cures of Spinal Cord Injury Paralysis. Guidelines for the conduct of clinical trials for spinal cord injury as developed by the ICCP Panel: clinical trial inclusion/exclusion criteria and ethics. Spinal Cord. 2007;45(3):222–31. https://doi.org/10.1038/sj.sc.3102009. Epub 2006 Dec 19.

10. James is a 34-year-old male with new incomplete tetraplegia without known brain injury or mental health concerns seen in your acute inpatient rehabilitation unit 2 weeks after his traumatic spinal cord injury. Which of the following characteristics makes James more likely to participate in effective shared decision making during his rehabilitation admission?

A. Gender
B. Age
C. Lack of mental health disorders
D. Incomplete neurologic Injury

Answer: C.

Tetraplegia, better physical health, and lack of mental health disorders were associated with more effective shared decision making. Veteran/civilian status and patient demographics were unrelated to shared decision making capacity. Interventions targeted to improve mental and physical health after spinal cord injury may improve shared decision making between the medical team and patient.

Locatelli SM, Etingen B, Heinemann A, Neumann HD, Miskovic A, Chen D, LaVela SL. Perceptions of shared decision making among patients with spinal cord injuries/disorders. Top Spinal Cord Inj Rehabil. 2016;22(3):192–202. https://doi.org/10.1310/sci2016-00027.

11. The short term and long-term cost related to care for persons with spinal cord injury are significant and may impact decisions by patients, families, and healthcare providers. Which of the following is true regarding healthcare costs in the final month and year before the end of life compared to 1-year prior for individuals with SCI?

   A. In the final year costs remain stable while in the final month costs increase more than twofold.
   B. In the final year costs increase more than twofold while in the final month costs increase more than fourfold.
   C. In the final year costs increase more than fourfold while in the final month costs increase more than tenfold.
   D. In the final year costs increase more than tenfold while in the final month costs increase more than 20-fold.

Answer: B.

In 2008, a study of veterans examined average healthcare costs near the end of life. The average annual cost was $24,900 in the second year before death and reached $61,900 in the final year. The average monthly cost accelerated during the final year from $3100 in month 12 to $14,600 in the final month. Cost of care is an ethical and practical concern in healthcare systems. Consideration of cost and risk vs. benefit should be considered in every medical decision and system policy.

Yu W, Smith B, Kim S, Chow A, Weaver FM. Major medical conditions and VA healthcare costs near end of life for veterans with spinal cord injuries and disorders. J Rehabil Res Dev. 2008;45(6):831–9. https://doi.org/10.1682/jrrd.2006.08.0102.

12. Which of the following is true regarding discussion of prognosis after spinal cord injury?

   A. Withholding clinical information is effective standard practice to protect the mental health of individuals early following SCI
   B. Providers are confident when confronted with prognostic conversations
   C. Discussions of prognosis should follow a predetermined structure determined by the medical team
   D. Failure to clearly explain the diagnosis and prognosis may interfere with a patient's process of coping and reduce their subjective well-being

Answer: D.

Evidence regarding prognostic discussion and breaking bad news after spinal cord injury is lacking. Most recommendations are adapted from other fields such as oncology. Overall, the timing and content of discussions should be customized to achieve the patient's individual goals and desires. There is currently no data to support that discussion of poor prognosis soon after injury causes depression or anxiety that may affect the patient's willingness to participate in comprehensive rehabilitation. In fact, failure to appropriately discuss prognosis can disrupt the rehabilitation process and have negative psychological effects.

Kirshblum S, Fichtenbaum J. Breaking the news in spinal cord injury. J Spinal Cord Med. 2008;31(1):7–12. https://doi.org/10.1080/10790268.2008.11753975.

13. Interdisciplinary clinicians who care for patients with spinal cord injury may experience heightened levels of workplace stress. Which of the following is FALSE regarding stress and burnout experienced by providers for this special population?

    A. Most providers who endorse burnout also report exhaustion.
    B. Self-reported personal health is not related to burnout.
    C. Clinicians report mostly positive attitudes towards their colleagues.
    D. Meaningfulness of work and intellectual stimulation is high.

Answer: B.

An international interdisciplinary survey of SCI providers demonstrated that most respondents reported feeling exhaustion (60.1%). Fewer reported feelings of burnout (41.1%) or work-life imbalance (31.9%). Personal health was significantly correlated with reported burnout along with various other metrics such as work-life balance, family life, ability to sleep, ability to stimulate your mind, financial situation, recreation, hobbies, and vacations. Spinal cord injury professionals reported high meaningfulness of work, positive impact from colleagues, and satisfaction with intellectual stimulation at work.

Slocum C, Stillman M, Capron M, Alexander S, Hultling C. International survey responses from an interdisciplinary cohort of spinal cord injury clinicians assessing professional burnout and meaning in work. Spinal Cord Ser Cases. 2019;5:59. https://doi.org/10.1038/s41394-019-0200-1.

14. In 2002, the American Board of Internal Medicine Foundation, in conjunction with the American College of Physicians Foundation and the European Federation of Internal Medicine authored Medical Professionalism in the New Millennium: A Physician Charter. The Charter articulates the professional commitments of physicians and health care professionals challenged by "increasing disparities among the legitimate needs of patients, the available resources to meet those needs, the increasing dependence on market forces to transform health care systems, and the temptation for physicians to forsake their traditional commitment to the primacy of patients' interests." Which of the following is NOT a fundamental principle laid out in the Charter?

A. Primacy of patient welfare
B. Patient autonomy
C. Social justice
D. Respect for institutional guidelines

Answer: D.

Institutional guidelines may vary based on the goals, interests, or structure of an individual group or system. The fundamental principles of the Physician Charter of Professionalism represent universal values and ideals of medical professionalism to be pursued by all physicians. They should supersede a physician's culture and national traditions as well as political, legal, and market forces. These principles mirror those described in the 1978 Belmont Report created to guide ethical research practices: respect for persons, beneficence, and justice.

ABIM Foundation, American Board of Internal Medicine, ACP-ASIM Foundation, American College of Physicians-American Society of Internal Medicine, European Federation of Internal Medicine. Medical professionalism in the new millennium: a physician charter. Ann Intern Med. 2002;136(3):243–6. https://doi.org/10.7326/0003-4819-136-3-200202050-00012.
Sabharwal S. Ethical issues in SCI practice. In: Essentials of spinal cord medicine. New York: Demos Medical; 2014. p. 444–52.

15. What course of action is recommended with regard to patients seeking unproven "cure" treatments for spinal cord injury?

    A. Physicians are obligated to perform treatments when risks are unproven based on the principle of autonomy
    B. Physicians have a greater than normal standard for informed consent when conducting cure-based research
    C. Physicians may decline to provide but must make reasonable efforts to refer patients to desired unproven cure treatments
    D. Physicians are mandated to report patients seeking potentially dangerous treatments to the National Institutes of Health

Answer: B.

Physicians should educate patients about the experimental nature of unproven treatments including the potential harms, design, validity, and regulatory oversight. Direct benefit to the subject is not the intent of research nor the expected outcome. Autonomy does not obligate physicians to provide or assist in unproven treatments though patients may independently pursue experimental therapies.

Sabharwal S. Ethical issues in SCI practice. In: Essentials of spinal cord medicine. New York: Demos Medical; 2014. p. 444–52.

16. A 68-year-old patient with Medicare falls and is admitted to an acute inpatient rehabilitation facility with new tetraplegia. By what day does the physician need to complete the post-admission physician evaluation (PAPE) and the individualized overall plan of care (IOPC)?

    A. PAPE by midnight of the day of admission and IOPC within 4 days
    B. PAPE within 24 h and IOPC within 4 days
    C. PAPE within 24 h and IOPC within 7 days
    D. PAPE within 72 h and IOPC within 7 days

    Answer: B.

    The Centers for Medicare & Medicaid Services (CMS) requires that a post-admission physician evaluation be performed within the first 24 h after admission to the Inpatient Rehabilitation Facility. This document must support medical necessity of admission, identify any relevant changes since the preadmission screening, include a history, physical exam, review of prior and current medical and functional conditions and comorbidities. This evaluation is not included as one of the three required rehabilitation physician face-to-face visits in the first week.

    The Centers for Medicare & Medicaid Services (CMS) requires that the individualized overall plan of care must be completed within the first 4 days of the IRF admission. The document must support medical necessity of admission, detail the patient's medical prognosis, anticipated interventions (including intensity, frequency, and total expected duration), functional outcomes, and discharge destination.

    Of note: the PAPE requirement was temporarily suspended during the COVID-19 pandemic. In 2021, CMS stated they will consider permanent removal of the PAPE after analyzing the temporary suspension.

    Medicare Benefit Policy Manual. Chapter 1—Inpatient hospital services covered under part A table of contents, Section 110.1.2–110.1.3, 2017. https://www.cms.gov/. Accessed 15 Jan 2021.

17. Insurance is denying coverage for admission to acute inpatient rehabilitation to a 71-year-old female with SCI and recommends referring her to a skilled nursing facility (SNF). You intend to complete a peer-to-peer evaluation to justify the need for acute inpatient rehabilitation facility (IRF). Which of the following is true regarding outcomes when comparing IRF to SNF rehabilitation?

    A. Patients discharged from IRF have greater increase in self-care FIM scores compared to those discharged from SNF
    B. Overall mortality is equivalent after IRF discharge compared to SNF
    C. Women benefit more than men from IRF admission
    D. Patients older than 70 years old do not benefit from admission to an IRF

    Answer: A.

Unfortunately, there is little research into outcomes of SCI after IRF vs SNF admissions. The work of Hong et al. (2019) compared functional status improvements in stroke patients after admissions to an IRF vs SNF. They found an increase in mobility and self-care scores that were significantly greater after IRF when compared to SNF. They found a reduced 30–365 day mortality rate after IRF when compared to SNF with multivariable analysis. There is no evidence that women benefit more than men from IRF. There are no firm age cutoffs for admission to IRF.

Hong I, Goodwin JS, Reistetter TA, Kuo YF, Mallinson T, Karmarkar A, Lin YL, Ottenbacher KJ. Comparison of functional status improvements among patients with stroke receiving postacute care in inpatient rehabilitation vs skilled nursing facilities. JAMA Netw Open. 2019;2(12):e1916646. https://doi.org/10.1001/jamanetworkopen.2019.16646.

18. Elizabeth is a 29-year-old patient who is preparing to discharge from acute inpatient rehabilitation following a non-traumatic spinal cord injury. Which of the following predicts increased risk of readmission to the acute care hospital?

    A. Acute care length of stay
    B. Hypertension
    C. Body max index greater than 30
    D. IV drug history

Answer: C.

The work of Robinson et al. (2018) evaluated causes for readmission to acute care in the non-traumatic SCI population and found 84% returned for medical reasons (infection, neurological, non-infectious respiratory) and 16% for surgical reasons (fractures and wound complications). Risk factors that were significant for predicting return to acute care included a lower FIM-motor subscore on admission, body mass index greater than 30, and paraplegia.

Robinson DM, Bazzi MS, Millis SR, Bitar AA. Predictors of readmission to acute care during inpatient rehabilitation for non-traumatic spinal cord injury. J Spinal Cord Med. 2018;41(4):444–9. https://doi.org/10.1080/10790268.2018.1426235. Epub 2018 Jan 22.

19. A patient 1 year removed from her injury presents for a follow up appointment in your clinic. She is interested in returning to work, however she is worried about the accommodations she needs preventing her from returning to the workplace. What advice can you give her about her rights to work accommodations?

    A. Recommend that employers have no obligation to provide accommodations so she should contact social services
    B. Recommend that employers will only provide accommodations following successful litigation so she should contact a lawyer

C. Recommend that employers must provide reasonable accommodations for qualified applicants and may be able to get help from her state vocational rehabilitation office

D. Recommend that employers must provide job retraining and any accommodations recommended by her physician

Answer: C.

The patient is protected under the "The Americans with Disabilities Act (ADA)" which became law in 1990. It is a civil rights law that prohibits discrimination against individuals with disabilities in all areas of public life, including jobs. Title I of the ADA and Section 501 and Section 504 of the Rehabilitation Act prohibits discrimination in employment and states that employers must provide reasonable accommodations to qualified applicants or employees. This is enforced by the "U.S. Equal Employment Opportunity Commission" and applies to employers with 15 or more employees. State offices of vocational rehabilitation can assist employees with disabilities to better know their rights and advocate on their behalf.

The United States Department of Justice Civil Rights Division. Title I of the The Americans with Disabilities Act (Public Law 101-336). 1990.

20. Which of the following is NOT a facilitating factor for self-management of individuals with traumatic SCI?

A. Caregiver support
B. Perceived sense of control
C. Household accessibility
D. Secondary complications

Answer: D.

The work of Munce et al. (2014) demonstrated that facilitating factors include physical and emotional caregiver support, peer support, perceived control/independence, and self-efficacy. Barriers include difficulty achieving positive outlook, caregiver burnout, physical limitations, secondary complications, lack of accessibility, and funding policies make significant contributions to the self-management of individuals with traumatic SCI.

Munce SE, Webster F, Fehlings MG, Straus SE, Jang E, Jaglal SB. Perceived facilitators and barriers to self-management in individuals with traumatic spinal cord injury: a qualitative descriptive study. BMC Neurol. 2014;14:48. https://doi.org/10.1186/1471-2377-14-48.

Community Living with Spinal Cord Injuries

21

Niña Carmela R. Tamayo, Heather Theobald, and Patricia L. Kiefer

Questions

1. The Americans with Disabilities Act of 1990 does all of the following EXCEPT:

    A. Ensures equal opportunities for persons with disabilities in employment, state, and local government activities and public accommodations
    B. Enforces standards for accessible design requiring specific building codes to improve accessibility and prevent discrimination
    C. Covers regulations for public transportation
    D. Determines regulations for air travel accessibility

    Answer: D.

    The Air Carrier Access of 1986 is responsible for governing accessibility regulations for the airline industry. It covers assistance in the airport including transportation of durable medical equipment and accessibility standards for aircrafts and airports. The Americans with Disabilities Act (ADA) was modeled after the Civil Rights Act of 1964 and is the most comprehensive disability

N. C. R. Tamayo (✉)
Department of Physical Medicine and Rehabilitation, Cleveland Clinic Edwin Shaw Rehabilitation Hospital; Tamayo Physiatry, LLC, Cleveland, OH, USA

H. Theobald
Department of Physical Medicine and Rehabilitation, Mercy Medical Center, Catholic Health Services of Long Island, Rockville Centre, NY, USA
e-mail: heather.theobald@chsli.org

P. L. Kiefer
Department of Medicine, Northeast Ohio Veteran Administration Healthcare System, Cleveland, OH, USA
e-mail: patricia.kiefer@va.gov

© The Author(s), under exclusive license to Springer Nature Switzerland AG 2022
B. A. Abramoff et al. (eds.), *The Essential Spinal Cord Injury Medicine Question Bank*, https://doi.org/10.1007/978-3-031-07796-8_21

rights law to date. It protects individuals who have a history of, or who are perceived to have a physical or mental impairment that substantially limits one or more major life activities. It also protects individuals who have a relationship or association with a disabled individual. Title I of the ADA covers employment and prohibits discrimination in recruitment, hiring, promotions, training, pay, social activities, and restricts questions about an applicant's disability before a job offer is presented. It requires employers to make reasonable accommodations based on the individual's limitations. Title II and III of the ADA cover public transportation services (city buses, subways, commuter rails) and public accommodations (restaurants, retail stores, hotels, movie theaters, private schools, recreation facilities, etc.) respectively. These entities must comply with nondiscrimination requirements, remove barriers, and follow specific accessibility design standards.

US Department of Justice. A guide to disability rights laws. Feb 2020. https://www.ada.gov/cguide.htm. Accessed 3 Nov 2020.

2. Which of the following was the first disability rights law prohibiting discrimination against persons with disabilities in programs and activities receiving federal funding?

A. The Architectural Barriers Act of 1968
B. The Rehabilitation Act of 1973
C. The Americans with Disabilities Act of 1990
D. The Affordable Care Act of 2010

Answer: B.

The Rehabilitation Act of 1973 was the first disability civil rights law to be enacted in the United States. It was the first piece of legislation to provide equal access for people with disabilities by removing architectural, employment, transportation, societal and environmental barriers, and creating opportunities through affirmative action programs. Section 504 specifically prohibits discrimination on the basis of disability and was modeled after Title VI of the Civil Rights Act of 1964. It states that "no qualified individual with a disability in the United States shall be excluded from, denied the benefits of, or be subjected to discrimination under any program receiving federal financial assistance." Entities including all government agencies, federally funded projects, K-12 schools, state colleges, universities, vocational training schools fall under this law. It has since been amended in 1978, 1986, 1992 and 2015.

The Architectural Barriers Act of 1968 was enacted by President Lyndon B. Johnson and requires that federal and federally funded buildings built, designed, or altered after August 12, 1968 be accessible. There Affordable

Care Act was an expansive health care reform law that was designed to control health care costs, improve health care deliver, and extend health care coverage to more individuals. The act also made it illegal for health insurances to deny coverage or charge more based on the existence of pre-existing conditions.

US Department of Justice. A guide to disability rights laws. Feb 2020. https://www.ada.gov/cguide.htm. Accessed 3 Nov 2020.

3. All of the following represent ADA requirements for accessibility in public spaces EXCEPT:

   A. Accessible routes need to be at least 36 in. wide.
   B. Interior doors that are open 90° must have a clear door opening width of at least 32 in. between the face of the door and the stop.
   C. Toilet stalls should have a grab bar at least 42 in. long on the side wall that is no more than 12 in. from the rear wall, and should be mounted no less than 33 in. and no greater than 36 in. above the floor to the top of the gripping surface.
   D. Floor surfaces in public spaces must be stable, firm, and slip resistant, and carpet is not allowed.

Answer: D.

All of the above statements are true except for D. In public spaces, pathways must be at least 36 in. wide, and floor surfaces should be stable, firm, and slip resistant, but carpeted paths should have carpet that is no higher than ½ in. and should be securely attached along the edges. Title III of the ADA follows four priorities for accessibility: (1) accessible approach and entrance, (2) access to goods and services, (3) access to public toilet rooms, and (4) access to other items such as water fountains and public telephones. The ADA created a checklist for public accommodations based on the 2010 ADA Standards for Accessible Design.

Institute for Human Centered Design. ADA checklist for facilities. 2016. https://www.ada-checklist.org/. Accessed 15 Dec 2020.

4. Which is the highest level of complete spinal cord injury that may allow an individual to drive a car?

   A. C3
   B. C5
   C. C7
   D. T1

Answer: B.

Individuals with complete C1–C4 injuries are unable to drive even with extensive vehicle adaptations as they need the use of at least one extremity. Individuals with C5–C7 complete injuries may be able to drive with modifications. Individuals with C8 and below may be able to drive with hand controls. Of note, the ability to transfer to the toilet can be used as a predictor of driving ability. It is also important to exclude other associated medical issues that may affect driving (cognitive dysfunction, spasticity, visual field or perception deficits).

Kiyono Y, Hashizume C, Matsui N, Ohtsuka K, Takaoka K. Car-driving abilities of people with tetraplegia. Arch Phys Med Rehabil. 2001;82(10):1389–92. https://doi.org/10.1053/apmr.2001.26089.

Norweg A, Jette AM, Houlihan B, Ni P, Boninger ML. Patterns, predictors, and associated benefits of driving a modified vehicle after spinal cord injury: findings from the National Spinal Cord Injury Model Systems. Arch Phys Med Rehabil. 2011;92(3):477–83. https://doi.org/10.1016/j.apmr.2010.07.234.

5. The driving evaluation is an essential component of a comprehensive Spinal Cord Injury (SCI) program. Components of the assessment include all of the following EXCEPT:

   A. Pre-driving assessment interview and clinical evaluation of muscle strength, balance, range of motion, seating evaluation and medications
   B. Visual, perception, and cognitive evaluation
   C. Static behind the wheel assessment and training including ability to accelerate, brake and use of secondary controls
   D. Confirmation of the strength and dexterity to control the pedals with at least one lower extremity.

Answer: D.

To test for driving fitness, an individual with SCI should seek out a certified driver rehabilitation specialist. A driving assessment is composed of undergoing a pre-driving assessment and behind the wheel (BTW) assessment, selecting the appropriate vehicle and equipment based on injury, obtaining medical clearance, and meeting license requirements. Driving rehabilitation services include testing visual acuity, range of motion, muscle strength and fine motor coordination, as well as cognitive-perceptual tests such as the trail making tests, motor free visual perception test-revised, and short cognitive screening tests. The BTW assessment, however, is the main factor in making a fitness-to-drive recommendation. There is no requirement for any strength in the lower extremities in order to drive.

Dickerson AE. Driving assessment tools used by driver rehabilitation specialists: survey of use and implications for practice. Am J Occup Ther. 2013;67(5):564–73. https://doi.org/10.5014/ajot.2013.007823.

6. Driving status is an important aspect of successful community participation and reintegration for individuals with spinal cord injury and is associated with health-related quality of life gains. Which of the following is a predictor of driving a modified vehicle following a SCI?

A. Single at the time of injury
B. Associates degree or higher-level education before time of injury
C. Female sex
D. Low functional independence measure score at the time of discharge

Answer: B.

Driving has a positive impact on quality of life, reintegration into the community, and increases the odds of an individual being employed at follow up. Factors that predict driving a modified vehicle post spinal cord injury include: married at injury, younger age at injury, associate's degree or higher before injury, paraplegia, a longer time since the injury, non-Hispanic race, white race, male sex, and using a wheelchair for more than 40 h a week after the injury, higher community integration scores, as well as higher activity of daily living independence at hospital discharge.

Norweg A, Jette AM, Houlihan B, Ni P, Boninger ML. Patterns, predictors, and associated benefits of driving a modified vehicle after spinal cord injury: findings from the National Spinal Cord Injury Model Systems. Arch Phys Med Rehabil. 2011;92(3):477–83. https://doi.org/10.1016/j.apmr.2010.07.234.

7. Studies on employment rates after spinal cord injury vary widely from 3% to 80% due to a variety of factors including the use of different definitions for employment, time since injury, sample characteristics, method of obtaining data, and time of measurement. Despite the variance of data, employment after SCI leads to improved quality of life, independence, social integration, and greater life satisfaction. Statistically, which of the following individuals is more likely to return to work status post SCI?

A. College educated white male who sustained injury 20 years ago
B. Female who sustained injury at age 55, and unable to live alone
C. Non-white male with C4 injury and a high school education
D. 33-year-old female with paraplegia and a history of depression and drug abuse

Answer: A.

Anderson et al. (2007) found that there are 11 key factors that are associated with returning to work for people with SCI: education, type of employment, disability severity, age, time since injury, sex, marital status and social support, vocational counseling, medical problems, employer role, environment, and professional interests. Characteristics that predicted return to work post SCI included:

Non-modifiable factors:
- Younger age at time of injury
- Greater number of years living with SCI (20–30 years)
- White race
- Male sex
- Paraplegia (compared to tetraplegia)

Modifiable factors:
- Education (strongest predictor of return to work for persons with SCI—college level and higher).
- Higher level of independence (using transportation independently, ability to live alone).
- Lower number of health complications.
- Environmental facilitators (increased social support, access to vocational rehabilitation and assistive technology, higher socioeconomic status and living in a suburban vs. urban area).
- Environmental barriers (financial disincentives, discrimination/ negative attitudes towards people with disabilities, accessibility in the workplace).

Anderson D, Dumont S, Azzaria L, Bourdais ML, Noreau L. Determinants of return to work among spinal cord injury patients: a literature review. J Voc Rehabil. 2007;27(1):57–68.

Ottomanelli L, Lind L. Review of critical factors related to employment after spinal cord injury: implications for research and vocational services. J Spinal Cord Med. 2009;32(5):503–31. https://doi.org/10.1080/10790268.2009.11754553.

Trenaman L, Miller WC, Querée M, Escorpizo R, SCIRE Research Team. Modifiable and non-modifiable factors associated with employment outcomes following spinal cord injury: a systematic review. J Spinal Cord Med. 2015;38(4):422–31. https://doi.org/10.1179/2045772315Y.0000000031. Epub 2015 May 20.

8. The Supportive Employment model is a non-traditional approach to vocational rehabilitation that has been increasingly utilized to help people with disabilities including the SCI population. Which of the following does NOT describe evidenced based supportive employment?

   A. Job finding and training can concurrently occur.
   B. The focus is competitive employment as the goal.
   C. There is a limited time frame due to losing benefits and other government entitlements.
   D. No one is excluded who wants to participate.

Answer: C.

Supportive Employment also known as the individualized placement and support model is a program that serves individuals with the most significant disabilities (zero exclusion policy) and focuses on helping individuals attain competitive integrated employment, including customized employment. It is a provision of the The Rehabilitation Act of 1973 and allows for services to be provided for persons with disability for whom competitive integrated employment has not historically occurred, or has been interrupted, and for whom intensive/ extended services are needed to perform the particular work due to the severity of an individual's disability. The aim is to find employment that is consistent with the individual's strengths, abilities, interests, and personal choice, and includes ongoing support services and counseling throughout the process to ensure individuals that there is no loss of benefits and entitlements. Job training can occur simultaneously with an individuals' job search. Supportive employment has a time frame of 24 months unless the individual has special circumstances where this has been agreed to be extended.

US Department of Justice. A guide to disability rights laws. Feb 2020. https://www.ada.gov/cguide.htm. Accessed 3 Nov 2020.
Bond GR. Supported employment: evidence for an evidence-based practice. Psychiatr Rehabil J. 2004;27(4):345–59. https://doi.org/10.2975/27.2004.345.359.
Thijssen DH, Heesterbeek P, van Kuppevelt DJ, Duysens J, Hopman MT. Local vascular adaptations after hybrid training in spinal cord-injured subjects. Med Sci Sports Exerc. 2005;37(7):1112–8. https://doi.org/10.1249/01.mss.0000170126.30868.fb.

9. State vocational rehab (VR) agencies under the State Department of Education have played a key role in promoting employment for persons with severe physical limitations and those with SCI. The services include all of the following EXCEPT:

A. Subsidizing education and vocational assessments
B. Covering transportation and personal care assistance costs
C. Assisting in purchasing equipment and other resources
D. Establishing eligibility for services prior to leaving the hospital

Answer: D.

Eligibility of State VR services is determined on the basis of disability. An individual is not able to be deemed eligible for services until they leave the hospital. Most SCI individuals by the nature of their injuries will meet eligibility criteria. Vocational rehabilitations' primary purpose is to assist and enable individuals with disabilities (including SCI) to increase their productivity as fully integrated and contributing members of society, usually through competitive employment. State VR agencies may arrange for specialized employment services or consultations with private and not-for-profit providers who also serve the needs of individuals with disabilities.

Rehabilitation Act of 1973. Pub. L. 93-112. http://www.usbr.gov/cro/pdfsplus/rehabact.pdf.
Ottomanelli L, Barnett SD, Goetz LL, Toscano R. Vocational rehabilitation in spinal cord injury: what vocational service activities are associated with employment program outcome? Top Spinal Cord Inj Rehabil. 2015;21(1):31–9. https://doi.org/10.1310/sci2101-31.

10. Which of the following has been cited as the top barrier for employment for both employed and unemployed individuals with SCI?

    A. Lack of insurance
    B. Lack of transportation
    C. No time off for health related issues
    D. Funds not compensating for benefits lost

Answer: B.

Fiedler et al. (2002) found that there are differing perceptions of barriers and factors helpful for employment between employed and unemployed individuals with SCI. Despite this, lack of transportation has been cited by both groups as the biggest barrier to employment. For employed SCI individuals, lack of Social Security benefits was considered a top barrier along with transportation. For those who are unemployed, no time off for health related issues, funds not compensating for benefit loss, and lack of insurance were also ranked highly. Other factors that were considered barriers included lack of workplace accommodation, no Medicaid/ Medicare coverage after supplemental security income stopped.

Fiedler I, Indermuehle D, Drobac W, Laud P. Perceived barriers to employment in individuals with spinal cord injury. Top Spinal Cord Inj Rehabil. 2002;7(3):73–82.

11. Patients with spinal cord injury often experience adverse effects to their pulmonary function. What pulmonary changes may be identified after participation in a long-term exercise program?

    A. Decreased peak exercise tolerance
    B. Improved vital capacity and increase in maximum volume of expired air during exercise
    C. Decreased Forced Expiratory Volume to Forced Vital Capacity (FEV_1/FVC) ratio
    D. No measurable changes to pulmonary function tests

Answer: B.

Injuries at or above C5 results in diaphragmatic dysfunction as the diaphragm is innervated by C3, C4, and C5. The internal and external intercostal muscles are innervated by the thoracic spinal cord. Thoracic spinal cord injury causes impaired function of expiratory muscles resulting in restrictive lung disease and subsequent reduction in vital capacity and lung capacity. Injuries to inspiratory muscles result in ventilation problems. Research indicates that there is improvement to pulmonary function after participation in long-term exercise programs. These improvements include increased peak exercise tolerance (Thijssen et al.

2005), improved vital capacity and maximum volume of expired air when exercising (Walker et al. 1989); and improved FVC, FEV_1, FEV_1/FVC and Forced Expiratory Flow (FEF) (Jung et al. 2014).

Thijssen DH, Heesterbeek P, van Kuppevelt DJ, Duysens J, Hopman MT. Local vascular adaptations after hybrid training in spinal cord-injured subjects. Med Sci Sports Exerc. 2005;37(7):1112–8. https://doi.org/10.1249/01.mss.0000170126.30868.fb.
Walker J, Cooney M, Norton S. Improved pulmonary function in chronic quadriplegics after pulmonary therapy and arm ergometry. Paraplegia. 1989;27(4):278–83. https://doi.org/10.1038/sc.1989.41.
Jung J, Chung E, Kim K, Lee BH, Lee J. The effects of aquatic exercise on pulmonary function in patients with spinal cord injury. J Phys Ther Sci. 2014;26(5):707–9. https://doi.org/10.1589/jpts.26.707. Epub 2014 May 29.

12. All of the following are part of an exercise regimen recommendation EXCEPT:

   A. Frequency
   B. Time
   C. Activity type
   D. Therapist specialty

Answer: D.

Four elements that should be included when developing an exercise program include: frequency, intensity, time, and physical activity (FITT). The four elements of the FITT protocol make up the exercise quantity needed to improve health similar to that of a pharmacologic intervention. According to guidelines by the American College of Sports Medicine and the American Heart Association, adults with spinal cord injuries should aim for at least 150 min/week of moderate-intensity or 75 min/week of vigorous-intensity per week. They should also complete muscle-strengthening exercises at least 2 days/week. Although the recommendations set a minimum guideline, patient's that are severely deconditioned like those with SCI may not be able to tolerate these minimum levels. Modifications to accommodate this deconditioning must be taken into account when prescribing an exercise regimen for this population.

Gaspar R, Padula N, Freitas TB, de Oliveira JPJ, Torriani-Pasin C. Physical exercise for individuals with spinal cord injury: systematic review based on the international classification of functioning, disability, and health. J Sport Rehabil. 2019;28(5):505–16. https://doi.org/10.1123/jsr.2017-0185. Epub 2019 Feb 19.
Billinger SA, Boyne P, Coughenour E, Dunning K, Mattlage A. Does aerobic exercise and the FITT principle fit into stroke recovery? Curr Neurol Neurosci Rep. 2015;15(2):519. https://doi.org/10.1007/s11910-014-0519-8.
Haskell WL, Lee IM, Pate RR, Powell KE, Blair SN, Franklin BA, Macera CA, Heath GW, Thompson PD, Bauman A, American College of Sports Medicine, American Heart Association. Physical activity and public health: updated recommendation for adults from the American College of Sports Medicine and the American Heart Association. Circulation. 2007;116(9):1081–93. https://doi.org/10.1161/CIRCULATIONAHA.107.185649. Epub 2007 Aug 1.

13. A patient with a complete T1 and higher injury can use all of the following methods to assess exercise intensity EXCEPT:

A. Max heart rate equation (220-age)
B. The Borg rating of perceived exertion (RPE) scale
C. 60–80% of measured peak VO_2
D. Centers for Disease Control Talk Test

Answer: A.

Those with complete lesions T1 and above will have a blunted HR response due to impaired sympathetic outflow below lesion. VO_2 max will continue to rise but HR will peak at 120 and will not give an accurate reflection of exercise intensity. Alternative approaches to measure exercise intensity include VO_2 peak measurement during an arm exercise and targeting 60–80% of this value, Borg RPE (although may not be linear with VO_2 max), and the Centers for Disease Control and Prevention Talk Test.

Goosey-Tolfrey V, Lenton J, Goddard J, Oldfield V, Tolfrey K, Eston R. Regulating intensity using perceived exertion in spinal cord-injured participants. Med Sci Sports Exerc. 2010;42(3):608–13. https://doi.org/10.1249/MSS.0b013e3181b72cbc.

Totosy de Zepetnek JO, Au JS, Hol AT, Eng JJ, MacDonald MJ. Predicting peak oxygen uptake from submaximal exercise after spinal cord injury. Appl Physiol Nutr Metab. 2016;41(7):775–81. https://doi.org/10.1139/apnm-2015-0670. Epub 2016 Mar 15.

Reed JL, Pipe AL. The talk test: a useful tool for prescribing and monitoring exercise intensity. Curr Opin Cardiol. 2014;29(5):475–80. https://doi.org/10.1097/HCO.0000000000000097.

14. Spinal cord injury causes widespread physical changes even on the molecular and cellular level. Exercise participation has been correlated with what physiologic benefit for an individual with a SCI?

A. Increased T- and B-cell function
B. Improved temperature regulation
C. Increased serum levels of brain-derived neurotrophic factor
D. Increased serum adrenaline levels

Answer: C.

Brain-derived neurotrophic factor (BDNF) protein has been shown to have many benefits including neuroprotection, neuroregeneration and promotion of both peripheral nervous system and central nervous system neural survival. Furthermore, it has been correlated with decreased food intake, improved glucose oxidation and improved insulin sensitivity. Nishimura et al. reported significant increases in BDNF protein in both lumbar SCI and cervical SCI after exercise. Those with cervical spinal cord injuries do not have increases in plasma adrenaline with exercise secondary to termination of the peripheral sympathetic nervous system in the spinal cord. T- and B-cell function is decreased with intense and prolonged exercise which may result in increased risk for infection; however, this response may be mitigated with consistent training intensities and durations and avoiding the stress associated with overtraining. Exercise has no benefit with regards to temperature regulation and may, in fact, place the patient at increased risk for hypothermia or hyperthermia based on the environment.

Banno M, Nakamura T, Furusawa K, Ogawa T, Sasaki Y, Kouda K, Kawasaki T, Tajima F. Wheelchair half-marathon race increases natural killer cell activity in persons with cervical spinal cord injury. Spinal Cord. 2012;50(7):533–7. https://doi.org/10.1038/sc.2011.188. Epub 2012 Jan 17.

Nieman DC. Marathon training and immune function. Sports Med. 2007;37(4–5):412–5. https://doi.org/10.2165/00007256-200737040-00036.

Nishimura Y, Nakamura T, Kamijo YI, Arakawa H, Umemoto Y, Kinoshita T, Sakurai Y, Tajima F. Increased serum levels of brain-derived neurotrophic factor following wheelchair half marathon race in individuals with spinal cord injury. J Spinal Cord Med. 2020:1–6. https://doi.org/10.1080/10790268.2020.1816402. Epub ahead of print.

15. Basketball wheelchairs include which of the following modifications to increase agility?

   A. Larger diameter hand rims
   B. Higher seat position
   C. Low-pressure pneumatic tires with decreased camber
   D. Heavy, rigid frame

Answer: A.

Basketball wheelchairs are made of ultra-lightweight rigid frames. Large hand rim diameter allows for greater time to apply propulsive forces and achieve greater levels of acceleration which aids in the start-stops demands of basketball. Lowering the seat results in decreased vertical distance between axle and shoulder making more of the hand rim available. High-pressure pneumatic tires with increased camber improve stability.

Churton E, Keogh JW. Constraints influencing sports wheelchair propulsion performance and injury risk. BMC Sports Sci Med Rehabil. 2013;5:3. https://doi.org/10.1186/2052-1847-5-3.

Mason BS, van der Woude LH, Goosey-Tolfrey VL. The ergonomics of wheelchair configuration for optimal performance in the wheelchair court sports. Sports Med. 2013;43(1):23–38. https://doi.org/10.1007/s40279-012-0005-x.

16. Many of the adverse health events related to spinal cord injury are secondary to prolonged immobility. Implementing a regular exercise regimen for this population is vital in preventing long-term sequelae of disease. Which of the following represents one of the benefits of a consistent fitness program for SCI?

A. Decreased bladder capacity, voiding efficiency and detrusor contraction time
B. Increased insulin resistance, and lipid lipoprotein profiles
C. Decreased shoulder pain from shoulder instability related to muscle weakness
D. Decreased forced vital capacity (FVC), Forced expiratory volume in the first second (FEV$_1$), and FEV$_1$/FVC

Answer: C.

There is consistent evidence that regular exercise for SCI individuals has positive effects on cardiorespiratory, metabolic, genitourinary, skin, musculoskeletal and psychosocial function. Some of these effects include:

- Improved lipid lipoprotein profiles, including decreased low-density lipoprotein and total cholesterol, decreased body fat and body mass index, and increased high-density lipoprotein.
- Improved peak exercise tolerance, vital capacity, and increased FVC, FEV$_1$, and FEV$_1$/FVC.
- Improved glucose homeostasis and insulin sensitivity (reduced insulin resistance).
- Increased bladder capacity, voiding efficiency and detrusor contraction time, as well as decreased voiding pressure and frequency of nocturia and urinary incontinence.
- Promoted maintenance of skin integrity and prevention of pressure ulcers.
- Improved bone mineral density and reduced osteoporosis.
- Reduction in stress, pain, anxiety, and depression, as well as increased energy, self-confidence, self-image, and improved overall quality of life.

Jung J, Chung E, Kim K, Lee BH, Lee J. The effects of aquatic exercise on pulmonary function in patients with spinal cord injury. J Phys Ther Sci. 2014;26(5):707–9. https://doi.org/10.1589/jpts.26.707. Epub 2014 May 29.

Hubscher CH, Herrity AN, Williams CS, Montgomery LR, Willhite AM, Angeli CA, Harkema SJ. Improvements in bladder, bowel and sexual outcomes following task-specific locomotor training in human spinal cord injury. PLoS One. 2018;13(1):e0190998. https://doi.org/10.1371/journal.pone.0190998.

Nightingale TE, Walhin JP, Thompson D, Bilzon JLJ. Impact of exercise on cardiometabolic component risks in spinal cord-injured humans. Med Sci Sports Exerc. 2017;49(12):2469–77. https://doi.org/10.1249/MSS.0000000000001390.

17. While the benefits of exercise are well documented for the SCI population, there are significant barriers to participation in the community. All of the following represent barriers to physical activity EXCEPT:

    A. Impaired thermoregulation, blunted sympathetic response, musculoskeletal overuse and injury
    B. Access to accessible gyms with wheelchair equipment, transportation to facilities, and awareness of adaptive sports programs
    C. Lack of motivation, depression, and reduced energy
    D. Loss of disability benefits by demonstrating independence with a physical activity program

Answer: D.

There are significant physical, psychological and environmental barriers to participating in regular exercise programs for SCI individuals. First, in addition to muscle paralysis, medical conditions including autonomic dysreflexia, blunted heart rate response, orthostatic hypotension, impaired temperature regulation, risk for fracture/dislocation and other musculoskeletal injuries as well as pressure injuries are physical factors that prevent participation. Psychosocial factors include lack of motivation, reduced energy, depression, lack of self-confidence, fear and concern about physical limitations which make participating in a fitness program difficult. These are further exacerbated by environmental factors like lack of accessible gyms with wheelchair equipment, lack of SCI experienced trainers at fitness centers, financial barriers, lack of transportation to gyms and exercise facilities, and general lack of awareness of exercise and adaptive sports programs. There is no direct relationship between being involved in a physical activity program and loss of benefits.

Cardinal BJ, Kosma M, McCubbin JA. Factors influencing the exercise behavior of adults with physical disabilities. Med Sci Sports Exerc. 2004;36(5):868–75. https://doi.org/10.1249/01.mss.0000126568.63402.22.

Lavis TD, Scelza WM, Bockenek WL. Cardiovascular health and fitness in persons with spinal cord injury. Phys Med Rehabil Clin N Am. 2007;18(2):317–31, vii. https://doi.org/10.1016/j.pmr.2007.03.003.

Scelza WM, Kalpakjian CZ, Zemper ED, Tate DG. Perceived barriers to exercise in people with spinal cord injury. Am J Phys Med Rehabil. 2005;84(8):576–83. https://doi.org/10.1097/01.phm.0000171172.96290.67.

18. A 22 year-old male with T6 ASIA A patient presents to your office for evaluation. He is a road paracyclist who is training for the 2021 Paralympic Games in Tokyo, Japan in August. He is concerned about potential problems that could affect his performance in comparison to other athletes participating at the games. He is at higher risk for which of the following potential complications in comparison to his SCI wheelchair basketball competitors?

A. Autonomic dysreflexia
B. Orthostatic hypotension
C. Heat illness
D. Sacral wounds

Answer: C.

Although all athletes with SCI are at risk for overuse injuries, skin breakdown/ wounds (abrasions, burns, blisters), falls, heat illness and orthostatic hypotension; this patient is at higher risk for heat illness. SCI resulting in tetraplegia or paraplegia at T6 or higher interrupts the autonomic nervous system and regular heat dissipation mechanisms resulting in impaired thermoregulation. This patient has a T6 injury and because he is a road paracyclist, he will be cycling outdoors in a potentially humid and hot environment increasing his risk for heat illness. Wheelchair basketball is usually performed indoors in a temperature-controlled environment reducing risk of heat illness in those athletes.

Zhang Y, Bishop PA. Risks of heat illness in athletes with spinal cord injury: current evidence and needs. Front Sports Act Living. 2020;1:68. https://doi.org/10.3389/fspor.2019.00068.

19. A 23-year-old female with T4 ASIA A SCI is interested in functional electrical stimulation (FES) of her lower extremities after reading online that it can help her walk again. After answering her questions, you review the risks associated with FES, which include all of the following EXCEPT:

A. Fracture
B. Rhabdomyolysis
C. Skin irritation or encapsulation
D. Autonomic dysreflexia

Answer: B.

Injury to the spinal cord results in disruption of communication between the brain and the body. In FES, a neuroprosthesis with either surface or implantable electrodes can be used to stimulate muscle contraction in SCI patients via electrical current to help prevent muscle atrophy, maintain range of motion, improve blood flow, reverse osteoporosis and reduce muscle spasm. As with all medical devices, there are risks or disadvantages which include fracture, local skin irritation with surface electrodes or encapsulation of implanted electrodes by scar tissue, autonomic dysreflexia (AD) from the noxious stimuli, infection after electrode implantation, and the high-cost of acquiring the device. Rhabdomyolysis is not a reported complication.

Krassioukov A, Warburton DE, Teasell R, Eng JJ, Spinal Cord Injury Rehabilitation Evidence Research Team. A systematic review of the management of autonomic dysreflexia after spinal cord injury. Arch Phys Med Rehabil. 2009;90(4):682–95. https://doi.org/10.1016/j.apmr.2008.10.017.

Ho CH, Triolo RJ, Elias AL, Kilgore KL, DiMarco AF, Bogie K, Vette AH, Audu ML, Kobetic R, Chang SR, Chan KM, Dukelow S, Bourbeau DJ, Brose SW, Gustafson KJ, Kiss ZH, Mushahwar VK. Functional electrical stimulation and spinal cord injury. Phys Med Rehabil Clin N Am. 2014;25(3):631–54, ix. https://doi.org/10.1016/j.pmr.2014.05.001.

Hartkopp A, Murphy RJ, Mohr T, Kjaer M, Biering-Sørensen F. Bone fracture during electrical stimulation of the quadriceps in a spinal cord injured subject. Arch Phys Med Rehabil. 1998;79(9):1133–6. https://doi.org/10.1016/s0003-9993(98)90184-8.

20. A 17-year-old male with a T6 ASIA B SCI sustained 16 months ago presents to your office for a pre-performance evaluation to participate in a community adaptive basketball team. His past medical history is significant for a distal femur fracture 1-year prior. Which of the following tests, if any, should be ordered?

A. Exercise stress test
B. Pulmonary function tests (PFTs)
C. Bone mineral density
D. No additional tests needed

Answer: C.

Currently there is no standardized preparticipation examination for those with SCI. Practitioners evaluating adaptive athletes must be aware of common issues related to the population, how to diagnose these issues, and whether these issues will preclude sports participation. Patients with SCI are at high risk for osteoporosis, overuse injuries, impaired thermoregulation, autonomic dysreflexia, skin breakdown, bowel and bladder dysfunction and spasticity. Osteoporosis is common amongst those with SCI which places them at increased risk for fractures, most commonly supracondylar femur fractures. Bone mineral density will need to be evaluated by dual energy X-ray absorptiometry (DEXA) scan to determine if the patient is safe for sport participation and if medical intervention is required. SCI patients may also need exercise stress tests or pulmonary function tests based on medical history, screening questions and physical exam findings.

Gaspar AP, Lazaretti-Castro M, Brandão CM. Bone mineral density in spinal cord injury: an evaluation of the distal femur. J Osteoporos. 2012;2012:519754. https://doi.org/10.1155/2012/519754. Epub 2012 Aug 28.

Hawkeswood JP, O'Connor R, Anton H, Finlayson H. The preparticipation evaluation for athletes with disability. Int J Sports Phys Ther. 2014;9(1):103–15.

De Luigi AJ, editor. Adaptive sports medicine: a clinical guide. Cham: Springer; 2017.

Sabharwal S. Medical complications and consequences of SCI: overview. In: Sabharwal S, editor. Essentials of spinal cord medicine. New York: Demos Medical Publishing/Springer; 2014. p. 229–31.

21. Community reintegration for people with SCI is an important aspect of the rehabilitation continuum, however, the heterogeneity of this population makes it difficult to identify the most effective approach to optimize adjustment back into society. Which of the following has been found to facilitate community reintegration for people with SCI?

   A. Cervical level of injury
   B. High self-efficacy and self-esteem
   C. Complete injury
   D. Reliance on federal disability support

Answer: B.

Gupta et al. (2019) studied injury related and personal factors and their impact on rehabilitation outcomes related to community reintegration for people with SCI. Their comprehensive review found there is level 1 evidence that social support, self-efficacy, and self-esteem facilitate community reintegration. Presence of psychological or medical complications decreased it (level 5 evidence). And the impact of injury-related factors (i.e. type and level of injury) on community integration revealed mixed results. It is important to note, however, that it is a combination of these factors interacting with each other that predicts community reintegration, and that none of these factors predict participation independently.

Gupta S, Jaiswal A, Norman K, DePaul V. Heterogeneity and its impact on rehabilitation outcomes and interventions for community reintegration in people with spinal cord injuries: an integrative review. Top Spinal Cord Inj Rehabil. 2019;25(2):164–85. https://doi.org/10.1310/sci2502-164.

Peter C, Müller R, Cieza A, Geyh S. Psychological resources in spinal cord injury: a systematic literature review. Spinal Cord. 2012;50(3):188–201. https://doi.org/10.1038/sc.2011.125. Epub 2011 Nov 29.

Mingaila S, Krisciūnas A. Occupational therapy for patients with spinal cord injury in early rehabilitation. Medicina (Kaunas). 2005;41(10):852–6.

Beedie A, Kennedy P. Quality of social support predicts hopelessness and depression post spinal cord injury. J Clin Psychol Med Settings. 2002;9(3):227–34.

22. There are various ways to measure an individual's participation, reintegration and quality of life (QOL) after a spinal cord injury. Which of the following utilizes a 100-point scale with 32 items measuring handicap based on 6 domains—physical dependence, cognitive independence, mobility, occupation, social integration and economic self-sufficiency?

   A. Assessment of Life Habits (LIFE-H)
   B. Impact on Participation and Autonomy (IPA)
   C. Craig Hospital Inventory of Environmental Factors (CHIEF)
   D. Craig Handicap Assessment and Reporting Technique (CHART)

Answer: D.

The Craig Handicap Assessment and Reporting Technique was developed in the 1980s by Craig Hospital to quantify the extent of handicap in individuals and is the most widely used instrument to assess participation in the community. CHART measures six separate areas of societal participation: physical dependence, cognitive independence, mobility, occupation, social integration and economic self-sufficiency. Each is scored on a one-hundred-point scale. There is a long version with 32 questions and a short form with 19 questions and has significant validity and reliability in the SCI community. While it was developed prior to the WHO International Classification of Functioning, Disability and Health (ICF) concept of participation, it still correlates with the ICF participation codes. In addition, it does not subjectively assess an individual's life roles nor their personal preferences.

LIFE-H is a qualitative measure of an individual's societal participation and considers the interaction of personal and environmental factors over 12 domains (nutrition, fitness, personal care, communication, housing, mobility, responsibility, interpersonal relation, community, education, employment, recreation). While it has been shown to be valid and reliable in the SCI population, it is not widely used.

Impact on Participation and Autonomy (IPA) measures participation and choice in decision making over five domains (autonomy indoors, autonomy outdoors, family role, social relations, paid work and education).

Craig Hospital Inventory of Environmental Factors (CHIEF) looks at environmental barriers to participation.

Whiteneck GG, Charlifue SW, Gerhart KA, Overholser JD, Richardson GN. Quantifying handicap: a new measure of long-term rehabilitation outcomes. Arch Phys Med Rehabil. 1992;73(6):519–26.

23. Which of the following is a multi-item scale that measures global life satisfaction as a cognitive judgmental process?

A. Diener Satisfaction with Life Scale (SWLS)
B. Short Form (SF-36)
C. Craig Hospital Inventory of Environmental Factors (CHIEF)
D. Sickness Impact Profile (SIP-68)

Answer: A.

The Diener Satisfaction with Life Scale is a short five item scale that asks subjects for an overall judgement of their life and is scored using a scale of 1–7. Scores range from extremely dissatisfied (5) to neutral (20) to extremely satisfied (35).

The Short Form 36 is one of the most widely used instruments to measure quality of life. It covers physical functioning, physical role limitations, emotional problems, bodily pain, general health, vitality, social functioning, and mental health. However, this was developed for non-disabled individuals, which does not take into account the limitations of people with SCI.

Diener E, Emmons RA, Larsen RJ, Griffin S. The satisfaction with life scale. J Pers Assess. 1985;49(1):71–5. https://doi.org/10.1207/s15327752jpa4901_13.

24. SCI is associated with significant indirect and direct health care costs that impact the individual and society. The average yearly health care and living expenses vary depending on the level of injury having important social, psychological, and economic implications. Which of the following is considered a direct cost attributed to spinal cord injuries:

    A. Cost of a caregiver
    B. Loss wages and productivity
    C. Transportation costs associated with medical appointments
    D. Rehospitalization for pressure injuries and urinary tract infections (UTIs)

Answer: D.

Direct costs are defined as the costs that are a direct result of the injury. This would include emergency medical services, rehospitalizations, nursing home/skilled nursing facility admissions, cost of medications, physician visits, equipment and supplies, therapies. Indirect costs include lost income and productivity, caregiver costs, transportation costs/vehicle repair or replacement. As of 2019, SCI care in the United States had lifetime direct costs ranging between 2.1 and 5.4 million dollars for individuals injured at age of 25. Lifetime indirect costs ranged from 0.5–2.3 million dollars for those injured at age 25, and 0.3–0.6 million dollars for those injured at age 50 and above.

Cao Y, Krause JS. Estimation of indirect costs based on employment and earnings changes after spinal cord injury: an observational study. Spinal Cord. 2020;58(8):908–13. https://doi.org/10.1038/s41393-020-0447-1. Epub 2020 Mar 5.

Cao Y, Chen Y, DeVivo M. Lifetime direct costs after spinal cord injury. Top Spinal Cord Inj Rehabil. 2011;16(4):10–6.

DeVivo M, Chen Y, Mennemeyer S, Deutsch A. Costs of care following spinal cord injury. Top Spinal Cord Inj Rehabil. 2011;16(4):1–9.

Chan B, McIntyre A, Mittmann N, Teasell R, Wolfe DL (2014). Economic evaluation of spinal cord injury. In: Eng JJ, Teasell RW, Miller WC, Wolfe DL, Townson AF, Hsieh JTC, Connolly SJ, Noonen VK, Loh E, McIntyre A, editors. Spinal cord injury rehabilitation evidence. Version 5.0. Vancouver, BC. p. 1–21.

25. Many health related, environmental and psycho-social factors dictate the participation of individuals with SCI in the community. Which of the following is false regarding barriers to community reintegration/ participation for individuals with SCI?

    A. Environmental barriers produce a sense of discrimination in individuals with SCI.
    B. Younger patients have a lower disability adjustment score, making reintegration more challenging.

C. Frequent rehospitalizations and wheelchair maintenance issues affect socialization for individuals with SCI.
D. Lack of knowledge of supportive government policies and laws interfered with community participation.

Answer: B.

There are health-related, environmental and psycho-social factors that affect an SCI individual's ability to actively participate in the community. Health related complications showed pain and pressure sores as top reasons hindering reintegration or participation, as well as bladder issues, spasticity, contractures, sleep problems, and lack of psychological support. Mobility problems like wheelchair maintenance issues, incapacity to transfer and inability to stand were other health related complications. Inaccessibility in public spaces, transportation were the main environmental barriers, and were accompanied by feelings of discrimination. Psychosocial factors like lack of support, social attitudes towards people with disabilities, financial security, and lack of involvement in social and leisure functions also influenced participation. Younger age was seen as being predictive of reintegration given better support and friends and family relationships and therefore led to increased ability to adjust to a spinal cord injury. Finally, while government policies especially in the US support reintegration, most individuals with SCI were not aware of their rights.

Barclay L, McDonald R, Lentin P, Bourke-Taylor H. Facilitators and barriers to social and community participation following spinal cord injury. Aust Occup Ther J. 2016;63(1):19–28. https://doi.org/10.1111/1440-1630.12241. Epub 2015 Nov 4.
Kashif M, Jones S, Darain H, Iram H, Raqib A, Butt AA. Factors influencing the community integration of patients following traumatic spinal cord injury: a systematic review. J Pak Med Assoc. 2019;69(9):1337–43.

Methods and Basic Science Considerations in Spinal Cord Injury Research

22

Felicia Skelton

Questions

1. According to the National Spinal Cord Injury Statistical Center's "Facts and Figures at a Glance 2020," there are approximately 294,000 people in the US currently living with spinal cord injury (SCI), and 17,810 new cases each year. 294,000 represents the _____ of SCI cases in the US, while 17,810 represents the _____ of cases.

    A. Incidence; prevalence
    B. Prevalence; count
    C. Prevalence; incidence
    D. Incidence; ratio

    Answer: C.

    Prevalence is defined as the existing new and old cases of a disease or health outcome at a given point in time. Incidence is the number of new cases of a disease or health outcome over a given time period. A count is a general description of cases of interest, and a ratio (or proportion) is the count relative to the size of the group from which the counts was calculated.

    Reid HM. Introduction to statistics: fundamental concepts and procedures of data analysis. 1st ed. New York: Sage Publishing; 2013.
    National Spinal Cord Injury Statistical Center. Spinal cord injury facts and figures at a glance: 2020 SCI data sheet. 2020. Available from: https://www.nscisc.uab.edu/Public/Facts%20 and%20Figures%202020.pdf.

F. Skelton (✉)
H. Ben Taub Department of Physical Medicine and Rehabilitation, Baylor College of Medicine, Houston, TX, USA
e-mail: felicia.skelton2@va.gov

© The Author(s), under exclusive license to Springer Nature Switzerland AG 2022
B. A. Abramoff et al. (eds.), *The Essential Spinal Cord Injury Medicine Question Bank*, https://doi.org/10.1007/978-3-031-07796-8_22

Jain NB, Ayers GD, Peterson EN, Harris MB, Morse L, O'Connor KC, Garshick E. Traumatic spinal cord injury in the United States, 1993–2012. JAMA. 2015;313(22):2236–43.
https://doi.org/10.1001/jama.2015.6250.
Lasfargues JE, Custis D, Morrone F, Carswell J, Nguyen T. A model for estimating spinal cord injury prevalence in the United States. Paraplegia. 1995;33(2):62–8. https://doi.
org/10.1038/sc.1995.16.

Please use the following information for questions 2 and 3.

In a randomized controlled trial exploring the effect of hydrophilic-coated urinary catheters on the incidence of urinary tract infection (UTI) Cardenas et al. (2011) reported that the daily risk of developing a UTI in the hydrophilic-coated catheter group compared to the usual treatment group was 0.666, with a 95% confidence interval of 0.453–0.978.

2. Which of the following statements is true?

    A. The measured hazard ratio statistic of the sample is 0.666 and there is a 95% certainty that the true population ratio is between 0.453–0.978.
    B. The use of hydrophilic catheters did not show a statistically significant reduction in the daily risk of developing a UTI.
    C. Use of a hydrophilic catheter decreased the daily risk of developing a UTI by 66%.
    D. The hydrophilic-coated catheter group was 66% more likely to develop a urinary tract infection.

3. Compared to the reported confidence interval, what is the meaning if the confidence interval was narrowed to 0.512–0.617?

    A. The measured ratio is less precise, and there is a high degree of error within this confidence interval.
    B. The measured ratio is more precise, and there is a low degree of error within this confidence interval.
    C. There is no meaningful change indicated by the narrower confidence interval compared to the original as long as the ratio remains the same.
    D. The measured ratio is no longer significant.

Answers: 2. A; 3. B.

Due to the impossibility to test an entire population you must take sample data and make inferences to the general population; a statistic is the measurement made from this sample data (in this instance, a hazard ratio). A confidence interval is the range of values that is suspected to contain the true population proportion. A confidence level is pre-selected and is a measure of the degree of reliability of the selected confidence interval. Typically, the confidence level is selected as a 5% chance that the range will not include the true population proportion or 95% certainty that your confidence interval contains the true population proportion. The statistic is considered significant if the confidence interval does not include 1. Therefore, there was a significant reduction in the daily risk of developing a UTI in this study. There was a 33% reduction in risk however (not 67%). A wider confidence interval indicates a higher degree of error within your chosen confidence interval, while a narrower confidence interval indicates a lower degree of error; this is correlated with a larger sample size, which yields a more precise estimate.

Cardenas DD, Moore KN, Dannels-McClure A, Scelza WM, Graves DE, Brooks M, Busch AK. Intermittent catheterization with a hydrophilic-coated catheter delays urinary tract infections in acute spinal cord injury: a prospective, randomized, multicenter trial. PM R. 2011;3(5):408–17. https://doi.org/10.1016/j.pmrj.2011.01.001.
Reid HM. Introduction to statistics: fundamental concepts and procedures of data analysis. 1st ed. New York: Sage Publishing; 2013.

Please use the following information for questions 4–6.

A study wants to determine the relationship between receiving midodrine (dosage in mg) and the presence of orthostatic hypotension (possible answers yes or no) through a survey of patients seen at an outpatient spinal cord injury clinic within the past 6 months. The researchers would like to determine the interaction of age, gender, race and completeness of injury on the presence of orthostatic hypotension as well.

4. Receiving midodrine is the _____, systolic blood pressure is the _____ and age, gender, race and completeness of injury are the _____.

   A. Exposure/independent variable; outcome/dependent variable; co-variates
   B. Co-variate; exposure/independent variable; outcome/dependent variable
   C. Outcome/dependent variable; exposure/independent variable; co-variates
   D. Exposure/independent variable; co-variates; outcome/dependent variable

5. The presence of orthostatic hypotension (yes/no) are what type of variables?

   A. Discrete
   B. Continuous
   C. Nominal
   D. Ordinal

6. Based on your answers above, the most appropriate regression model to answer this question is:

   A. Logistic regression
   B. Log-binomial regression
   C. Cox proportional hazard regression
   D. Linear regression

Answers: 4. A; 5. C; 6. A.

The exposure/independent variable is the variable that you expect may influence the outcome/dependent variable. So, during your study, you will alter the exposure variable to measure what changes occur in the outcome variable. In this case, the researchers are investigating whether the patient received midodrine to see what effect it has on the systolic blood pressure. Co-variates are characteristics of the participants in the experiment (excluding the actual exposure variable) that are expected to change (vary) the outcome. Age, gender, race and completeness of injury are co-variates in this scenario.

Variables can be classified into two types. Categorical variables are finite—"either you have it or not" examples of categorical variables are ordinal variables (where there is a meaningful order or rank, like a Likert scale) and nominal, where there is no order (i.e. gender, race, disease or treatment present yes/no). Numerical variables are ongoing; examples include discrete variables, which include a finite number of values (i.e. 7 comorbidities, 1 hospitalization in a year, etc.) and continuous variables, which could contain an infinite number of values (such as blood pressure or drug doses).

Regression models are a statistical model used to measure the interaction between variables and co-variates. The choice of model to use is first determined by whether the outcome is numerical or categorical, then the temporal relationship of the exposure to the outcome. The outcome in this case is categorical, so a logistic regression, log-binomial regression or a Cox Proportional Hazard regression may be appropriate. However, we are uncertain of when the exposure (receiving midodrine) occurred in relationship to the outcome (diagnosis of orthostatic hypotension) due to the chart review nature of the study, so a logistic regression is the most appropriate test in this case.

Reid HM. Introduction to statistics: fundamental concepts and procedures of data analysis. 1st ed. New York: Sage Publishing; 2013.

7. A research team would like to determine the impact of decompression surgery on survival after acute traumatic spinal cord injury in a prospective trial. The most appropriate measure of association to use to answer this question is:

   A. Logistic regression
   B. Log-binomial regression
   C. Cox proportional hazard regression
   D. Linear regression

Answer: C.

The outcome in this scenario is survival (which is inherently nominal-yes or no). Given that the outcome is categorical, a logistic regression, log-binomial regression or a Cox Proportional Hazard regression may be appropriate. We know the exposure (decompression surgery) occurred prior to the outcome (survival), so a log-binomial regression or cox proportional hazard regression could be used in this case. A cox proportional hazard regression, however, incorporates a survival analysis (time to survival) in addition to exploring whether the outcome occurred, so it is the most appropriate test in this case.

Reid HM. Introduction to statistics: fundamental concepts and procedures of data analysis. 1st ed. New York: Sage Publishing; 2013.

8. A study team observes 80 SCI patients receiving baclofen for spasticity management and records the following:

	Receiving baclofen (n)	Not receiving baclofen (n)
Reports spasticity (n)	10	30
Does not report spasticity (n)	30	10

What statistical test could be used to determine the significance of these findings?

A. t-test
B. Paired t-test
C. ANOVA
D. Chi square test

Answer: D.

The first step in deciding the statistical model is by determining the nature of the variables. Both variables in this scenario are categorical (disease yes/no and treatment yes/no). Therefore, the most appropriate test would be a chi-square test. All the other choices are used when the outcome is quantitative.

Reid HM. Introduction to statistics: fundamental concepts and procedures of data analysis. 1st ed. New York: Sage Publishing; 2013.

9. A research team distributes a survey to 100 SCI physicians about their use of telehealth during the COVID-19 study. This is an example of a:

A. Cross-sectional study
B. Retrospective cohort study
C. Prospective cohort study
D. Randomized controlled trial

Answer: A.

Cross-sectional and cohort studies are types observational studies—the researcher examines the study population but does not influence the exposure or outcome in any way (like in a randomized controlled trial). A cross-sectional study measures the exposure and outcome at a single point in time; survey studies are a good example of cross-sectional studies. Their advantage is that they are inexpensive and can help quantify the magnitude of a problem. Their disadvantage is that it cannot establish cause-effect relationships nor measure risk in any way. Cohort studies are either prospective (exposure is identified and then the cohort is followed over time to measure the outcome) or retrospective (exposure is measured at a point in time after the outcome has already occurred).

Reid HM. Introduction to statistics: fundamental concepts and procedures of data analysis. 1st ed. New York: Sage Publishing; 2013.

10. A study team identifies 100 patients with SCI and issues them an exoskeleton walking device. The team follows these 100 patients over the next 5 years, and measures how frequently they use device and any adverse effects. This is an example of a:

    A. Cross-sectional study
    B. Retrospective cohort study
    C. Prospective cohort study
    D. Randomized controlled trial

    Answer: C.

    This scenario is an example of a prospective cohort trial. The exposure (use of an exoskeleton walking device) is defined a priori to the outcomes of interest (frequency of use, adverse effects). The cohort is then followed prospectively to determine when the outcome occurs. This is not a randomized control trial due to the absence of randomization with a control and treatment group.

Reid HM. Introduction to statistics: fundamental concepts and procedures of data analysis. 1st ed. New York: Sage Publishing; 2013.

11. A new drug is being developed for neuropathic pain after spinal cord injury. The research team has reached the clinical trial step of the drug discovery process. They are currently testing the safety and tolerability of the drug in human subjects, along with the pharmacokinetics of the drug in the human body. This is considered a:

    A. Phase 1 drug trial
    B. Phase 2 drug trial
    C. Phase 3 drug trial
    D. Phase 4 drug trial

    Answer: A.

    See answer to question 12.

12. A drug used to treat orthostatic hypotension after spinal cord injury has been used in the general population for 7 years. Post-marketing surveillance for adverse effects and efficacy are ongoing. This is considered a:

A. Phase 1 drug trial
B. Phase 2 drug trial
C. Phase 3 drug trial
D. Phase 4 drug trial

Answer: D.

Step 1 of drug trials includes discovery and development of novel therapeutic agents. Step 2 includes pre-clinical research in animal models to identify potential harmful effects. Step 3 involves human clinical trials and is broken into 4 phases. Phase 1 includes identifying if the therapeutic agent is safe and tolerable in humans, initial considerations on dosing, and human pharmacokinetics. Phase 2 determines efficacy in humans. Phase 3 determines comparative effectiveness versus the current gold standard treatment. Phase 4 includes post-marketing surveillance after the drug is in use in the general population.

Reid HM. Introduction to statistics: fundamental concepts and procedures of data analysis. 1st ed. New York: Sage Publishing; 2013.

13. _____ data collection methods typically involve numerical data collection and results are easy to summarize, compare and generalize.

A. Qualitative
B. Quantitative
C. Ecologic
D. Random

Answer: B.

See answer to question 14.

14. _____ data collection methods use techniques aimed at gaining understanding of underlying reasons, opinions and motivation of patients. It is not intended to be precisely measured.

A. Qualitative
B. Quantitative
C. Ecologic
D. Random

Answer: A.

This is a description of quantitative data collection. Types of quantitative data collection include questionnaires and physiologic measurements (either through direct measurement or self-report). Qualitative measurement uses techniques aimed at gaining understanding of reasons, opinions, and measurements of the subject, and are often hypothesis generating rather than hypothesis testing. Ecologic studies are population studies, and identify correlations that could be observed between exposure and disease rates among different groups of populations.

Reid HM. Introduction to statistics: fundamental concepts and procedures of data analysis. 1st ed. New York: Sage Publishing; 2013.

15. An investigator is eager to start a randomized controlled trial looking at the efficacy of a new drug on motor recovery in chronic spinal cord injury compared to traditional rehabilitation. However, after reviewing the protocol, The Institutional Review Board (IRB) of record questioned the ethics of proceeding due to the fact that there had not been studies showing efficacy of the drug in humans, and there were some adverse effects noted in animal trials. The two ethical principles used in this decision were:

    A. Autonomy and beneficence
    B. Beneficence and non-maleficence
    C. Justice and autonomy
    D. Justice and beneficence

    Answer: B.

    The ethical principles most at play here are those of beneficence and non-maleficence. Autonomy is defined as respect for the individual's right to choose their own treatments. Beneficence is doing what is in the best interest of the patient, and appropriately balancing risks versus benefits. Non-maleficence is avoiding unnecessarily risky treatments that could make things worse. Justice is defined as fairness for all and equitable allocation of resources.

    Holm S. Not just autonomy—the principles of American biomedical ethics. J Med Ethics. 1995;21(6):332–8. https://doi.org/10.1136/jme.21.6.332.
    Donovan WH. Ethics, health care and spinal cord injury: research, practice and finance. Spinal Cord. 2011;49(2):162–74. https://doi.org/10.1038/sc.2010.106. Epub 2010 Sept 14.

16. In animal and human models of acute spinal cord injury, _____ infiltration at the injury site is noted within hours of injury and peaking within 1–3 days.

    A. Macrophage
    B. Natural killer (NK) cell
    C. Neutrophil
    D. CD8 lymphocyte

    Answer: C.

Neutrophils are the first inflammatory cells noted in the most proximal zone closest to the acute spinal cord injury. Macrophages appear within weeks and were noted months after injury. CD8 lymphocytes were noted sporadically at different timepoints after acute injury. NK cells were not noticed on histological evaluation.

Fleming JC, Norenberg MD, Ramsay DA, Dekaban GA, Marcillo AE, Saenz AD, Pasquale-Styles M, Dietrich WD, Weaver LC. The cellular inflammatory response in human spinal cords after injury. Brain. 2006;129(Pt 12):3249–69. https://doi.org/10.1093/brain/awl296. Epub 2006 Oct 28.

17. Which of the following is not a secondary injury after acute traumatic spinal cord injury from inflammation, vascular injury and production of toxic reactive oxygen species and neurotransmitters can continue weeks to months after the initial injury.

    A. Activation of an ischemic cascade
    B. Inflammation due to lymphocyte infiltration in to the spinal lesion
    C. Production of toxic reactive oxygen species
    D. Shearing of neurons in the spinal cord

Answer: D.

Primary injury includes cell death at the site of injury and hemorrhage during the immediate post-injury period. In contrast, the ischemic, inflammatory and excitotoxicity cascade that results from these injuries can be propagated for months after injury. Targets that reduce inflammation and minimize excitotoxicity (and the resultant apoptosis) have been targets of therapeutic agents being investigated for neuroprotection after SCI.

Fleming JC, Norenberg MD, Ramsay DA, Dekaban GA, Marcillo AE, Saenz AD, Pasquale-Styles M, Dietrich WD, Weaver LC. The cellular inflammatory response in human spinal cords after injury. Brain. 2006;129(Pt 12):3249–69. https://doi.org/10.1093/brain/awl296. Epub 2006 Oct 28.

18. Compounds that block excess _____ release have been suggested to be neuroprotective in animal spinal cord injury models.

    A. GABA
    B. Serotonin
    C. Dopamine
    D. Glutamate

Answer: D.

Glutamate release has been implicated in the vicious cycle of excitotoxicity and cell death seen after acute traumatic spinal cord injury, mediated through NMDA and AMPA/kainate receptors. The other neurotransmitters listed are not implicated in this process.

Sadowsky C, Volshteyn O, Schultz L, McDonald JW. Spinal cord injury. Disabil Rehabil. 2002;24(13):680–7. https://doi.org/10.1080/09638280110110640.
Wrathall JR, Teng YD, Choiniere D. Amelioration of functional deficits from spinal cord trauma with systemically administered NBQX, an antagonist of non-N-methyl-D-aspartate receptors. Exp Neurol. 1996;137(1):119–26. https://doi.org/10.1006/exnr.1996.0012.

19. Excitotoxicity results from excessive cellular levels of _____, mediated in part by N-methyl-D aspartate (NMDA) receptors.

    A. Calcium
    B. Sodium
    C. Phosphate
    D. Potassium

Answer: A.

Excess intracellular calcium starts the cascade towards apoptosis, or programmed cell death, seen after acute spinal cord injury and other inflammatory neurodegenerative diseases.

Guzmán-Lenis MS, Navarro X, Casas C. Drug screening of neuroprotective agents on an organotypic-based model of spinal cord excitotoxic damage. Restor Neurol Neurosci. 2009;27(4):335–49. https://doi.org/10.3233/RNN-2009-0482.

20. Inflammatory cytokines that have been implicated in suppression of the hypothalamus, pituitary, adrenal (HPA) axis after acute traumatic spinal cord injury include all the following EXCEPT

    A. Interleukin-1
    B. TNF-alpha
    C. Interleukin-6
    D. Interleukin-12

Answer: D.

IL-1, IL-6 and TNF-alpha have all been implicated in the inflammatory cascade that results in suppression of the HPA axis and relative immunodeficiency. These are drug targets in other inflammatory conditions, and are being explored in as neuroprotective and anti-inflammatory agents after SCI.

Allison DJ, Ditor DS. Immune dysfunction and chronic inflammation following spinal cord injury. Spinal Cord. 2015;53(1):14–8. https://doi.org/10.1038/sc.2014.184. Epub 2014 Nov 4.

21. Pointillart et al. (2000) conducted a randomized controlled trial of _____ in promoting neurological recovery in acute SCI through calcium channel blockade. It was not found to be effective.

A. Naloxone
B. Nimodipine
C. Losartan
D. Tirilazad mesylate

Answer: B.

Of the choices listed, only nimodipine is a calcium channel blocker. Naloxone is a mu opioid receptor antagonists. Losartan is an angiotensin receptor blocker. Tirilazad mesylate is an antioxidant (specifically against lipid peroxidation) that has been trialed in stroke and SCI recovery.

Pointillart V, Petitjean ME, Wiart L, Vital JM, Lassié P, Thicoipé M, Dabadie P. Pharmacological therapy of spinal cord injury during the acute phase. Spinal Cord. 2000;38(2):71–6. https://doi.org/10.1038/sj.sc.3100962.

22. Two small studies administering _____ have shown promising results in promoting neural recovery after acute SCI through its anti-inflammatory, free radical scavenger and axon regenerative properties.

A. Erythropoietin
B. Cholecalciferol
C. Prednisone
D. Naloxone

Answer: A.

Erythropoietin (given with methylprednisolone) has shown promise as a neuroprotective agent after acute traumatic SCI. Cholecalciferol is a form of vitamin D and has not been shown to be neuroprotective. Steroids (usually IV preparations, not oral preparations such as prednisone) and naloxone have both been studied in spinal cord injury recovery and have not been shown to be effective.

Alibai E, Zand F, Rahimi A, Rezaianzadeh A. Erythropoietin plus methylprednisolone or methylprednisolone in the treatment of acute spinal cord injury: a preliminary report. Acta Med Iran. 2014;52(4):275–9.
Xiong M, Chen S, Yu H, Liu Z, Zeng Y, Li F. Neuroprotection of erythropoietin and methylprednisolone against spinal cord ischemia-reperfusion injury. J Huazhong Univ Sci Technol Med Sci. 2011;31(5):652. https://doi.org/10.1007/s11596-011-0576-z. Epub 2011 Oct 25.

23. Granulocyte-colony stimulating factor (G-CSF) has shown promise in one cohort study and one prospective controlled trial in promoting motor and sensory recovery after SCI through inhibition of _____, or programmed cell death.

A. Agenesis
B. Neurogenesis
C. Apoptosis
D. Wallerian degeneration

Answer: C.

Apoptosis is programmed cell death and can occur as part of normal neural development or after severe catastrophic injury to a cell. Wallerian degeneration is the active process of nerve fiber degeneration after injury. Agenesis is defined as the failure of an organ to develop completely during development. Neurogenesis denotes new neuron formation.

Schneider A, Kuhn HG, Schäbitz WR. A role for G-CSF (granulocyte-colony stimulating factor) in the central nervous system. Cell Cycle. 2005;4(12):1753–7. https://doi.org/10.4161/cc.4.12.2213. Epub 2005 Dec 27.

Kamiya K, Koda M, Furuya T, Kato K, Takahashi H, Sakuma T, Inada T, Ota M, Maki S, Okawa A, Ito Y, Takahashi K, Yamazaki M. Neuroprotective therapy with granulocyte colony-stimulating factor in acute spinal cord injury: a comparison with high-dose methylprednisolone as a historical control. Eur Spine J. 2015;24(5):963–7. https://doi.org/10.1007/s00586-014-3373-0. Epub 2014 Jun 25.

Takahashi H, Yamazaki M, Okawa A, Sakuma T, Kato K, Hashimoto M, Hayashi K, Furuya T, Fujiyoshi T, Kawabe J, Yamauchi T, Mannoji C, Miyashita T, Kadota R, Ito Y, Takahashi K, Koda M. Neuroprotective therapy using granulocyte colony-stimulating factor for acute spinal cord injury: a phase I/IIa clinical trial. Eur Spine J. 2012;21(12):2580–7. https://doi.org/10.1007/s00586-012-2213-3. Epub 2012 Mar 6.

24. One cohort study has shown that _____ may be effective in promoting long term motor or sensory recovery after acute spinal cord injury through blocking sodium channels, and thus an osmotic response that causes cellular swelling.

A. Riluzole
B. Minocycline
C. Nimodipine
D. Prednisone

Answer: A.

This question describes the proposed mechanism of riluzole, and the rationale behind studying it as a neuroprotective agent after spinal cord injury. Minocycline is a tetracycline antibiotic that has been studied for recovery after spinal cord injury but has not been shown to be effective. Nimodipine is a calcium channel blocker. Prednisone is a glucocorticoid that has not been shown to be effective for neurorecovery.

Grossman RG, Fehlings MG, Frankowski RF, Burau KD, Chow DS, Tator C, Teng A, Toups EG, Harrop JS, Aarabi B, Shaffrey CI, Johnson MM, Harkema SJ, Boakye M, Guest JD, Wilson JR. A prospective, multicenter, phase I matched-comparison group trial of safety, pharmacokinetics, and preliminary efficacy of riluzole in patients with traumatic spinal cord injury. J Neurotrauma. 2014;31(3):239–55. https://doi.org/10.1089/neu.2013.2969. Epub 2013 Oct 11.

Casha S, Zygun D, McGowan MD, Bains I, Yong VW, Hurlbert RJ. Results of a phase II placebo-controlled randomized trial of minocycline in acute spinal cord injury. Brain. 2012;135(Pt 4):1224–36. https://doi.org/10.1093/brain/aws072.

25. Which of the following has NOT been proposed and researched as potential treatments for traumatic spinal cord injuries:

   A. Epidural electrical stimulation
   B. Implantation of mesenchymal stem cells into the spinal cord lesion
   C. Use of the genetic therapy, nusinersen
   D. Intermittent hypoxia

Answer: C.

All of the answer choices are currently being investigated for use in individuals with traumatic spinal cord injury with the exception of nusinersen. Nusinersen (brand name: Spinraza™) is a genetic therapy used in individuals with spinal muscular atrophy.

Eisdorfer JT, Smit RD, Keefe KM, Lemay MA, Smith GM, Spence AJ. Epidural electrical stimulation: a review of plasticity mechanisms that are hypothesized to underlie enhanced recovery from spinal cord injury with stimulation. Front Mol Neurosci. 2020;13:163. https://doi.org/10.3389/fnmol.2020.00163.

Cofano F, Boido M, Monticelli M, Zenga F, Ducati A, Vercelli A, Garbossa D. Mesenchymal stem cells for spinal cord injury: current options, limitations, and future of cell therapy. Int J Mol Sci. 2019;20(11):2698. https://doi.org/10.3390/ijms20112698.

Navarrete-Opazo A, Alcayaga J, Sepúlveda O, Rojas E, Astudillo C. Repetitive intermittent hypoxia and locomotor training enhances walking function in incomplete spinal cord injury subjects: a randomized, triple-blind, placebo-controlled clinical trial. J Neurotrauma. 2017;34(9):1803–12. https://doi.org/10.1089/neu.2016.4478. Epub 2016 Jul 19.

Index